VISUAL DIAGNOSIS AND TREATMENT IN PEDIATRICS

Second Edition

Editor-in-Chief
ESTHER K. CHUNG, MD, MPH
Associate Professor
Department of Pediatrics
Jefferson Medical College of Thomas Jefferson University
Jefferson Pediatrics/Nemour's Children's Health Program
Philadelphia, Pennsylvania
Alfred I. duPont Hospital for Children
Wilmington, Delaware

Associate Editors
LEE R. ATKINSON-McEVOY, MD
Associate Residency Program Director
HS Associate Clinical Professor
Director of UCSF Parnassus Pediatric Primary Care Clinic
Associate Chief of Outpatient General Pediatrics
Department of Pediatrics
University of California, San Francisco School of Medicine
San Francisco, California

JULIE A. BOOM, MD
Associate Professor
Department of Pediatrics
Baylor College of Medicine
Director
Infant and Childhood Immunization
Center for Vaccine Awareness and Research
Texas Children's Hospital
Houston, Texas

PAUL S. MATZ, MD
Advocare Haddon Pediatric Group
Haddon Heights, New Jersey

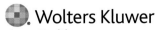
Wolters Kluwer | Lippincott Williams & Wilkins
Health

Philadelphia · Baltimore · New York · London
Buenos Aires · Hong Kong · Sydney · Tokyo

Acquisitions Editor: Sonya Seigafuse
Product Manager: Nicole Walz
Vendor Manager: Alicia Jackson
Senior Manufacturing Manager: Benjamin Rivera
Marketing Manager: Lisa Lawrence
Design Coordinator: Holly Reid McLaughlin
Production Service: SPi Technologies

Second Edition

Two Commerce Square
2001 Market Street
Philadelphia, PA 19103 USA
LWW.com

Library of Congress Cataloging-in-Publication Data
   Visual diagnosis and treatment in pediatrics/editor-in-chief, Esther K. Chung ; associate editors,
Lee R. Atkinson-McEvoy, Julie A. Boom, Paul S. Matz. — 2nd ed.
        p. ; cm.
   Rev. ed. of: Visual diagnosis in pediatrics.
   Includes bibliographical references and index.
   ISBN 978-1-60547-546-2
   1. Children—Diseases—Diagnosis—Handbooks, manuals, etc. 2. Children—Medical examinations—Handbooks, manuals, etc. I. Chung, Esther K. II. Visual diagnosis in pediatrics.
   [DNLM: 1. Pediatrics—Handbooks. 2. Child. 3. Diagnosis, Differential—Handbooks. 4. Medical History Taking—Handbooks. 5. Physical Examination—Handbooks. WS 39 V834 2010]
   RJ50.V57 2010
   618.92'075—dc22
                                                                                        2010001258

To purchase additional copies of this book, call our customer service department at (800) 638-3030 or fax orders to (301) 223-2320. International customers should call (301) 223-2300.

Visit Lippincott Williams & Wilkins on the Internet: at LWW.com. Lippincott Williams & Wilkins customer service representatives are available from 8:30 am to 6 pm, EST.

10 9 8 7 6 5 4 3 2 1

We dedicate this book to:

My parents, Drs. Okhyung Kang and Ed Baik Chung; my husband, Dennis; and my daughters,
Marissa and Emma
—*Esther*

My parents, Patrick and Beverly Atkinson, my husband Michael, and my children Amara, Mason, and Noah
—*Lee*

My husband, Marc, and my children, Kathryn, John, and Janie
—*Julie*

Miriam, Rebecca, and Eliana
—*Paul*

Photo Credits

Joyce Adams, MD
Clinical Professor of Pediatrics
Division of Adolescent Medicine
University of California
San Diego, California

Ben Alouf, MD
Department of General Pediatrics
Alfred I. duPont Hospital for Children
Wilmington, Delaware

Lee R. Atkinson-McEvoy, MD
Associate Residency Program Director
HS Associate Clinical Professor
Director of UCSF Parnassus Pediatric Primary
Care Clinic
Associate Chief of Outpatient General
Pediatrics
Department of Pediatrics
University of California, San Francisco School
of Medicine
San Francisco, California

M. Douglas Baker, MD
Pediatric Emergency Medicine
Yale-New Haven Children's Hospital
New Haven, Connecticut

**Benjamin Barankin Dermatology
Collection**
Dermatologist
Dermatology Center
Toronto, Ontario

Douglas A. Barnes, MD
Shriners Hospital for Children
Houston, Texas

Dean John Bonsall, MD, MS, FACS
Associate Professor
Department of Ophthalmology
University of Cincinnati
Associate Professor
Division of Pediatric Ophthalmology
Cincinnati Children's Hospital
Cincinnati, Ohio

Julie A. Boom, MD
Associate Professor
Department of Pediatrics
Baylor College of Medicine
Director
Infant and Childhood Immunization
Center for Vaccine Awareness and
Research
Texas Children's Hospital
Houston, Texas

Mary L. Brandt, MD
Baylor College of Medicine
Houston, Texas

Gerardo Cabrera-Meza, MD
Baylor College of Medicine
Houston, Texas

Esther K. Chung, MD, MPH
Associate Professor
Department of Pediatrics
Jefferson Medical College of Thomas Jefferson
University
Jefferson Pediatrics/Nemour's Children's
Health Program
Philadelphia, Pennsylvania
Alfred I. duPont Hospital for Children
Wilmington, Delaware

Sophia M. Chung, MD
Associate Professor
Department of Ophthalmology
St. Louis University School of Medicine
St. Louis, Missouri

Jayme Coffman, MD
Medical Director, CARE Team
Cook Children's Medical Center
Fort Worth, Texas

Steven P. Cook, MD
Chief
Division of Pediatric Otolaryngology
Alfred I. duPont Hospital for Children
Wilmington, Delaware

Kathleen Cronan, MD
Associate Professor
Department of Pediatrics
Jefferson Medical College
Philadelphia, Pennsylvania
Attending Physician
Department of Pediatrics
Division of Pediatric Emergency Medicine
Nemors/Alfred I. duPont Hospital for Children
Wilmington, Delaware

Carrie Ann Cusack, MD
Department of Dermatology
Drexel University College of Medicine
Philadelphia, Pennsylvania

George A. Datto, III, MD
Instructor
Department of Pediatrics
Jefferson Medical College of Thomas Jefferson
University
Philadelphia, Pennsylvania
Pediatrician
Department of Pediatrics
Alfred I. duPont Hospital for Children
Wilmington, Delaware

Allan R. De Jong, MD
Clinical Professor of Pediatrics
Department of Pediatrics
Jefferson Medical College
Thomas Jefferson University
Philadelphia, Pennsylvania
Director
Children at Risk Evaluation (CARE) Program
Department of Pediatrics
Nemors/Alfred I. duPont Hospital for Children
Wilmington, Delaware

Christopher D. Derby, MD
Cardiothoracic Surgeon
Nemours Cardiac Center
Alfred I. duPont Hospital for Children
Wilmington, Delaware

Ellen Deutsch, MD
Division of Otolaryngology
Alfred I. duPont Hospital for Children
Wilmington, Delaware

Michael C. Distefano, MD
Assistant Professor
Department of Pediatrics
Section of Pediatric Emergency Medicine
Baylor College of Medicine
Staff Physician
Department of Pediatrics
Section of Pediatric Emergency Medicine
Texas Children's Hospital
Houston, Texas

Jan Edwin Drutz, MD
Professor of Pediatrics
Department of Pediatrics
Baylor College of Medicine
Director of the Continuity Clinic Teaching
Program
Department of Pediatrics
Texas Children's Hospital
Houston, Texas

T. Ernesto Figueroa, MD, FAAP, FACS
Clinical Associate Professor
Department of Urology
Thomas Jefferson University
Philadelphia, Pennsylvania
Chief
Division of Pediatric Urology
Alfred I. duPont Hospital for Children
Wilmington, Delaware

Christine Finck, MD
Section of General Surgery
St. Christopher's Hospital for Children
Philadelphia, Pennsylvania

Susan A. Fisher-Owens, MD, MPH
Assistant Clinical Professor
Department of Pediatrics
University of California
San Francisco, California

Brian Forbes, MD
The Children's Hospital of Philadelphia
Philadelphia, Pennsylvania

Lourdes Forster, MD, FAAP
Assistant Professor of Clinical Pediatrics
Department of Pediatrics
University of Miami, Miller School of Medicine
Miami, Florida

Martin Fried, MD
Jersey Shore Medical Center
Neptune, New Jersey

Ilona J. Frieden, MD
Director of Pediatric Dermatology
University of California
San Francisco, California

John A. Germiller, MD, PhD
Assistant Professor
Division of Pediatric Otolaryngology
The Children's Hospital of Philadelphia
Philadelphia, Pennsylvania

Amy Gilliam, MD
Dermatolgist
Department of Dermatology
Palo Alto Medical Foundation
Freemont, California

Scott Goldstein, MD
Oculoplastic and Aesthetic
Surgeon
Wills Eye Institute
Philadelphia, Pennsylvania

Vani V. Gopalareddy, MD
Division of Gastroenterology
Levine Children's Hospital
Carolinas Medical Center
Charlotte, North Carolina

Bettina Gyr, MD
Staff Orthopaedic Surgeon
Shriners Hospitals for Children
Twin Cities Unit
Minneapolis, Minnesota

Steven D. Handler, MD, MBE
Division of Pediatric Otolaryngology
The Children's Hospital
of Philadelphia
Philadelphia, Pennsylvania

Fernando L. Heinen, MD
Deutsches Hospital of Buenos Aires
Buenos Aires, Argentina

Lior Heller, MD
Associate Professor
Division of Plastic Surgery
Michael E. DeBakey Department of
Surgery
Baylor College of Medicine

Larry H. Hollier, Jr., MD, FACS
Professor and Program Director
Department of Plastic Surgery
Baylor College of Medicine
Professor
Department of Plastic Surgery
Texas Children's Hospital
Houston, Texas

David A. Horvath, MD
Plastic Surgeon
Horvath Plastic and Cosmetic Surgery
Center
Abington, Pennsylvania

Glenn Isaacson, MD
Temple University Health System
Temple University Children's Medical
Center
Philadelphia, Pennsylvania

Douglas Katz, MD
Section of General Surgery
St. Christopher's Hospital
for Children
Philadelphia, Pennsylvania

Hans B. Kersten, MD
Associate Professor of Pediatrics
Department of Pediatrics
Drexel University College of Medicine
Attending Physician
Section of General Pediatrics
St. Christopher's Hospital for Children
Philadelphia, Pennsylvania

Aida Z. Khanum, MD
Fellow
Academic General Pediatrics
Baylor College of Medicine
Texas Children's Hospital
Houston, Texas

Shirley P. Klein, MD, FAAP
Clinical Assistant Professor
Department of Pediatrics
Jefferson Medical College of Thomas
Jefferson University
Philadelphia, Pennsylvania
Director
Pediatric Practice Program
Wilmington Hospital Health Center
Christiana Care Health System
Wilmington, Delaware

Naline Lai, MD
Attending Physician
Buckingham Pediatrics
Buckingham, Pennsylvania
Attending Physician
Department of Pediatrics
Doylestown Hospital
Doylestown, Pennsylvania

Kevin P. Lally, MD
University of Texas Medical Sciences
Center
Houston, Texas

Michael Lemper, DDS
Department of Pediatric Dental Medicine
St. Christopher's Hospital for Children
Philadelphia, Pennsylvania

Moise L. Levy, MD
Baylor College of Medicine
Houston, Texas

John Loiselle, MD
Associate Professor of Pediatrics
Jefferson Medical College
Thomas Jefferson University
Philadelphia, Pennsylvania

Joseph Lopreiato, MD
Uniformed Services University of Health
Sciences
Bethesda, Maryland

Steven Manders, MD
Department of Dermatology
Cooper University Hospital
Cherry Hill, New Jersey

Gary Marshall, MD
University of Louisville
Louisville, Kentucky

Paul S. Matz, MD
Advocare Haddon Pediatric Group
Haddon Heights, New Jersey

James W. McManaway, III, MD
Hershey Pediatric Ophthalmology Associates
Hershey, Pennsylvania

Denise W. Metry, MD
Associate Professor
Department of Dermatology and Pediatrics
Baylor College of Medicine
Chief
Department of Dermatology
Texas Children's Hospital
Houston, Texas

Tony Olsen, MD
Senior Consultant
Department of Pediatrics
Naestved Hospital
Naestved, Denmark

Barry Oppenheim, MD
Bucks County Eye Group
Wrightstown, Pennsylvania

Parul B. Patel, MD, MPH
Assistant Professor
Department of Pediatrics
Feinberg School of Medicine
Northwestern University
Attending Physician
Department of Pediatric Emergency Medicine
Children's Memorial Hospital
Chicago, Illinois

William Phillips, MD
Baylor College of Medicine
Houston, Texas

Joseph Piatt, MD
Section of Neurosurgery
St. Christopher's Hospital for Children
Philadelphia, Pennsylvania

Hannah Ravreby, BS
Temple University School of Medicine
Center for Urban and Bioethics and Humanities
Philadelphia, Pennsylvania

Kenneth Rosenbaum, MD
Children's National Medical Center
Children's Hospital
Washington, DC

Amy Ross, MD
Department of Dermatology
Drexel University College of Medicine
Philadelphia, Pennsylvania

Denise A. Salerno, MD, FAAP
Associate Professor
Department of Pediatrics
Drexel University College of Medicine
Attending Pediatrician
Department of Pediatrics
Saint Christopher's Hospital for Children
Philadelphia, Pennsylvania

Steven M. Selbst, MD, FAAP
Professor
Department of Pediatrics
Jefferson Medical College
Thomas Jefferson University
Philadelphia, Pennsylvania
Pediatric Residency Program Director
Attending Physician
Department of Pediatrics
Division of Emergency Medicine
Alfred I. duPont Hospital
for Children
Wilmington, Delaware

Philip Siu, MD
Chinatown Pediatric Services
Philadelphia, Pennsylvania

Julia L. Stevens, MD
Department of Ophthalmology
University of Kentucky
Lexington, Kentucky

Valarie Stricklen, MD, FAAP
Pediatrician
University of Toledo Medical Center
Toledo, Ohio

Sidney Sussman, MD
Department of Pediatrics
Cooper University Hospital
Cherry Hill, New Jersey

Daniel R. Taylor, DO
Assistant Professor
Department of Pediatrics
Drexel University College of Medicine
General Pediatrician
General Pediatrics
St. Christopher's Hospital for Children
Philadelphia, Pennsylvania

Tom Thacher, MD
Department of Family Medicine
Jos University Teaching Hospital
Jos, Nigeria

E. Douglas Thompson, Jr., MD
Assistant Professor
Department of Pediatrics
Drexel University College of Medicine
Director
Pediatric Generalist Service
Department of Pediatrics
St. Christopher's Hospital for Children
Philadelphia, Pennsylvania

Sujata R. Tipnis, MD
Voluntary Faculty
Department of Pediatrics
University of Miami Miller School of
Medicine
Miami, Florida
Staff Pediatrician
Department of Pediatrics
Sheridan Children's Healthcare Services
Parkway Regional Medical Center
North Miami, Florida

David Tunkel, MD
Associate Professor
Departments of Otolaryngology-Head
and Neck
Surgery and Pediatrics
Johns Hopkins University School of
Medicine

Scott VanDuzer, MD
Section of Plastic Surgery
St. Christopher's Hospital for Children
Philadelphia, Pennsylvania

Mark A. Ward, MD
Baylor College of Medicine
Houston, Texas

Evan J. Weiner, MD, FAAP
Assistant Professor of Pediatrics and
Emergency Medicine
Drexel University College of Medicine
Attending Physician
Department of Emergency Medicine
St. Christopher's Hospital for Children
Philadelphia, Pennsylvania

D'Juanna White-Satcher, MD, MPH
Assistant Professor
Department of Pediatrics
Baylor College of Medicine
Attending Physician
Section of Academic General Pediatrics
Texas Children's Hospital
Houston, Texas

Michael J. Wilsey, Jr., MD, FAAP
Affiliate Assistant Professor
Department of Pediatrics
Associate Director
Pediatric Residency Training Program
University of South Florida College of
Medicine
Attending Physician
Department of Pediatric
Gastroenterology
All Children's Hospital
St. Petersburg, Florida

Jeoffrey K. Wolens, MD
Staff Physician
Department of General Medicine
Texas Children's Hospital
Houston, Texas

Terri L. Young, MD
Professor
Departments of Ophthalmology and
Pediatrics
Duke University Medical Center
Duke University Hospital
Duke University Eye Center
Durham, North Carolina

Robert L. Zarr, MD, MPH, FAAP
Assistant Clinical Professor
School of Medicine and Health Services
George Washington University
Washington, DC

Seth Zwillenberg, MD
Department of Otolaryngology
St. Christopher's Hospital for Children
Philadelphia, Pennsylvania

Contributors

Bethlehem L. Abebe, MD
HS Assistant Clinical Professor
Department of Pediatrics
University of California
San Francisco, California

Angela M. Allevi, MD
Assistant Professor
Department of Pediatrics
Thomas Jefferson University
Faculty
Department of Pediatrics
Thomas Jefferson University Hospital and Alfred I. duPont
Hospital for Children
Philadelphia, Pennsylvania

Lee R. Atkinson-McEvoy, MD
Associate Residency Program Director
HS Associate Clinical Professor
Director of UCSF Parnassus Pediatric Primary Care Clinic
Associate Chief of Outpatient General Pediatrics
Department of Pediatrics
University of California, San Francisco School of Medicine
San Francisco, California

Barbara W. Bayldon, MD
Assistant Professor
Feinberg School of Medicine
Northwestern University
Head
Section of Primary Care, General Academic Pediatrics
Department of Pediatrics
Children's Memorial Hospital
Chicago, Illinois

Robert L. Bonner, Jr., MD
Assistant Professor
Department of Pediatrics
Drexel University School of Medicine
Medical Director, General Pediatric
Outpatient Services
Department of General Pediatrics
St. Christopher's Hospital for Children
Philadelphia, Pennsylvania

Dean John Bonsall, MD, MS, FACS
Associate Professor
Department of Ophthalmology
University of Cincinnati
Associate Professor
Division of Pediatric Ophthalmology
Cincinnati Children's Hospital
Cincinnati, Ohio

Julie A. Boom, MD
Associate Professor
Department of Pediatrics
Baylor College of Medicine
Director
Infant and Childhood Immunization
Center for Vaccine Awareness and Research
Texas Children's Hospital
Houston, Texas

Anthony E. Burgos, MD, MPH
Assistant Professor of Pediatrics
Department of Pediatrics
Stanford University
Medical Director, Well Baby Nursery
Department of Pediatrics
Lucile Packard Children's Hospital
Palo Alto, California

Esther K. Chung, MD, MPH
Associate Professor
Department of Pediatrics
Jefferson Medical College of Thomas
Jefferson University
Jefferson Pediatrics/Nemour's Children's
Health Program
Philadelphia, Pennsylvania
Alfred I. duPont Hospital for Children
Wilmington, Delaware

Patrick D. Cole, MD
Resident Physician
Department of Plastic Surgery
Baylor College of Medicine
Houston, Texas

Kathleen Cronan, MD
Associate Professor
Department of Pediatrics
Jefferson Medical College
Philadelphia, Pennsylvania
Attending Physician
Department of Pediatrics
Division of Pediatric Emergency Medicine
Nemours/Alfred I. duPont Hospital for Children
Wilmington, Delaware

Kathryn R. Crowell, MD
Assistant Professor of Pediatrics
Department of Pediatrics
Penn State University School of Medicine
Assistant Professor of Pediatrics
Department of Pediatrics
Penn State University Children's Hospital
Hershey, Pennsylvania

Mario Cruz
Assistant Professor
Department of Pediatrics
Drexel University College of Medicine
Attending Physician
Ambulatory Pediatrics
St. Christopher's Hospital for Children
Philadelphia, Pennsylvania

Allan R. De Jong, MD
Clinical Professor of Pediatrics
Department of Pediatrics
Jefferson Medical College of Thomas Jefferson University
Philadelphia, Pennsylvania
Director
Children at Risk Evaluation (CARE) Program
Department of Pediatrics
Nemours/Alfred I. duPont Hospital for Children
Wilmington, Delaware

Lisa E. De Ybarrondo, MD
Assistant Professor
Department of Pediatrics
University of Texas Health Science Center
Director of Lyndon B. Johnson Pediatric Clinic
Department of Pediatrics
Lyndon B. Johnson General Hospital
Houston, Texas

Ami D. Dharia, MD
Physician
Department of Pediatrics
Harris County Hospital District
Houston, Texas

Michael C. Distefano, MD
Assistant Professor
Department of Pediatrics
Section of Pediatric Emergency Medicine
Baylor College of Medicine
Staff Physician

Department of Pediatrics
Section of Pediatric Emergency Medicine
Texas Children's Hospital
Houston, Texas

Jan Edwin Drutz, MD
Professor of Pediatrics
Department of Pediatrics
Baylor College of Medicine
Director of the Continuity Clinic Teaching Program
Department of Pediatrics
Texas Children's Hospital
Houston, Texas

Gary A. Emmett, MD, FAAP
Professor
Department of Pediatrics
Thomas Jefferson University
Director of Hospital Pediatrics
Thomas Jefferson University Hospital
Philadelphia, Pennsylvania

T. Ernesto Figueroa, MD, FAAP, FACS
Clinical Associate Professor
Department of Urology
Thomas Jefferson University
Philadelphia, Pennsylvania
Chief
Division of Pediatric Urology
Alfred I. duPont Hospital for Children
Wilmington, Delaware

Darren M. Fiore, MD
Assistant Clinical Professor
Department of Pediatrics
University of California
San Francisco, California

Susan A. Fisher-Owens, MD, MPH
Assistant Clinical Professor
Department of Pediatrics
University of California
San Francisco, California

Lourdes Forster, MD, FAAP
Assistant Professor of Clinical Pediatrics
Department of Pediatrics
University of Miami
Miller School of Medicine
Miami, Florida

Johnnie P. Frazier, MD, MEd, FAAP
Associate Professor
Department of Pediatrics
University of Texas Medical School at Houston
Medical Director
Power Medical Center
Department of Pediatrics
University of Texas Medical School at Houston
Houston, Texas

Vani V. Gopalareddy, MD
Division of Gastroenterology
Levine Children's Hospital
Carolinas Medical Center
Charlotte, North Carolina

William R. Graessle, MD
Associate Professor
Department of Pediatrics
UMDNJ-Robert Wood Johnson Medical School
Director
Pediatric Medical Education
Department of Pediatrics
Cooper University Hospital
Camden, New Jersey

Maryellen E. Gusic, MD
Associate Dean for Clinical Education
Penn State College of Medicine
Professor of Pediatrics
Division of General Pediatrics
Penn State Hershey Children's Hospital
Hershey, Pennsylvania

Keith Herzog, MD
Assistant Professor of Pediatrics
Drexel University College of Medicine
Section of General Pediatrics
St. Christopher's Hospital for Children
Philadelphia, Pennsylvania

Larry H. Hollier, Jr., MD, FACS
Professor and Program Director
Department of Plastic Surgery
Baylor College of Medicine
Professor
Department of Plastic Surgery
Texas Children's Hospital
Houston, Texas

Karina Irizarry, MD, FAAP
Affiliate Assistant Professor
Department of Pediatrics
University of South Florida College of Medicine
Attending Physician
Department of Pediatric Gastroenterology
All Children's Hospital
St. Petersburg, Florida

Shonul Agarwal Jain, MD
Assistant Clinical Professor
Department of Pediatrics
University of California
Assistant Clinical Professor
Department of Pediatrics
San Francisco General Hospital
San Francisco, California

Shareen F. Kelly, MD
Assistant Professor of Pediatrics
Department of Pediatrics
Drexel College of Medicine
Attending Physician
Ambulatory Pediatrics
St. Christopher's Hospital for Children
Philadelphia, Pennsylvania

Brandi M. Kenner, MD
Pediatric Dermatology Fellow
Departments of Pediatrics and Dermatology
Northwestern University
Feinberg School of Medicine
Pediatric Dermatology Fellow
Division of Pediatric Dermatology
Children's Memorial Hospital
Chicago, Illinois

Hans B. Kersten, MD
Associate Professor of Pediatrics
Department of Pediatrics
Drexel University College of Medicine
Attending Physician
Section of General Pediatrics
St. Christopher's Hospital for Children
Philadelphia, Pennsylvania

David M. Krol, MD, MPH, FAAP
Team Director and Senior Program Officer
Robert Wood Johnson Foundation
Princeton, New Jersey

Naline Lai, MD
Attending Physician
Buckingham Pediatrics
Buckingham, Pennsylvania
Attending Physician
Department of Pediatrics
Doylestown Hospital
Doylestown, Pennsylvania

Tomitra Latimer, MD
Clinical Assistant Professor
Department of Pediatrics
Northwestern Feinberg School of Medicine
Attending Physician
General Academic Pediatrics
Children's Memorial Hospital
Chicago, Illinois

Kelly R. Leite, DO
Associate Professor
Department of Pediatrics
Penn State College of Medicine
Director
Pediatric Residency Program
Department of Pediatrics
Penn State Hershey Children's Hospital
Hershey, Pennsylvania

Paul S. Matz, MD
Advocare Haddon Pediatric Group
Haddon Heights, New Jersey

Liana K. McCabe, MD
Clinical Instructor
Department of Pediatrics
UCSF
San Francisco, California

Devendra I. Mehta, MBBS, MS, MRCP
Associate Professor
Florida State University College of Medicine
Tallahassee, Florida
Head, Outcome and Translational Research
Pediatric Subspecialty Practice
Arnold Palmer Hospital for Children
Orlando, Florida

Denise W. Metry, MD
Associate Professor
Department of Dermatology and Pediatrics
Baylor College of Medicine
Chief
Department of Dermatology
Texas Children's Hospital
Houston, Texas

Colette C. Mull, MD
Assistant Professor in Pediatrics and Emergency
Medicine
Director, Pediatric Emergency Medicine Fellowship
Department of Emergency Medicine
Drexel University School of Medicine
St. Christopher's Hospital for Children
Physician Faculty Member
Department of Emergency Medicine
St. Christopher's Hospital for Children
Philadelphia, Pennsylvania

Julieana Nichols, MD, MPH
Assistant Professor
Department of Pediatrics
Baylor College of Medicine
Assistant Professor
Department of Pediatrics
Texas Children's Hospital
Houston, Texas

Christopher O'Hara, MD
Assistant Professor
Department of Pediatrics
Drexel University College of Medicine
Attending Physician
Department of Pediatrics
St. Christopher's Hospital for Children
Philadelphia, Pennsylvania

Parul B. Patel, MD, MPH
Assistant Professor
Department of Pediatrics
Feinberg School of Medicine
Northwestern University
Attending Physician
Department of Pediatric Emergency Medicine
Children's Memorial Hospital
Chicago, Illinois

Charles A. Pohl, MD
Professor
Department of Pediatrics
Jefferson Medical College
Philadelphia, Pennsylvania

David M. Pressel, MD, PhD
Associate Professor
Department of Pediatrics
Jefferson Medical College of Thomas Jefferson University
Philadelphia, Pennsylvania
Director
General Pediatrics Inpatient Service
Department of Pediatrics
Alfred I. duPont Hospital for Children
Wilmington, Delaware

Amy Renwick, MD
Assistant Professor
Department of Pediatrics
Jefferson Medical College of Thomas Jefferson University
Philadelphia, Pennsylvania
Attending Physician
Department of General Pediatrics
Alfred I. duPont Hospital for Children
Wilmington, Delaware

Denise A. Salerno, MD, FAAP
Professor of Clinical Pediatrics
Pediatric Clerkship Director
Department of Pediatrics
Temple University School of Medicine
Attending Physician
Department of Neonatology
Temple University Hospital
Philadelphia, Pennsylvania

Harold V. Salvati, MD
Attending Pediatrician
Virtua Hospital
Carnie Boulevard
Voorhees, New Jersey
General Pediatrician
Advocare-DelGiorno Pediatrics
Blackwood, New Jersey

Lee M. Sanders, MD, MPH
Associate Professor
Department of Pediatrics
University of Miami
Holtz Children's Hospital
Miami, Florida

Steven M. Selbst, MD, FAAP
Professor
Department of Pediatrics
Jefferson Medical College of Thomas Jefferson University
Philadelphia, Pennsylvania
Pediatric Residency Program Director
Attending Physician
Department of Pediatrics
Division of Emergency Medicine
Alfred I. duPont Hospital for Children
Wilmington, Delaware

Beth A. Shortridge, MD, FAAP
Attending Physician
Department of Pediatrics
Alfred I. duPont Hospital for Children
Nemours Children's Clinic
Wynnewood, Pennsylvania

Laura E. Smals, MD
Associate Professor of Pediatrics
Department of Pediatrics
Penn State University College of Medicine
Section of General Pediatrics
Milton S. Hershey Medical Center Children's Hospital
Hershey, Pennsylvania

Nancy D. Spector, MD
Associate Professor
Department of Pediatrics
Drexel University College of Medicine
Associate Chair of Education and Faculty Development
Associate Residency Program Director
Department of Medical and Academic Affairs
St. Christopher's Hospital for Children
Philadelphia, Pennsylvania

Valarie Stricklen, MD, FAAP
Assistant Professor
Department of Pediatrics
University of Toledo
Toledo, Ohio

Daniel R. Taylor, DO
Assistant Professor
Department of Pediatrics
Drexel University College of Medicine
General Pediatrician
Department of Pediatrics
St. Christopher's Hospital for Children
Philadelphia, Pennsylvania

E. Douglas Thompson, Jr., MD
Assistant Professor
Department of Pediatrics
Drexel University College of Medicine
Director
Pediatric Generalist Service
Department of Pediatrics
St. Christopher's Hospital for Children
Philadelphia, Pennsylvania

Renee M. Turchi, MD, MPH, FAAP
Assistant Professor
Department of Community Health and Prevention
Drexel University School of Public Health
Medical Director, Special Programs
Department of Pediatrics
St. Christopher's Hospital for Children
Philadelphia, Pennsylvania

Daniel T. Walmsley, DO
Clinical Assistant Professor
Department of Pediatrics
Thomas Jefferson University
Philadelphia, Pennsylvania
Pediatrician
Department of Pediatrics
Alfred I. duPont Hospital for Children
Wilmington, Delaware

Evan J. Weiner, MD, FAAP
Assistant Professor of Pediatrics and Emergency Medicine
Drexel University College of Medicine
Attending Physician
Department of Emergency Medicine
St. Christopher's Hospital for Children
Philadelphia, Pennsylvania

D'Juanna White-Satcher, MD, MPH
Assistant Professor
Department of Pediatrics
Baylor College of Medicine
Attending Physician
Section of Academic General Pediatrics
Texas Children's Hospital
Houston, Texas

Michael J. Wilsey, Jr., MD, FAAP
Affiliate Assistant Professor
Department of Pediatrics
Associate Director
Pediatric Residency Training Program
University of South Florida College of Medicine
Attending Physician
Department of Pediatric Gastroenterology
All Children's Hospital
St. Petersburg, Florida

Jeoffrey K. Wolens, MD
Staff Physician
Department of General Medicine
Texas Children's Hospital
Houston, Texas

Mary Elizabeth Wroblewski, MD, FAAP
Assistant Professor
Department of Pediatrics
The University of Toledo
Toledo, Ohio

Serena Yang, MD, MPH
Assistant Clinical Professor
Department of Pediatrics
UCSF Fresno Medical Education Program
Fresno, California
Assistant Clinical Professor
Department of Pediatrics
Children's Hospital Central California
Madera, California

Foreword

A second edition of a book is somewhat like having grandchildren, more fun, fewer issues, and a chance to learn from the first effort. The second edition is an opportunity to build on the structure of the first edition, learning what readers liked and what they thought could be improved as well as adding new information. The objective of the first edition was to produce a fresh and focused visual compendium of pediatric conditions that allowed the reader to enter into the diagnostic process in an efficient way. Since the concept and design of the first edition were very well planned and executed, the second edition required only minor polishing of the contents, making some alterations to the content and organization, and adding new topics. This new edition accomplishes all of these objectives.

The new section "When to Consider Further Evaluation or Treatment" is such an example of how this second edition has been improved. No book would be complete without another table or two, so the new table on differential diagnosis is a welcomed addition. Improved legends for the illustrations will also help the reader use the information to make a diagnosis of a lesion or rash.

Dr. Chung and her editorial staff should be congratulated for continuing the high standards that they established in their first book. Again they present a consultative book that will help the reader quickly make a diagnosis and begin treatment. That, of course, is the goal of a good reference.

M. William Schwartz, MD
Emeritus Professor of Pediatrics
University of Pennsylvania School of Medicine
Senior Physician Emeritus, The Children's Hospital of Philadelphia

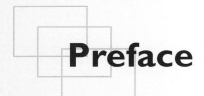

Preface

The making of the first edition of *Visual Diagnosis in Pediatrics* was an exciting adventure, filled with endless possibilities. On the one hand, we wanted to produce a book that added something new to the existing library of diagnostic books available to clinicians. On the other hand, we had to keep in mind that clinicians today are busier than ever, with little time to seek guidance from a book, and are in need of quick, well-organized information. To address these needs, we developed a user-friendly format with differential diagnoses for a problem listed in a single table and photographs of these diagnoses placed side by side for comparison. We focused on providing pearls and approaches, rather than providing exhaustive descriptions or detailed lists. The final product surpassed anyone's expectations. Available worldwide, this book has been translated into two different languages, Chinese and Portuguese.

The new and improved second edition of this book has a number of new features including the following: (1) improved readability with respect to format and layout, (2) a new section for each chapter called "When to Consider Further Evaluation or Treatment," and (3) a new column added to the Differential Diagnoses table that addresses Treatment Guidelines. All of the chapters pertaining to the newborn are now organized into a single section, "Visual Diagnoses in the Newborn." A new addition is a chapter on breastfeeding images that demonstrates proper latch and contains essential photographs to help clinicians promote and support breastfeeding.

A major goal for this edition and the first was to include photographs demonstrating the breadth of pediatrics and the ethnic diversity of patients living in the United States and abroad. We have photographs demonstrating marks found after "coining," a practice performed by some East Asian cultures, and we show classic "Mongolian" spots that are found in many people with pigmented skin. Bear in mind that these photographs are of people—someone's child, grandchild, nephew, or niece—to whom we are indebted. This book would not have been possible without them and the generosity of their families, who allowed us to care for and take photographs of them.

I am grateful for a second opportunity to work with such a talented group of dedicated and experienced clinicians. Their willingness to gather photographs and to write chapters stems from their commitments to education and to improving the clinical care of patients. Our contributors, from academic medicine and private practice, have spent hours that extended well into the night. I am grateful that two very talented and committed associate editors, Drs. Julie A. Boom and Paul S. Matz, returned to make our second edition better than the first. Dr. Lee R. Atkinson-McEvoy, our newest associate editor, was a true asset to our team. Special thanks are due to Dr. Steven Handler who provided many of the otolaryngology photographs in both editions of this book. Dr. George A. Datto, who helped conceptualize the first edition of this book and whose photographs are found throughout both editions, deserves special recognition.

Lippincott Williams & Wilkins, our publisher, continues to produce books of the highest quality, thanks to their well-trained and professional staff. Sonya Seigafusa, our acquisitions editor, who is highly professional and forward thinking, made producing a book of this scope easy. Nicole Walz, our product manager, made the final stages of production run smoothly and stress free!

Medical books continue to be an important source of information even during a time when many medical facts can be found by simply entering a few words into a computer search engine. We hope that you find this visual diagnosis book to be a valuable addition to the resources used in your clinical practice.

Table of Contents

Visual Diagnoses
in the Newborn

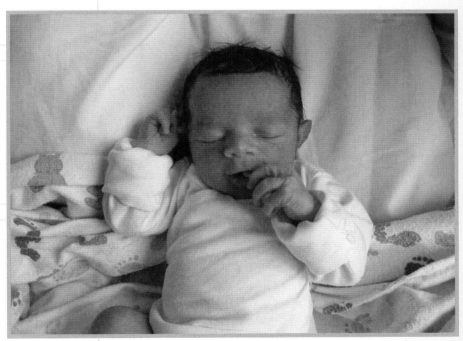

(Courtesy of Lee R. Atkinson-McEvoy, MD.)

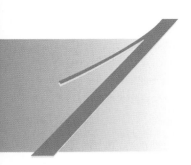

LOURDES FORSTER
AND LEE M. SANDERS

Breastfeeding

APPROACH TO THE PROBLEM

Assessing a nursing infant requires careful attention to the mother and the child during each clinical encounter. Effective diagnosis and treatment of breastfeeding problems cannot be accomplished without the clinician's observation of the infant at the mother's breast.

Unlike most other pediatric encounters, the mother becomes an important subject of a focused history and physical examination. In the mother's medical and social history, critical findings can help the clinician identify easily treatable conditions or more difficult challenges to successful breastfeeding. Similarly, examination of the mother's breast can reveal tell-tale signs of underlying problems. First-time mothers will usually feel their milk "come in" by 72 hours after delivery. Infrequent or inadequate drainage of the breasts in the first days of life can result in greater pain from engorgement and ultimately affect the volume of milk produced.

While the infant is breastfeeding or attempting to breastfeed, the clinician can observe critical features—including infant feeding cues, position, and latch—that can help diagnose common problems or determine the need for further assistance from a lactation consultant.

The clinician's goals should be three-fold: (1) to encourage breastfeeding for all mothers and infants; (2) to assess and treat breastfeeding-related problems early; and (3) to provide a positive, nonjudgmental environment for promoting infant nutrition and growth.

KEY POINTS IN THE HISTORY

Mother

- **Delivery Complications**. C-section incisions are often associated with increased pain during breastfeeding.

- **Medications**. Sedatives, antihistamines, diuretics, or exogenous estrogen (oral contraceptives) contribute to low milk synthesis. Even a single dose of barbiturates during labor (often given for a C-section delivery for failure to progress) has been shown to impede the milk intake of infants in the first days of life.

- *Medical History*. Hypothyroidism, peripartum infection, or retained placenta may impair breastfeeding success. Mothers who were overweight or obese (Body Mass Index >24) prior to pregnancy are less likely to initiate breastfeeding or to continue breastfeeding through 6 months. Preexisting or pregnancy-related back pain or hemorrhoids may also complicate the pain associated with certain breastfeeding positions.

- *Surgical History*. Breast reduction surgery may lead to a significant reduction in milk production. By contrast, most mothers who have breast implants can successfully nurse.

- *Tobacco Use*. Smoking has been shown to interfere with the milk let-down reflex. There is a direct relationship between the amount a woman smokes and decreased milk production.

- *Maternal Support*. Traditionally, women have relied on their spouses, mothers and grand-mothers for support and instruction. If these support figures are not available, mothers are more likely to benefit from thorough lactation instruction and support.

- *Depressive Symptoms*. Peripartum depression is common, often undiagnosed, and a significant contributor to other common maternal stressors in the first months of an infant's life. Depression and anxiety may impede milk production and successful infant latch.

Infant

- *Gestational Age*. Preterm and near-term (<37 weeks' gestation) infants are at higher risk for breastfeeding difficulty because of problems with latch and coordinated suckling.

- *Apgar Scores*. A 5-minute Apgar score less than 6 has been associated with decreased rates of successful breastfeeding initiation.

- *Medical History*. Significant metabolic, renal, or cardiac disorders may increase infant losses or metabolic demand. In addition to impairing adequate weight gain, these conditions may make breastfeeding more difficult for the infant or require supplementation with high-calorie formulas. Infants with Trisomy 21 syndrome often exhibit impaired oromotor skills that may make breastfeeding more challenging.

- *Feeding Pattern*. Infrequent feedings because of mother-infant separation, pacifier use, or supplementation with water, teas, or juices will interfere with milk production. Diaphoresis or tiring with feedings may be a sign of an undiagnosed cardiac or metabolic disease.

- *Use of Infant Formula*. Use of infant formula in the newborn nursery is a predictor of early discontinuation of breastfeeding and considered a red flag for insufficient milk production.

| KEY POINTS IN THE PHYSICAL EXAMINATION | |

Mother

- *Nipple*. Cracks or fissures of the nipple may indicate problems (see below). Nipple inversion is a common problem that may be corrected with the use of a nipple shield.

- *Maternal Mood*. Fatigue and stress are the most common causes of inadequate milk supply. Maternal-infant emotional attachment is crucial for the breastfeeding dyad to succeed. The mother's ability to identify and respond to her infant's feeding cues will ensure frequent and timely feeds. This, in turn, promotes continued milk production.

Nursing Process

- *Infant Feeding Cues*. Common infant feeding cues include wriggling with eyes wide open, hands to mouth or face, rooting with an open mouth, and smacking lips. Assess the mother's facility in identifying and acting on these cues.

- *Infant Feeding Position*. Four common positions (cradle hold, football hold, cross-cradle hold, and lying) are illustrated in the figures 1-1 to 1-4 below. Assess the mother's comfort and confidence in trying at least two different positions to accommodate her and her infant.

- *Infant Latch*. Nipple cracks, fissures, and pain may be caused by superficial latches that do not reach the infant's soft palate, where the infant's lower lip is curled inward, where mother is taking the infant off the breast without breaking suction or leading with the baby's nose instead of the chin. Appropriate infant latch should include the following:
    a. a wide-open mouth immediately prior to bringing the baby to breast
    b. the baby's lips should be flanged, "fish-like"
    c. the mother holds her breast with her thumb on top and four fingers beneath ("C" hold)
    d. audible or visible swallowing, with about two to three sucks per swallow

- *Maternal Comfort*. During effective breastfeeding, the mother may experience tingling within the breast, but she should not experience sharp pains. After nursing, her breasts should feel softer without any soreness. Pain during breastfeeding is one of the most common causes of poor milk production and discontinuation of breastfeeding.

Infant

- Normal weight gain is a good sign of successful breastfeeding. Weight loss of greater than 10% from birth weight or other signs of failure to thrive merit further investigation, including increased attention to the breastfeeding history and examination of the nursing process.

- Moist mucous membranes, flat anterior fontanelle, and adequate peripheral perfusion are good signs of adequate oral hydration.

- Cleft lip or palate, high-arched palate, tight lingual frenulum, or micrognathia may impair a successful latch. Absence of a strong suck reflex may indicate poor oromotor development or an underlying neurologic abnormality that would impair breastfeeding.

- Abnormal motor tone or reflexes may indicate an underlying neurologic abnormality that may also impair oromotor development and, therefore, breastfeeding.

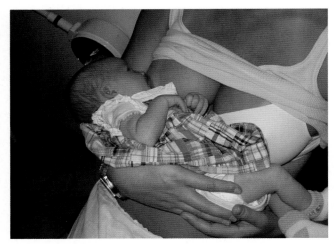

Figure 1-1 Cradle hold.
(Courtesy of Lourdes Forster, MD, FAAP.)

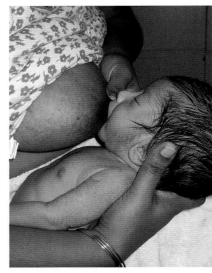

Figure 1-2 Football hold.
(Courtesy of Lourdes Forster, MD, FAAP.)

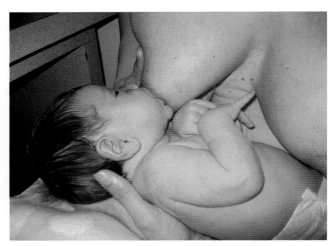

Figure 1-3 Cross-cradle hold.
(Courtesy of Lourdes Forster, MD, FAAP.)

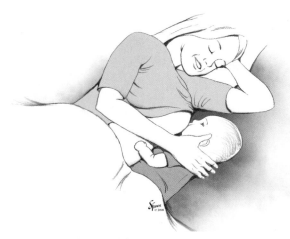

Figure 1-4 Lying position.
(Drawing by Satyen Tripathi, MA.)

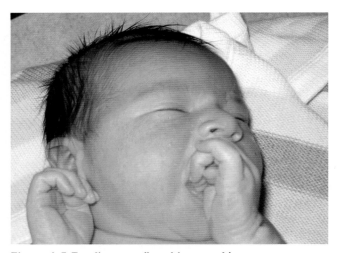

Figure 1-5 Feeding cue (hand in mouth).
(Courtesy of Lourdes Forster, MD, FAAP.)

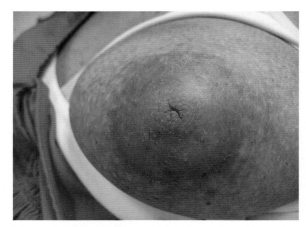

Figure 1-6 Nipple fissure. Note fissure from 2 o'clock to 8 o'clock position. Such a fissure indicates an improper latch (i.e., "nipple latch").
(Courtesy of Lourdes Forster, MD, FAAP.)

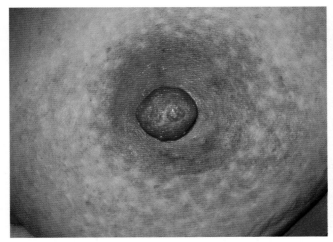

Figure 1-7 Nipple fissure. Note fissure from 11 o'clock to 5 o'clock position. Such a fissure indicates an improper latch (i.e., "nipple latch").
(Courtesy of Lourdes Forster, MD, FAAP.)

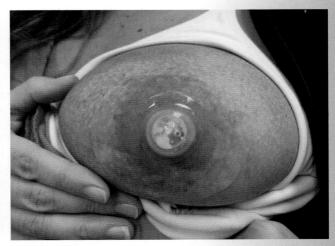

Figure 1-8 Infant nursing on a retracted nipple covered with a nursing shield.
(Courtesy of Lourdes Forster, MD, FAAP.)

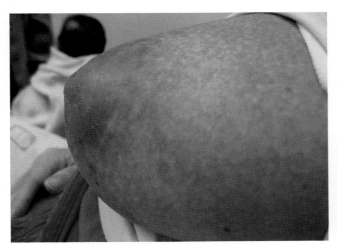

Figure 1-9 Breast engorgement. Signs of breast engorgement include a flat nipple.
(Courtesy of Lourdes Forster, MD, FAAP.)

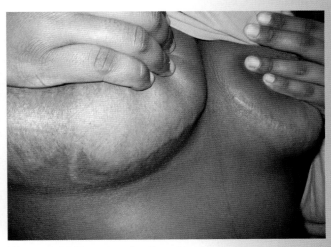

Figure 1-10 Breast reduction. Note scars from breast reduction surgery.
(Courtesy of Lourdes Forster, MD, FAAP.)

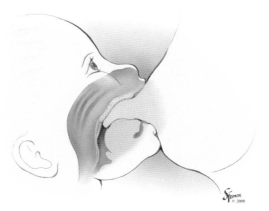

Figure 1-11 Cross section of infant latch. Note two critical features of a successful latch: the nipple protrudes to make contact with the infant's soft palate, and the infant's lower lip is folded outward.
(Drawing by Satyen Tripathi, MA.)

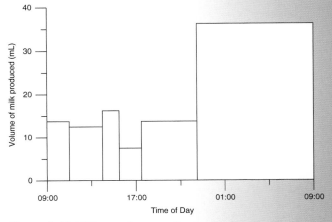

Figure 1-12 Milk supply, over time.
(Drawing by Satyen Tripathi, MA.)

DIFFERENTIAL DIAGNOSIS

DIAGNOSIS	ICD-9	CHARACTERISTICS	DURATION
Nipple, Burning Pain, Hyperesthesia	782.0	Nipple fissure, cracking	Variable
Nipple, Cracks or Fissures	676.14	Usually in first week, often worsening	Variable
Nipple, Sore	676.34	First indication of poor latch Up to 96% of mothers	Variable
Nonnutritive Sucking/ Feeding Problem of Newborn	779.3	Poor weight gain, fussy Decreased stool and urine output	Variable
Breast Engorgement	676.24	Congestion or distension of the breast tissue Up to 85% of mothers	Peaks at 3–4 days after birth but can last up to 14 days

ASSOCIATED FINDINGS	COMPLICATIONS	PRECIPITATING FACTORS	TREATMENT GUIDELINES
Pain	Infection	Fissures or cracks	Pain management Evaluate latch
Pain, bleeding	Mastitis Abscess	Poor latch, position	Counseling, repositioning
Scabbing of the nipple	Infrequent feeds	Poor latch, position	Counseling, repositioning
Apparently normal latch without rhythmic suck/swallow	Poor weight gain Failure to thrive	Near-term infant Oral-motor dysfunction	Lactation consultant referral Supplement with expressed breast milk
Breast tissue is tight and shiny. Milk flow is difficult.	Mastitis Decreased milk production	Supplemental feeding Infrequent feedings Mother-infant separation	Frequent feedings Heat application Cold therapy

Maternal Causes of Poor Milk Supply

- Peripartum depression
- Retained placenta
- Post-partum hemorrhage
- Eating disorder
- Primary mammary glandular insufficiency
- Polycystic ovary syndrome
- Systemic lupus erythematosus
- Autoimmune disease or connective tissue disorder
- Other chronic illness

Infant Diagnoses that May Impair Breastfeeding

- Viremia/Viral syndrome
- Serious bacterial illness including urinary tract infection, pneumonia, enteritis, sepsis, and meningitis
- Gastroesophageal reflux
- Prematurity
- Cleft lip or palate
- Gastroesophageal malformations
- Metabolic disorder
- Renal disease
- Hypocalcemia
- Hypothyroidism
- Oral-motor dysfunction
- Central nervous system abnormality

WHEN TO
CONSIDER
FURTHER
EVALUATION
OR TREATMENT

Failure to thrive is the most important indication for further evaluation by the pediatrician in partnership with a lactation consultant. Concerns for failure to thrive would include

- Weight loss of greater than 10% in the first week of life

- Failure to regain birth weight by day 14

- Average daily weight gain of less than 20 g/day

- Infrequent stools, less than 4 stools/day, by the end of the first week

- Concentrated urine, less than 6 wet diapers/day, by the end of the first week

SUGGESTED READINGS

Ahluwalia IB, Morrow B, Hsia J. Why do women stop breastfeeding? Findings from the Pregnancy Risk Assessment and Monitoring System. *Pediatrics.* 2005;116:1408–1412.

Brent N, Rudy SJ, Redd B, et al. Sore nipples in breast-feeding women. *Arch Pediatric Adolesc Med.* 1998;152:1077–1082.

Ip S, Chung M, Raman G, et al. Breastfeeding and maternal and infant health outcomes in developed countries. Evidence Report/Technology Assessment No. 153 (Prepared by Tufts-New England Medical Center Evidence-based Practice Center, under Contract No. 290–02–0022). AHRQ Publication No. 07-E007. Rockville, MD: Agency for Healthcare Research and Quality; 2007.

Lawrence RA, Lawrence RL. *Breastfeeding—A guide for the medical profession.* Philadelphia, PA: Elsevier Mosby; 2005.

Neifert MR. Clinical aspects of lactation. Promoting lactation success. *Clin Perinatol.* 1999;26:281–306.

Riordan J. *Breastfeeding and human lactation.* Sudbury: Jones and Bartlett; 2005.

HANS B. KERSTEN

Scalp Swellings in Newborns

APPROACH TO THE PROBLEM

Most scalp swellings unique to newborns are related to the forces exerted on the head during the infants' passage through the birth canal. These problems are usually self-limited, and they resolve within a couple of days to weeks, although some may require close monitoring. Fixed abnormalities in the skull shape may represent synostosis (see Chapter 4).

KEY POINTS IN THE HISTORY

- Molding and caput succedaneum are usually evident right after birth, but a cephalohematoma or subgaleal hemorrhage may take hours to form or become evident.

- Caput succedaneum results from local subcutaneous edema and fluid collection, most commonly in the parieto-occipital region following a vaginal birth.

- Caput succedaneum and molding usually resolve in the first few days of life.

- Cephalohematoma, a hemorrhage that occurs between the periosteum and the skull bone, may take weeks to resolve.

- Five percent to twenty-five percent of patients with cephalohematomas may have an accompanying skull fracture.

- Subgaleal hemorrhage is bleeding under the galea aponeurotica that may occur with significant birth trauma.

- There is an increased incidence of subgaleal hemorrhage with vacuum extraction.

KEY POINTS IN THE PHYSICAL EXAMINATION

- The swelling in caput succedaneum crosses suture lines because it is above the cranium in the subcutaneous tissue.

- Caput succedanea, unlike cephalohematomas, tend to have pitting edema.

- Cephalohematomas are boggy and do not extend across suture lines because they are limited by the boundaries of the periosteum.

- There is no discoloration of the scalp with a cephalohematoma unless there is an overlying caput or bruising in the subcutaneous tissue.

- Subgaleal hematomas are considered fluctuant masses that cross suture lines, may be associated with a fluid wave or ecchymoses behind the ear, and may extend to other areas of the scalp.

- The ecchymoses that may be associated with caput succedaneum and the bleeding seen with cephalohematomas and subgaleal hematomas may contribute to neonatal jaundice.

- A cranial meningocele and an encephalocele are pulsatile midline masses, and this may differentiate them from other causes of scalp swelling.

PHOTOGRAPHS OF SELECTED DIAGNOSES

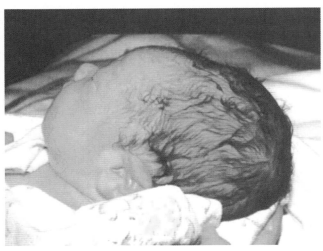

Figure 2-1 Molding. Note the superior and posterior displacement of the skull bones.
(Courtesy of Joseph Piatt, MD.)

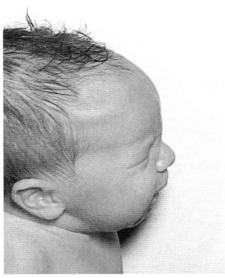

Figure 2-2 Caput succedaneum. Caput succedaneum shows pitting on pressure.
(Used with permission from O'Doherty N. *Atlas of the newborn*. Philadelphia, PA: JB Lippincott Co.; 1979:136.)

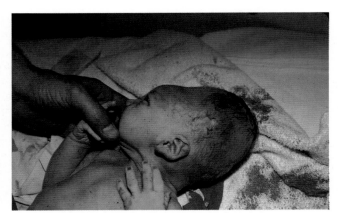

Figure 2-3 Caput succedaneum. Large soft swelling over the vertex, not confined to suture lines.
(Courtesy of the late Peter Sol, MD.)

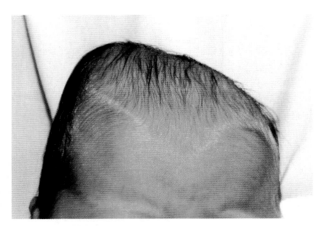

Figure 2-4 Cephalohematoma. Note the swelling over the right parietal area.
(Used with permission from Fletcher MA. *Physical diagnosis in neonatology*. Philadelphia, PA: Lippincott–Raven Publishers; 1998:185.)

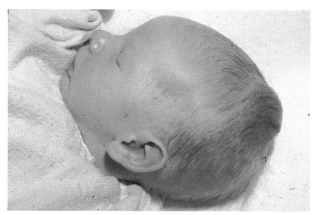

Figure 2-5 Cephalohematoma. Well-demarcated swelling over the left parietal bone.
(Courtesy of the late Peter Sol, MD.)

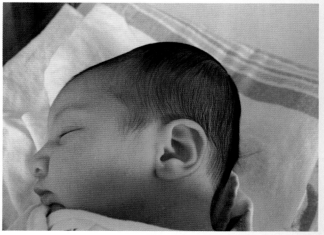

Figure 2-6 Cephalohematoma. Note the prominence of the left parietooccipital area in this newborn with a cephalohematoma.
(Courtesy of Esther K. Chung, MD, MPH.)

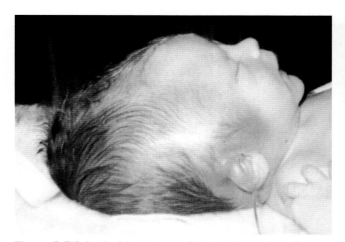

Figure 2-7 Subgaleal hematoma. Discoloration and swelling extends across suture lines onto the neck, even onto the ear, causing protuberance of the pinna.
(Used with permission from Fletcher MA. *Physical diagnosis in neonatology.* Philadelphia, PA: Lippincott–Raven Publishers; 1998:185.)

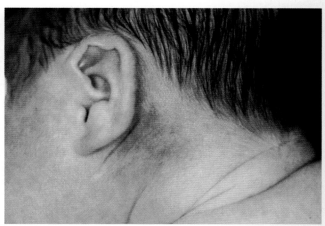

Figure 2-8 Ecchymosis after subgaleal hemorrhage. The bilateral location of this blood collection away from the site of forceps application suggests a wide area of involvement typical of a moderately large subgaleal hematoma.
(Used with permission from Fletcher MA. *Physical diagnosis in neonatology.* Philadelphia, PA: Lippincott–Raven Publishers; 1998:128.)

DIFFERENTIAL DIAGNOSIS

DIAGNOSIS	ICD-9	DISTINGUISHING CHARACTERISTICS	DISTRIBUTION
Molding	767.3	Overlapping bones along suture lines	Along suture lines
Caput Succedaneum	767.1	Soft-tissue swelling that crosses suture lines	Parieto-occipital or diffuse swelling May see dependent edema on one side
Cephalohematoma	767.1	Subperiosteal hemorrhage Swelling that does not cross suture lines Boggy feeling	Focal swelling Usually the parietal area May be bilateral
Subgaleal Hematoma	767.11	Fluctuant to tense swelling that crosses suture lines	Focal or diffuse swelling Fluid wave
Cranial Meningocele	742	CSF-filled meningeal sac Pulsatile Increased pressure when crying	Midline cranium
Cranial Encephalocele	742	CSF-filled meningeal sac plus cerebral cortex, cerebellum, and/or portions of the brain stem	Midline cranium, most commonly at the occiput

ASSOCIATED FINDINGS	COMPLICATIONS	PREDISPOSING FACTORS	TREATMENT GUIDELINES
Caput succedaneum	Hemorrhage Fracture	Vaginal birth	Observation Resolves in first few weeks of life Rare cause of shock requiring blood transfusion
Swelling develops during birth process Scalp ecchymoses Discoloration and distortion of the face with face presentations	Hemorrhage Fracture Jaundice	Vaginal delivery Vertex delivery Vacuum suctioning	Observation Usually resolves in the first few days of life Monitor for neonatal jaundice.
Palpable rim Swelling develops hours after birth Calcifications may develop Rare association with skull fracture, coagulopathy, and intracranial hemorrhage	Hemorrhage Skull fracture Jaundice Calcification	Vaginal delivery Vacuum suctioning	Observation May take 2 weeks to 3 months to resolve Monitor for neonatal jaundice.
Swelling Ecchymosis develops shortly after birth. Ecchymoses behind ear	Hemorrhage Shock Severe anemia Death	Vacuum suctioning	Observation Requires observation in an NICU for progressive enlargement and associated anemia, hypovolemia, shock, or jaundice
Fluctuant midline mass Transilluminates Occasional tethering, syringomyelia, and diastematomyelia	Good prognosis	Embryologic defect causing herniation of meninges through defect in the skull/cranial sutures	X-ray of the skull and cervical spine to define anatomy
Elevated α-fetoprotein levels in utero, midline mass, hydrocephalus due to aqueductal stenosis Chiari malformation or Dandy Walker syndrome	Poorer prognosis with visual problems, mental retardation, craniofacial anomalies, and epilepsy occurring	Embryologic defect causing herniation of meninges and other neural tissues through defect in the skull/cranial sutures	X-ray of the skull and cervical spine to define anatomy Ultrasound or neuroimaging to determine the contents and extent of the sac Neurosurgery consultation to assess need for removal or decompression

OTHER
DIAGNOSES
TO CONSIDER

- Plagiocephaly

- Skull fractures

- Porencephalic or leptomeningeal cyst

- Cranial meningocele

- Cranial encephalocele

WHEN TO
CONSIDER
FURTHER
EVALUATION
OR TREATMENT

- Subgaleal hematomas are important to consider, as they will require observation in an NICU for progressive enlargement and associated anemia, hypovolemia, shock, or jaundice.

- A cephalohematoma with an accompanying skull fracture may need to have neuroimaging and a neurosurgical consultation.

- Cephalohemotomas, subgaleal hematomas, and caput succedaneums may be complicated by anemia or jaundice requiring phototherapy or blood transfusions.

- If a cranial meningocele is a consideration, an x-ray must be done to confirm if there is a skull defect, and other neuroimaging should be done to see if there are any associated complications.

- If a cranial encephalocele is a consideration, prompt neurosurgical consultation should be arranged for possible decompression.

SUGGESTED READINGS

Bates B, ed. *A guide to physical examination and history taking*. 5th ed. Philadelphia, PA: JB Lippincott Co. 1991:586–589.

Behrman RE, Kliegman RM, Jenson HB, eds. *Nelson textbook of pediatrics*. 16th ed. Philadelphia, PA: WB Saunders; 2000:488–489.

Fletcher MA. *Physical diagnosis in neonatology*. Philadelphia, PA: Lippincott–Raven Publishers; 1998:128, 173–185.

McMillan JA, DeAngelis CD, Feigin RD, Warshaw JB, eds. *Oski's pediatrics: principles and practice*. 3rd ed. Philadelphia, PA: Lippincott Williams & Wilkins; 1999:163, 610–611.

O'Doherty N. *Atlas of the newborn*. Philadelphia, PA: JB Lippincott Co.; 1979:136.

Rudolph CD, Rudolph AM, Hostetter MK, Siegel NJ, eds. *Rudolph's pediatrics*. 21st ed. New York: McGraw-Hill; 2003: 87, 186–187.

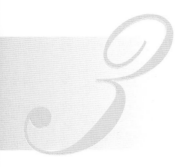

SHAREEN F. KELLY
AND LAURA E. SMALS

Newborn Facial Lesions

APPROACH TO THE PROBLEM

Lesions on the face of a newborn may be the result of congenital malformations, birthmarks, or common skin rashes such as seborrhea and neonatal acne. These lesions are usually benign, but, at times, they may represent underlying pathology. Familiarity with the appearance of various newborn facial lesions will enable the physician to allay parental fears and to provide appropriate recommendations.

KEY POINTS IN THE HISTORY

- A reddish lesion that has been present since birth indicates a congenital lesion such as a nevus simplex (also known as salmon patch, stork bite, angel's kiss) or a nevus flammeus (port-wine stain).

- Most nevus simplex lesions fade and become less noticeable over time.

- Nevus flammeus lesions usually do not fade.

- Neonatal acne is often not present at birth but appears within the first 1 or 2 weeks of life.

- Pruritus or scaliness of the skin suggests infantile eczema.

- When assessing lesions that have been present since birth, it is essential to ask about the infant's delivery to determine whether incidental trauma or trauma from the use of forceps may be a contributing factor.

- Forceps marks generally resolve over time.

- A rash that spreads from the scalp to the face in early infancy may indicate seborrhea (also known as *cradle cap*).

KEY POINTS IN THE PHYSICAL EXAMINATION

- A flat, blanching erythematous patch on the forehead, eyelids, or nape of the neck is likely to be a nevus simplex.

- A flat deep red-purplish patch is most likely to be a nevus flammeus, or port-wine stain.

- Erythematous pustules on the cheeks at 2 to 4 weeks of life suggest neonatal acne.

- Yellowish, shiny plaques on the scalp and face, particularly involving the brow, are most likely seborrhea.

- Dry, scaly pustules, papules, and plaques are seen in infantile eczema.

- In young infants with eczema, a circular collection of papules may be seen and, at times, be mistaken for tinea corporis.

- Eczema tends to spare the nasolabial folds and skin folds behind the ear, but seborrhea does not.

- Multiple small, yellow papules on the nose of a newborn are likely sebaceous hyperplasia, a self-limited benign finding often mistaken for milia.

PHOTOGRAPHS OF SELECTED DIAGNOSES

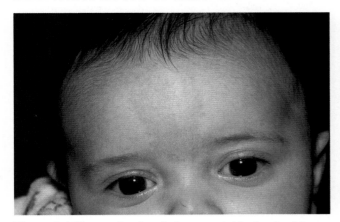

Figure 3-1 Nevus simplex (salmon patch). A pale pink, blanching macule on the face of an infant.
(Used with permission from Goodheart HP. *Goodheart's photoguide of common skin disorders.* 2nd ed. Philadelphia, PA: Lippincott Williams & Wilkins; 2003:1.)

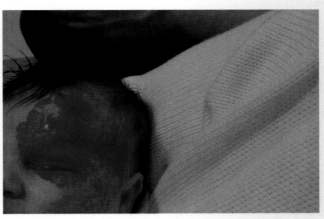

Figure 3-2 Nevus flammeus (port-wine stain). The involvement of the ophthalmic division of the trigeminal nerve necessitates brain imaging in this neonate.
(Courtesy of Brian Forbes, MD.)

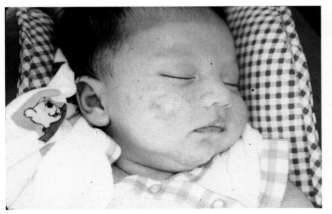

Figure 3-3 Neonatal acne. Mild facial acne commonly seen in the first 2 months of life.
(Courtesy of Amy Ross, MD.)

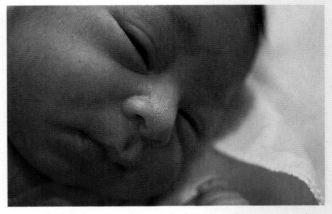

Figure 3-4 Sebaceous hyperplasia. Note the numerous tiny yellow-white papules on this infant's nose.
(Courtesy of George A. Datto, III, MD.)

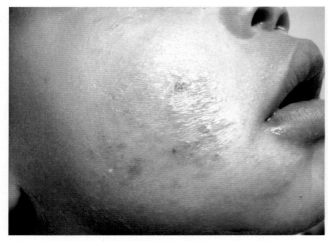

Figure 3-5 Infantile eczema. Dry excoriated skin progressing to weeping lesions is common in neonatal acne.
(Courtesy of Paul S. Matz, MD.)

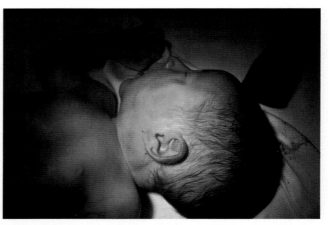

Figure 3-6 Forceps marks. Forceps marks are generally seen on the head and face and may mimic the shape of the forceps themselves.
(Courtesy of the late Peter Sol, MD.)

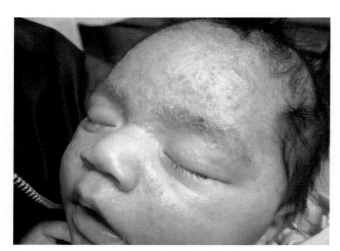

Figure 3-7 Seborrhea. Note the yellow crusting overlying the salmon-colored lesions on this African American infant.
(Courtesy of Paul S. Matz, MD.)

DIFFERENTIAL DIAGNOSIS

DIAGNOSIS	ICD-9	DISTINGUISHING CHARACTERISTICS	DISTRIBUTION	ASSOCIATED FINDINGS	COMPLICATIONS	TREATMENT GUIDELINES
Nevus Simplex (Salmon Patch)	757.38	Erythematous macular patch present at birth that generally fades with time Represents dilated capillaries	Nape of the neck, forehead, and eyelids	Will darken in color with Valsalva maneuver (crying, etc.)	None	No treatment needed
Nevus Flammeus (Port-Wine Stain)	757.32	Begins as pink-red macular patch that darkens and becomes more purple (port-wine colored) with time Dilated superficial and deep capillaries	Most commonly the face and neck, but may occur anywhere Typically unilateral	Nevus flammeus in the ophthalmic division of the trigeminal nerve may be associated with Sturge-Weber syndrome Ipsilateral glaucoma	None	Depending on the size and location of the lesion, no treatment may be needed or pulsed dye laser may be used. Brain imaging if occurs in ophthalmic division of the trigeminal nerve
Neonatal Acne	706.1	Closed comedones, occasionally open comedones, pustules, and papules	Forehead, nose, and cheeks	Secondary to maternal hormone stimulation	None	Treatment rarely required beyond normal cleansing
Sebaceous Hyperplasia	706.9	1–2 mm yellow papules Resolves spontaneously within 4–6 months	Nose and cheeks of young infants	Secondary to stimulation by maternal hormones	None	No treatment needed
Infantile Eczema	690.12	Erythematous papules, pustules, plaques, with crusting and scale	Face, scalp, anywhere on the body—tends to spare the diaper area	Pruritus and excoriation	Superinfection	Moisturizing skin products Steroid creams
Forceps Marks	763.2	Linear or curvilinear marks	Sides of the face and skull	Indentation Abrasion	Very rarely may be associated with skull fracture	Usually no treatment is needed.
Seborrhea	706.3	Yellowish, greasy plaques with scale Erythematous papules	Scalp, face, behind ears, and in folds of neck	Irritation	Superinfection	Topical corticosteroids may be used to reduce inflammation. Antifungal shampoos may be used on the scalp. Selenium sulfide or other selenium-containing shampoos

OTHER
DIAGNOSES
TO CONSIDER

- Milia

- Miliaria rubra or crystallina

- Herpes simplex virus infection

- Telangiectasia

- Subcutaneous fat necrosis

WHEN TO
CONSIDER
FURTHER
EVALUATION
OR TREATMENT

- Nevus flammeus lesions occurring in the ophthalmic area of the trigeminal nerve should prompt an evaluation for Sturge-Weber syndrome (including magnetic resonance imaging of the brain looking for intracranial vascular malformations).

- Nevus flammeus lesions may also be associated with Klippel-Trenaunay-Weber, Beckwith-Wiedemann, and Cobb syndromes.

- Infantile eczema, which does not improve with topical steroid treatment, should be evaluated for possible low-grade superinfection and/or exacerbation from possible allergens (often food).

SUGGESTED READINGS

Cohen B. *Pediatric dermatology.* 3rd ed. St. Louis, MO: Elsevier; 2005:15–66.

Conlon JD, Drolet BA. Skin lesions in the neonate. *Pediatr Clin North Am.* 2004;51:863–888.

Goodheart HP. *Goodheart's photoguide of common skin disorders.* 2nd ed. Philadelphia, PA: Lippincott Williams & Wilkins; 2003:1.

Habif TP. *Clinical dermatology: a color guide to diagnosis and therapy.* 4th ed. St. Louis, MO: C.V. Mosby; 2003:819–823.

Hurwitz S. *Clinical pediatric dermatology: a textbook of skin disorders of childhood and adolescence.* 3rd ed. St. Louis, MO: Elsevier; 2006:17–27, 49–72, 322–327.

MARIO CRUZ
AND LAURA E. SMALS

Abnormal Head Shape

APPROACH TO THE PROBLEM

Abnormal head shape may be the result of genetic disorders, metabolic abnormalities, or improper positioning of the head. The infant skull is a moldable structure composed of seven unfused cranial plates that are separated by suture lines. Shaping of the skull can be disrupted by internal, external, or intrinsic forces. *Internal* forces include abnormalities of the brain and surrounding tissues such as abnormally poor brain growth and hydrocephalus. External forces include intrauterine compression and prolonged positioning of the head against a firm surface. *Intrinsic* forces include craniosynostosis (premature closure of one or more cranial sutures). Craniosynostosis can interfere with the growth of the brain and other intracranial structures, resulting in increased intracranial pressure and vision and hearing problems. Positional plagiocephaly ("flattened head") is the most common cause of abnormal head shape and is frequently due to molding from supine sleep positioning and congenital torticollis.

KEY POINTS IN THE HISTORY

- Prematurity may lead to dolichocephaly because of positional molding in the hospital.

- Perinatal injury or trauma may cause intracranial bleeding and can lead to hydrocephalus.

- Prolonged labor can result in severe, although transient, molding of the skull.

- History of intrauterine fibroids or oligohydramnios can lead to cranial compression and abnormal head shape at birth.

- Developmental delays may indicate abnormal brain development as a cause of abnormal head shape.

- History of vomiting, lethargy, and poor head control may be signs of increased intracranial pressure.

- History of head tilt with flattening of one side of the head may be a sign of congenital torticollis.

- A history of prolonged supine head position may be associated with positional plagiocephaly.

- A family history of genetic syndromes may help to identify the etiology of an abnormal head shape.

KEY POINTS IN THE PHYSICAL EXAMINATION

- When assessing the head shape, it is best to look at the skull from multiple angles: the top of the head from above, upward from below the chin, from the side (profile), and from the front and back.

- Symmetry of the forehead, eyes, nose, cheeks, mouth, and ears should be evaluated. Facial asymmetry may be noted in positional plagiocephaly or craniosynostosis.

- Measure head circumference to see whether macrocephaly or microcephaly is present in addition to the abnormal head shape. Assess the anterior fontanelle for evidence of increased intracranial pressure or premature closure.

- Alopecia along a "flattened" area of the skull may be seen, especially in positional plagiocephaly.

- Congenital torticollis is suspected when the child has a palpable nodule within the sternocleidomastoid muscle, a preference to look in one direction, and decreased range of rotation at the neck.

- In craniosynostosis, the smaller or flattened side of the skull is where the suture has prematurely fused (Fig. 4-2). A palpable ridge may be appreciated over the fused suture line. Cloverleaf skull (kleeblattschädel; Figure 4-11) occurs as the result of multiple suture synostosis and is rare.

- Dysmorphic facial features or extremities may indicate a genetic syndrome as the cause of craniosynostosis.

- Unilateral lambdoid craniosynostosis and positional plagiocephaly may be difficult to distinguish clinically. Positional plagiocephaly is common and associated with anterior positioning of the ipsilateral forehead and ear. Lambdoid craniosynostosis is rare and associated with posterior positioning of the ipsilateral ear and prominence of the contralateral forehead and parieto-occipital region (Fig. 4-4).

PHOTOGRAPHS OF SELECTED DIAGNOSES

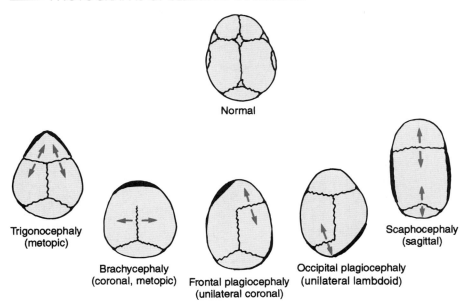

Figure 4-1 Skull shapes associated with craniosynostosis. The heavy line denotes
the area of maximal flattening. The arrows indicate the direction of continued growth across
the sutures that remain open. Growth perpendicular to the fused suture line is halted.
(Used with permission from Fletcher MA. *Physical diagnosis in neonatology*. Philadelphia, PA:
Lippincott–Raven; 1998:186.)

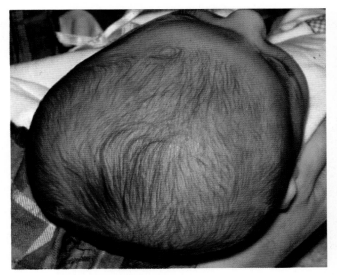

Figure 4-2 Positional plagiocephaly. Flattening of the right
posterior skull and anterior positioning of the ipsilateral forehead
and ear.
(Courtesy of Joseph Piatt, MD.)

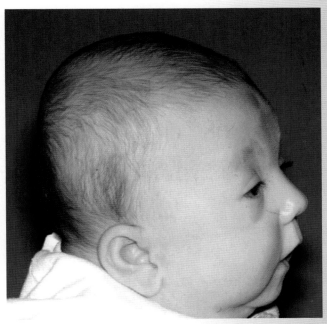

Figure 4-3 Brachycephaly. The short AP skull diameter results
in shallow orbits and subsequent proptosis.
(Courtesy of Joseph Piatt, MD.)

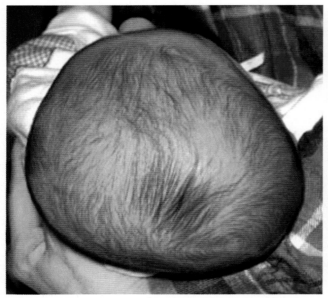

Figure 4-4 Unilateral lambdoid craniosynostosis, left sided. Prominence of the contralateral forehead and parieto-occipital region.
(Courtesy of Joseph Piatt, MD.)

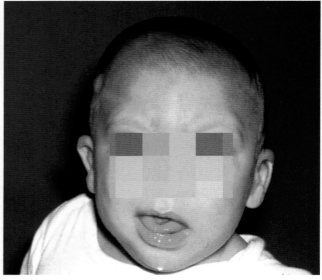

Figure 4-5 Metopic synostosis. Vertical ridge along the fused metopic suture line.
(Courtesy of Joseph Piatt, MD.)

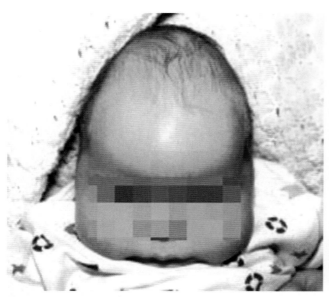

Figure 4-6 Sagittal synostosis. Narrow biparietal diameter.
(Courtesy of Joseph Piatt, MD.)

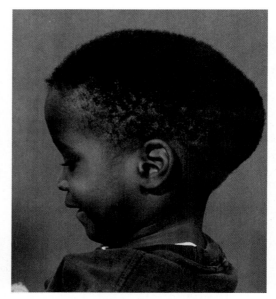

Figure 4-7 Sagittal synostosis. Severe, untreated presentation at 29 months.
(Used with permission from Sabry MZ, Wornom IL, Ward JD. Results of cranial vault reshaping. *Ann Plast Surg.* 2001;47(2):123.)

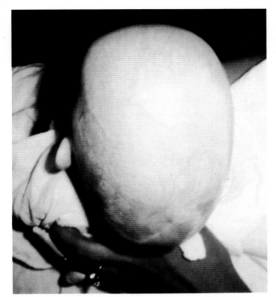

Figure 4-8 Dolichocephaly (scaphocephaly), top view. Marked increase in head length with narrowed width resulting from premature fusion of the sagittal suture. Premature infants allowed to remain with the head in a side-lying position develop scaphocephalic changes but with more flattening of the sides of the skull.
(Used with permission from Fletcher MA. *Physical diagnosis in neonatology*. Philadelphia, PA: Lippincott–Raven; 1998:186.)

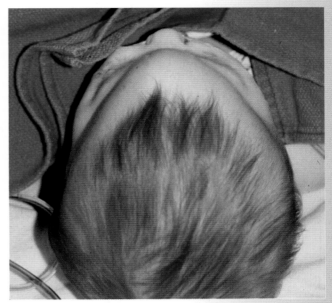

Figure 4-9 Trigonocephaly. Prominent ridge at the metopic suture line.
(Courtesy of Scott VanDuzer, MD.)

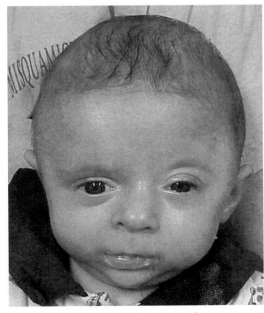

Figure 4-10 Left coronal synostosis. Compensatory growth of the right forehead with marked facial asymmetry.
(Used with permission from Lui Y, Kadlub N, da Silva Freitas R, et al. The misdiagnosis of craniosynostosis as deformational plagiocephaly. *J Craniofac Surg.* 2008;19(1):133.)

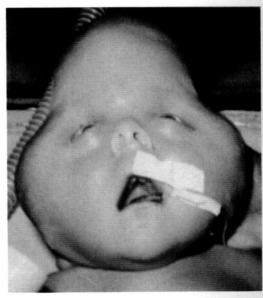

Figure 4-11 Cloverleaf skull (kleeblattschädel). Caused by craniosynostosis of all sutures forcing brain growth through the anterior and temporal fontanels. This most severe form of restricted skull growth has the poorest prognosis because of a combination of craniostenosis and hydrocephalus.
(Used with permission from Fletcher MA. *Physical diagnosis in neonatology*, Philadelphia: Lippincott—Raven; 1998:186.)

DIAGNOSIS	ICD-9	DISTINGUISHING CHARACTERISTICS	DISTRIBUTION	ASSOCIATED FINDINGS	COMPLICATIONS	TREATMENT GUIDELINES
Positional Plagiocephaly	754.0	Flattened area of the skull with history of lying with the head in one position routinely	Usually posterior occiput Can be unilateral, especially when associated with torticollis	Alopecia in area of flattening Congenital torticollis	Facial asymmetry Poor cosmetic appearance	"Tummy time," prone positioning in the infant when awake only Repositioning of the head Physical therapy Molding helmets
Brachycephaly	756.0	Broad head with recessed forehead secondary to premature closure of the coronal suture	Shortened anteroposterior (AP) diameter	More common in girls Associated with syndromes, especially if bilateral	If untreated, can compromise orbits and globes resulting in vision loss	Skull radiography (x-ray or CT scan) Neurosurgery, ophthalmology and/or otolaryngology referral Consider genetics consult if other anomalies are present.
Craniosynostosis	756.0	Abnormal head shape secondary to premature closure of one or more cranial sutures	Will vary with type Sagittal synostosis is most common	Mental retardation when complete (all sutures affected) May be associated with certain syndromes (e.g., Apert syndrome)	Increased ICP, mental retardation, visual and hearing deficits	Skull radiography (x-ray or CT scan) Neurosurgery, ophthalmology and/or otolaryngology referral Consider genetics consult if other anomalies are present.
Dolichocephaly	754.0	Long and narrow skull secondary to premature closure of the sagittal suture or positional molding	Elongation of the AP diameter with narrow biparietal width	More common in boys May occur in premature infants without synostosis because of positional molding	Poor cosmetic appearance	Skull radiography (x-ray or CT scan) Observe if synostosis is not suspected, otherwise needs neurosurgical evaluation.
Trigonocephaly	756.0	Triangular-shaped head secondary to premature closure of the metopic suture	Frontal forehead area	Hypotelorism	May also be associated with mental retardation, urinary tract abnormalities, cleft palate, coloboma, and holoprosencephaly	Skull radiography (x-ray or CT scan) Neurosurgical evaluation

OTHER
DIAGNOSES
TO CONSIDER

- Dandy-Walker malformation

- Cerebral agenesis

- Hydrocephalus

Diseases associated with craniosynostosis:

- Ataxia-telangiectasia

- Hyperthyroidism

- Mucopolysaccharidoses

- Rickets

- Sickle cell disease

- Thalassemia major

Syndromes associated with craniosynostosis:

- Antley Bixler

- Apert

- Baller Gerold

- Carpenter

- Crouzon

- Pfeiffer

WHEN TO
CONSIDER
FURTHER
EVALUATION
OR TREATMENT

- Positional plagiocephaly does not require imaging. Repositioning of the head away from the flattened side and "tummy time," prone positioning of the infant when awake only, should resolve the deformity over several weeks to months. Refractory cases may respond to molding helmets.

- Physical therapy consultation and range of motion exercises for the neck are helpful in congenital torticollis.

- When craniosynostosis is suspected, imaging with a skull x-ray or CT scan is indicated.

- Neurosurgical evaluation for craniosynostosis should take place promptly, within the first few months of life, to minimize the risk of severe complications, such as increased intracranial pressure, impaired brain development, severe cosmetic deformity, and vision and hearing loss.

- Severe cases of craniosynostosis, especially when syndromic in etiology, require a multidisciplinary approach, which may include consultation with neurosurgery, otolaryngology, maxillofacial surgery, plastic surgery, ophthalmology, genetics, orthopedics, social work, developmental pediatrics, psychiatry, and other subspecialties.

SUGGESTED READINGS

Fletcher MA. *Physical diagnosis in neonatology*. Philadelphia, PA: Lippincott–Raven; 1998:186.

Gartner JC, Zitelli BJ. *Common and chronic symptoms in pediatrics*. St. Louis: C.V. Mosby; 1997:102–109.

Peitsch WK, Keefer CH, LaBrie RA, et al. Incidence of cranial asymmetry in healthy newborns. *Pediatrics*. 2002;110:72.

Ridgway EB, Weiner HL. Skull deformities. *Pediatr Clin North Am*. 2004;51(2):359–387.

Rohan AJ, Golombek SG, Rosenthal AD. Infants with misshapen skulls: when to worry. *Contemp Pediatr*. 1999;16:47–70.

Sloan GM, Wells KC, Raffel C, et al. Surgical treatment of craniosynostosis: outcome analysis of 250 consecutive patients. *Pediatrics*. 1997;100:e2.

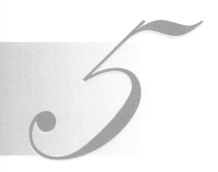

Newborn Lower Extremity Abnormalities

APPROACH TO THE PROBLEM

To understand torsional and angular deformities of the newborn lower extremity, one must first recognize the typical positioning of the lower extremities in utero, where the feet are in contact with the posterolateral portion of the contralateral thigh. In addition, the feet are in slight equinus and are supinated; the knees are flexed with the lower legs internally rotated; and the hips are flexed, abducted, and externally rotated. Abnormal positional deformities result when the fetus is unable to kick, which is crucial to the normal development of the lower extremities. Deformities may result from intrinsic factors such as central nervous system defects and muscle degeneration or extrinsic factors related to fetal crowding that occurs with breech presentation or oligohydramnios.

KEY POINTS IN THE HISTORY

- Infants who were breech in utero are at increased risk of hip dysplasia and valgus abnormalities of the foot.

- The risk of caudal regression syndrome, which includes sacral agenesis, in infants of mothers with insulin-dependent diabetes mellitus has been estimated to be 200 times that of infants in the general population, but this syndrome is rare.

- When a skeletal dysplasia is suspected in a newborn, it is essential to obtain a family history that assesses for skeletal dysplasias, consanguinity, and short stature.

- Heterozygous achondroplasia is the most common form of chondrodysplasia and follows an autosomal dominant inheritance pattern.

- The newborn lower extremity may appear bowed because of the combination of an externally rotated hip and an internally rotated tibia.

- The calcaneovalgus deformity, typically self-correcting in the first 2 to 3 months of life, is characterized by hyperdorsiflexion, hindfoot valgus, and forefoot abduction.

- Congenital vertical talus (also known as "rocker bottom foot" or congenital convex pes valgus) presents with a convex plantar surface, forefoot abduction, rigid plantar flexion of the talus, and fixed dorsiflexion of the midfoot. Most of these infants may have additional findings, such as multiple joint contractures consistent with arthrogryposis multiplex or an underlying neurologic disorder such as a meningomyelocele.

- The examination findings of sacral agenesis vary depending on the severity of the agenesis (unilateral versus bilateral, partial versus complete, extent of spinal cord involvement). The most severely affected infants may have lack of growth in the caudal region, hip flexion and abduction, and popliteal webs because of the lack of movement.

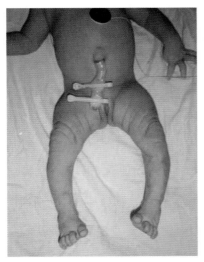

Figure 5-1 Physiologic bowing of legs. Legs of a newborn appear bowed because of externally rotated hips and internally rotated tibia.
(Courtesy of Gerardo Cabrera-Meza, MD.)

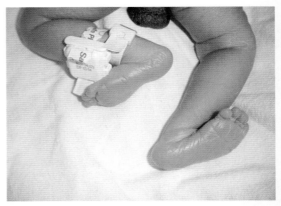

Figure 5-2 Calcaneovalgus foot. Right foot is in hyperdorsiflexion, with the forefoot abducted.
(Courtesy of Gerardo Cabrera-Meza, MD.)

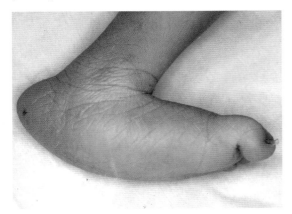

Figure 5-3 Congenital vertical talus (rocker bottom foot). Forefoot is abducted and dorsiflexed and has a convex planter surface.
(Courtesy of Gerardo Cabrera-Meza, MD.)

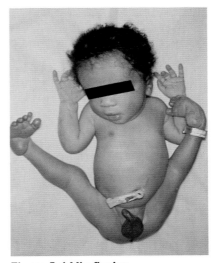

Figure 5-4 Hip flexion contracture. A newborn presents with bilateral hip flexion contracture after breech presentation.
(Courtesy of Gerardo Cabrera-Meza, MD.)

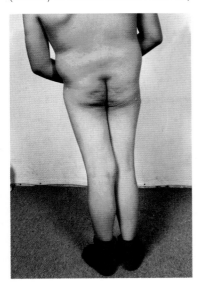

Figure 5-5 Sacral agenesis. This 8-year old with complete sacral agenesis (absent sacrum) has flattened buttocks, a shortened gluteal cleft, and a narrowed pelvis.
(Courtesy of Shriners Hospitals for Children, Houston, Texas.)

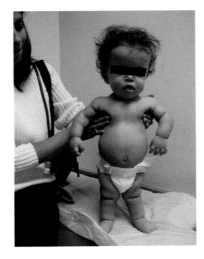

Figure 5-6 Achondroplasia. This infant with achondroplasia has tibial bowing, frontal bossing, rhizomelia (the proximal limb segment is shorter than the distal segment), and brachydactyly (short fingers).
(Courtesy of Paul S. Matz, MD.)

DIFFERENTIAL DIAGNOSIS

DIAGNOSIS	ICD-9	DISTINGUISHING CHARACTERISTICS	DURATION/ CHRONICITY	ASSOCIATED FINDINGS	PREDISPOSING FACTORS	TREATMENT GUIDELINES
Physiologic Bowing of Legs	754.43	Legs appear bowed because of a combination of externally rotated hips and internally rotated tibia	Resolves after 6 to 12 months of independent walking	N/A	Secondary to in utero positioning	Spontaneously resolves
Pes Calcaneovalgus	754.69	Hyperdorsiflexion, forefoot abduction, and hindfoot valgus	Resolves during first 6 months of life	External tibial torsion	Secondary to in utero positioning	Spontaneously resolves Gentle stretching if mild limitation in range of motion Casting if severe limitation in range of motion (rare)
Congenital Vertical Talus (Rocker Bottom Foot)	754.79	Convex plantar surface, forefoot abduction, and dorsiflexion	Most require surgical correction at 6–12 months	Arthrogryposis multiplex Meningomyelocele Trisomy 18	N/A	Casting and surgery
Lower Limb Abnormalities Associated with Breech Presentation	763.0	Developmental dysplasia of the hip (DDH) Valgus foot deformities	Varies with diagnosis	Breech deformation sequence also includes torticollis, facial asymmetry, and bathrocephaly (a step-like posterior projection of the skull)	N/A	DDH: Pavlik harness (newborn), spica cast (ages 6 months to 2 years), open reduction, and possible femoral shortening (older than age 2 years)
Sacral Agenesis	756.13	Partial, symmetric sacral agenesis (the most common type of agenesis); bilateral hip subluxation and foot deformities because of loss of lower sacral innervation Complete sacral agenesis (absent sacrum); flattened buttocks, shortened gluteal cleft, narrowed pelvis	N/A	Bowel and/or urinary incontinence and lower extremity neurologic deficits Renal anomalies Imperforate anus Cleft lip and palate Microcephaly Meningomyelocele Kyphosis	Infants of mothers with insulin-dependent diabetes mellitus	Management of associated findings Surgical repair of spine and lower limbs
Achondroplasia (Heterozygous)	756.4	Tibial bowing Rhizomelia (the proximal limb segment is shorter than the distal segment) Brachydactyly (short fingers)	Increased mortality in first 5 years of life (particularly in first year) because of sudden death from cervicomedullary compression	Frontal bossing and head circumference greater than 97th percentile Hypotonia Normal intelligence Hydrocephalus Spinal cord compression Pulmonary hypertension Sleep-disordered breathing	Autosomal dominant inheritance 90% of cases arise de novo, likely to be exclusively inherited from the father and associated with advanced paternal age	Management of associated findings

<table>
<tr>
<td>

OTHER
DIAGNOSES
TO CONSIDER

</td>
<td>

- Steinert myotonic dystrophy

- Werdnig-Hoffman disease

- Congenital posteromedial tibial angulation

- Congenital anterolateral tibial angulation

</td>
</tr>
<tr>
<td>

WHEN TO
CONSIDER
FURTHER
EVALUATION
OR TREATMENT

</td>
<td>

- Further evaluation for congenital vertical talus should be conducted if a foot's valgus abnormality is not flexible or corrected with manipulation.

- All newborns with a positive Ortolani or Barlow sign (signs of hip instability) should be referred for the treatment and prevention of long-term complications of DDH.

</td>
</tr>
</table>

SUGGESTED READINGS

Dugoff L, Thieme G, Hobbins JC. Skeletal anomalies. *Clin Perinatol.* 2000:27(4):979–1005.

Hosalkar HS, Gholve PA, Wells L. Torsional and angular deformities. In: Kliegman RM, Behrman RE, Jensen HB, Stanton BF, eds. *Nelson textbook of pediatrics.* 18th ed. Philadelphia, PA: WB Saunders; 2007:2784–2791.

Hosalkar HS, Spiegel DA, Davidson RS. The foot and toes. In: Kliegman RM, Behrman RE, Jensen HB, Stanton BF, eds. *Nelson textbook of pediatrics.* 18th ed. Philadelphia, PA: WB Saunders; 2007:2776–2784.

Jones KL. Achondroplasia. *Smith's recognizable patterns of human malformation.* 6th ed. Philadelphia, PA: Elsevier Saunders; 2006:390–391.

Kasser JR. The foot. In Morrissy RT, Weinstein SL, eds. *Lovell and Winter's pediatric orthopaedics.* 6th ed. Philadelphia, PA: Lippincott Williams & Wilkins; 2006:1258–1328.

Raffel LJ, Goodarzi MO, Rotter JI. Diabetes mellitus. In: Rimon DL, Connor JM, Pyeritz RE, eds. *Emery and Rimoin's principles and practice of medical genetics.* 5th ed. Philadelphia, PA: Churchill Livingstone Elsevier; 2007:1980–2022.

Imperforate Anus

APPROACH TO THE PROBLEM

The imperforate anus, also termed anorectal malformation, is a congenital anomaly that occurs with an incidence of 1 in 5,000 live births. Most of these anomalies are evident at birth and result from faulty development in utero of the anus, lower rectum, and urogenital tract. The exact cause is unknown, though the defect usually occurs during the fifth to seventh weeks of fetal development. Furthermore, these anomalies are often part of a malformation complex. The imperforate anus may be classified into three main categories based on the position of the rectum relative to the puborectalis muscle. The rectum ends above the puborectalis muscle in high anomalies. Intermediate malformations develop at the same level or just below the puborectalis muscle. The low anomalies terminate below the level of the puborectalis muscle. The classification of these malformations is significant since the high anomalies are more often associated with other congenital anomalies compared to the low lesions. There is a higher incidence of genitourinary and lower spinal abnormalities in patients with imperforate anus.

KEY POINTS IN THE HISTORY

- When evaluating an infant during the neonatal period, it is important to check the delivery record to note if there was meconium present in the amniotic fluid.

- Affected infants often present with delayed passage of meconium, greater than 24 hours after birth, in the neonatal period.

- Severe anorectal anomalies usually present with signs and symptoms of intestinal obstruction, such as abdominal distension and lack of stooling, within 72 hours of birth.

- Diagnosis beyond the neonatal period may occur in low anorectal malformations that may present as chronic constipation, usually prior to 12 months of age, and overflow incontinence.

- Malformations associated with fistulas extending from the rectum to the urethra or bladder may present with a urinary tract infection.

KEY POINTS IN THE PHYSICAL EXAMINATION

- Fistulas may present with discharge of meconium from the perineum, scrotum, vagina, or urethra.

- A prominent midline groove and anal dimple indicate a low-level anomaly.

- The perineum appears flat with the absence of a midline groove and anal dimple with a high-level anomaly.

- Higher defects may present with a poorly formed or absent sacrum.

- It is important to detect the presence of other congenital anomalies on examination, such as musculoskeletal anomalies, cardiovascular anomalies, and dysmorphic features.

PHOTOGRAPHS OF SELECTED DIAGNOSES

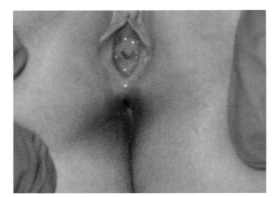

Figure 6-1 Perineal fistula. Opening into the perineum just posterior to the fourchette. (Courtesy of Christine Finck, MD.)

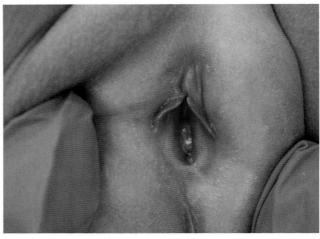

Figure 6-2 Rectovestibular fistula. While there may be a normal appearing vagina and urethra, the rectum opens through the vestibule and causes meconium to pass through the vagina. There is no visible anal orifice. (Courtesy of Mary L. Brandt, MD.)

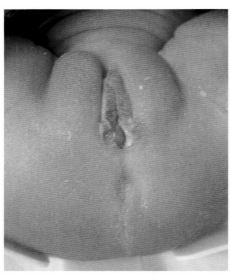

Figure 6-3 Rectovestibular fistula. The rectum opens through the posterior fourchette, and there is no visual anal orifice. (Courtesy of Mary L. Brandt, MD.)

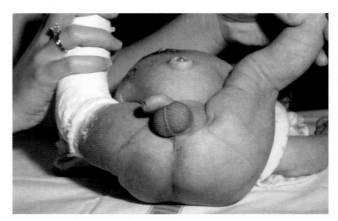

Figure 6-4 Rectourethral fistula. Meconium is passed through a fistula opening into the urethra, and there is no visible anal orifice. (Courtesy of Kevin P. Lally, MD.)

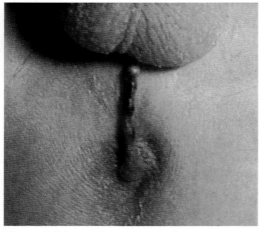

Figure 6-5 Imperforate anus without fistula. The visible meconium streak along the raphe is consistent with a low imperforate anus. (Courtesy of Kevin P. Lally, MD.)

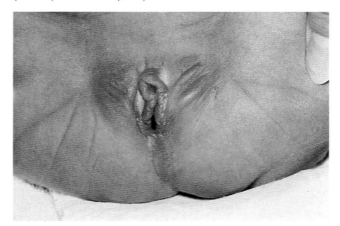

Figure 6-6 Cloaca is a high-level anomaly with the vagina, urethra, and rectum sharing a single perineal opening. (Courtesy of Kevin P. Lally, MD.)

DIFFERENTIAL DIAGNOSIS

DIAGNOSIS	ICD-9	DISTINGUISHING CHARACTERISTICS	ASSOCIATED FINDINGS	COMPLICATIONS	TREATMENT GUIDELINES
Perineal Fistula	565.1	Small orifice in the perineum, anterior to the external sphincter	"Bucket-handle" or "black ribbon"-like structure, which is a subepithelial fistula filled with meconium	Associated defects are rare.	Anoplasty during the newborn period by a pediatric surgeon
Rectovestibular Fistula	619.1	Rectum opens through the vestibule, outside the hymenal orifice	Meconium is passed through the vagina.	Urologic defects	Referral to a pediatric surgeon for surgical correction
Rectourethral Fistula	619.1	Rectum opens through the lower (bulbar) urethra or upper (prostatic) urethra	Meconium is passed through the urethra.	Urologic defects	Referral to a pediatric surgeon and urologist for surgical correction
Rectovesical Fistula	596.1	Rectum opens through the bladder neck	Meconium is passed through the urethra.	Urologic defects	Referral to a pediatric surgeon and urologist for surgical correction
Rectal Atresia	751.2	Externally normal appearing anus	Failure to pass meconium	Associated defects are rare.	Referral to a pediatric surgeon for surgical correction
Cloaca	751.5	Single orifice behind the clitoris for the rectum, vagina, and urethra	Abnormally large vagina filled with mucous secretions	Urologic defects	Referral to a pediatric surgeon for surgical correction

OTHER
DIAGNOSES
TO CONSIDER

- VATER—vertebral defects, anal atresia, tracheoesophageal fistula with esophageal atresia, and radial and renal dysplasia

- VACTERL—above anomalies as well as additional cardiac and limb anomalies

- Congenital heart defects

- Tracheal and esophageal defects

- Urinary tract malformations

- Spinal abnormalities, such as hemivertebra, tethered spinal cord, and sacral agenesis

- Limb defects

WHEN TO
CONSIDER
FURTHER
EVALUATION
OR TREATMENT

- All anorectal malformations require a referral to a pediatric surgeon for correction.

- These malformations may require one or more surgeries, and the surgical technique depends on the type of malformation.

SUGGESTED READINGS

Cho S, Moore SP, Fangman T. One hundred three consecutive patients with anorectal malformations and their associated anomalies. *Arch Pediatr Adolesc Med.* 2001;155:587–591.

Colorectal Center, Cincinnati Children's Hospital Medical Center. Anorectal Malformations. http://www.cincinnatichildrens.org/health/info/surgery/anorectal-malformations-imperforate-anus.htm. Accessed August 15, 2008.

Da Silva GM, Jorge JM, Belin B, et al. New surgical options for fecal incontinence in patients with imperforate anus. *Dis Colon Rectum.* 2004;47:204–209.

Di Lorenzo C, Benninga MA. Pathophysiology of pediatric fecal incontinence. *Gastroenterology.* 2004;126:S33–S40.

Kim HL, Gow KW, Penner JG, et al. Presentation of low anorectal malformations beyond the neonatal period. *Pediatrics.* 2000;105:E68.

Rintala RJ, Pakarinen MP. Imperforate anus: long-and short-term outcome. *Semin Pediatr Surg.* 2008;17:79–89.

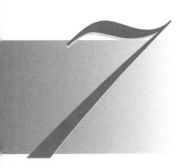

DENISE A. SALERNO

Newborn Skin Abnormalities

APPROACH TO THE PROBLEM

A thorough inspection of the skin for rashes and skin abnormalities is an essential part of the newborn examination. Most skin findings are transient and very rarely require treatment, but it is important to distinguish benign skin lesions from cutaneous manifestations of more serious disorders. New parents are often concerned about their baby's skin. Skin issues are a common "chief complaint" during the initial newborn visit in the hospital and the outpatient setting. Knowledge and recognition of common, benign lesions of the newborn are important for counseling parents about the natural course of these dermatological lesions.

KEY POINTS IN THE HISTORY

- A maternal history of primary active genital herpes infection perinatally puts the infant at the highest risk for developing herpes neonatorum. A negative maternal history does not exclude the possibility of this diagnosis.

- A history of cyanosis of the hands and feet is often benign, while cyanosis of the lips and mouth is a sign of hypoxia.

- Physiologic cutis marmorata, a transient rash brought on by exposure to cold or distress, resolves once the baby is warmed. Cutis marmorata telangiectatica is always visible.

- Mongolian spots are present at birth in more than 90% of African Americans, 80% of Asians, and rarely in Caucasians.

- The lesions of epidermolysis bullosa heal slowly, while sucking blisters often heal within 48 hrs.

KEY POINTS IN THE PHYSICAL EXAMINATION

- Infants who appear ill should have skin lesions cultured to rule out viral, bacterial, or yeast infections.

- Mongolian spots are nontender, gray-blue macular lesions primarily located on the lumbosacral area, but may be seen over the entire back and on the shoulders and extremities. Familiarity with these lesions will enable a clinician to distinguish these from ecchymoses.

- Miliaria crystallina are pinpoint vesicles containing clear fluid. The lesions are easily denuded with pressure.

- The lesions of erythema toxicum are often not present at birth and will often appear during the first few days of life.

- Erythema toxicum spares the palms and soles, while pustular melanosis may involve the palms and soles.

- Pustular melanosis may present at birth with small hyperpigmented macular lesions if the pustular phase occurred in utero.

- Milia are white pinhead-sized papules that usually occur on the face.

- Initially, neonatal acne may resemble milia, but the lesions become larger and pustular in the first month of life.

- Acropustulosis of infancy consists of extremely pruritic lesions concentrated on the palms and soles.

- Neonatal seborrhea usually involves the ears, back of neck, and shoulders. Neonatal eczema spares these areas.

- The vesicles of herpes simplex virus infection often occur on the presenting body part of the infant during birth.

- Cultures of pustular or vesicular lesions can help distinguish benign cutaneous lesions from those of infectious etiology.

PHOTOGRAPHS OF SELECTED DIAGNOSES

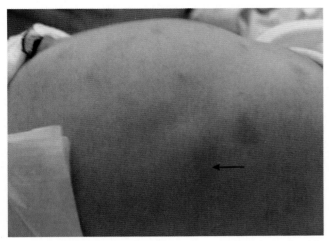

Figure 7-1 Erythema toxicum. Note the central papule with surrounding erythema.
(Courtesy of Esther K. Chung, MD, MPH.)

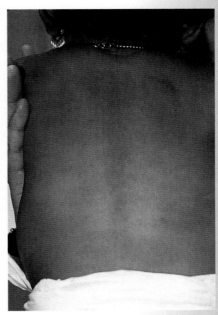

Figure 7-2 Mongolian spots. Bluish-gray macular pigmentation on the back of a neonate.
(Courtesy of George A. Datto, III, MD.)

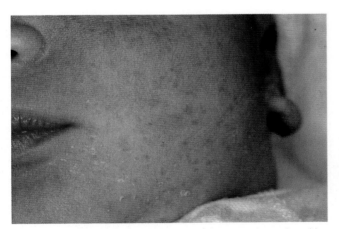

Figure 7-3 Pustular melanosis. Hyperpigmented macules with adherent white scale seen after the pustular lesions have ruptured.
(Courtesy of Paul S. Matz, MD.)

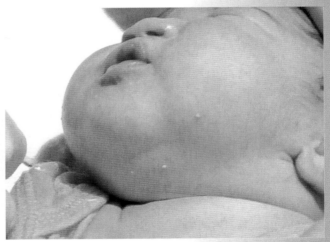

Figure 7-4 Pustular melanosis. Pustular phase of pustular melanosis located on the chin of a newborn.
(Courtesy of Denise A. Salerno, MD, FAAP and Hannah Ravereby, BS.)

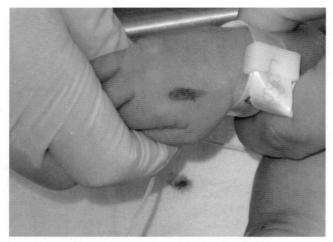

Figure 7-5 Sucking blister. The lesion on the left hand of this
newborn is the result of sucking that occurred in utero.
(Courtesy of Denise A. Salerno, MD, FAAP.)

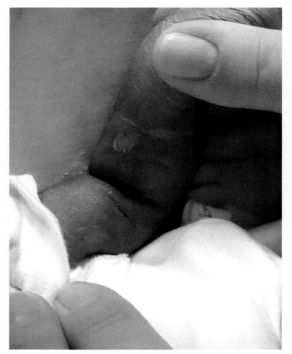

Figure 7-6 Sucking blister. The lesion on the right
arm of this newborn resulted from sucking in utero.
(Courtesy of Denise A. Salerno, MD, FAAP and
Hannah Ravreby, BS.)

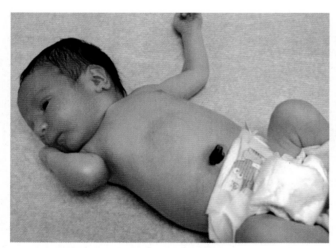

Figure 7-7 Jaundice. Physiologic jaundice.
(Courtesy of Denise A. Salerno, MD, FAAP.)

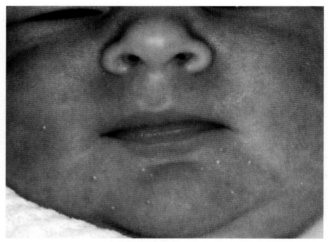

Figure 7-8 Milia. Milia on the cheek and chin of a newborn.
(Courtesy of Denise A. Salerno, MD, FAAP.)

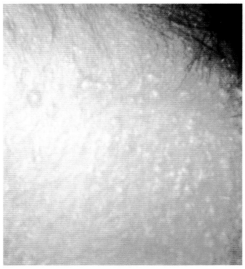

Figure 7-9 Miliaria crystallina alba.
(Used with permission from Fletcher MA. *Physical diagnosis in neonatology*. Philadelphia, PA: Lippincott Williams & Wilkins; 1998:124.)

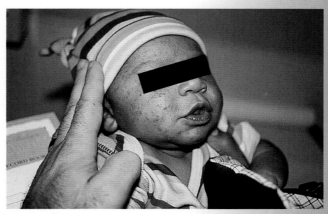

Figure 7-10 Neonatal acne. Erythematous pustular rash on cheeks of a 3-week-old neonate.
(Courtesy of George A. Datto, III, MD.)

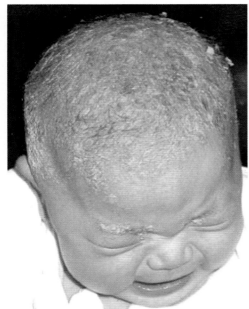

Figure 7-11 Seborrhea. Greasy, scaly lesions of scalp and eyebrows.
(Courtesy of the Benjamin Barankin Dermatology Collection.)

DIFFERENTIAL DIAGNOSIS

DIAGNOSIS	ICD-9	DISTINGUISHING CHARACTERISTICS	DISTRIBUTION
Erythema Toxicum	778.8	Small white-yellow papules with surrounding flare of erythema	Trunk Arms Legs Face Palms and soles spared Few to several hundred
Mongolian Spots	757.33	Bluish-gray macular lesions Varying sizes Resulting from accumulation of melanocytes Incidence varies with ethnicity No risk of malignancy	Lumbosacral area Extensor surfaces Spares face, palms, and soles Single or multiple
Pustular Melanosis	782.1	Pustules present in utero or at birth Pustules unroof leaving brown macules surrounded by scale (a "collarette" of peeling skin)	Chin Face Lower back Nape of neck
Sucking Blister	959.09	Bullous lesion or erosion	Finger Hand Wrist Lip
Neonatal Jaundice (Physiologic)	774.6	Usually noted at 48–72 hrs Yellow discoloration of skin Spreads cephalo-caudally as the bilirubin level increases	Skin Mucous membranes Sclera
Cutis Marmorata (Physiologic)	782.61	Reticulated mottling of skin Disappears with re-warming	Arms Legs Torso
Milia (Epidermal Inclusion Cyst)	706.2	Results from retention of keratin and sebaceous material within sebaceous glands Grouped whitish pinhead-sized papules Not denuded by pressure	Forehead Chin Cheeks Nose
Miliaria	705.1	Crystallina • Clear pinpoint vesicles • Appear as early as first day of life Rubra • Erythematous papules or vesicles • Appear after first week	Around hairline Face Nape of neck Upper trunk Intertriginous areas Occluded areas
Acne Neonatal	706.1	Comedones	Cheeks Forehead
Seborrhea	706.3 Infantile—690.12 Dermatitis—690.10	Greasy Red scaling Yellow crusting Non-pruritic	Scalp Diaper area Face Postauricular area Shoulder
Acropustulosis of Infancy	696.1	Pruritic papulopustules or vesiculopustules Appear in crops Recur every few weeks	Hands Feet Wrists Ankles

DURATION/ CHRONICITY	ASSOCIATED FINDINGS	COMPLICATIONS	PRECIPITATING FACTORS	TREATMENT GUIDELINES
Self-limited Few days to few weeks	None	None	More common in full-term infants	Gram stain from fluid in lesions shows eosinophils. No treatment necessary
Fade during childhood Seldom last into adulthood	None	None	N/A	No treatment necessary
Pustular phase—24–48 hrs Melanosis stage—Few weeks to few months	None	None	N/A	Gram stain from fluid in pustules shows neutrophils. No treatment necessary
Resolves in 24–48 hrs	None	None	Results from vigorous sucking on affected body part in utero	No treatment necessary
Depends on severity	May be associated with polycythemia, ABO incompatibility, Rh incompatibility, infection, or liver disease	Kernicterus—if level of bilirubin gets too high	ABO or Rh incompatibility Excessive bruising Breastfeeding	Depends on level of bilirubin and age of infant Resolution can be accelerated by phototherapy AAP published guidelines can be found at: http://aappolicy.aappublications.org/cgi/content/full/pediatrics;114/1/297
Lasts until 6 months of life	None	None	Physiologic response to chilling	No treatment necessary
Few weeks to few months	None	None	N/A	No treatment necessary
Resolves with elimination of excessive heat	None	None	Hot, humid weather Over-bundled infants	No treatment necessary
Resolves spontaneously over a few months	None	None	Placental transfer of maternal androgens	No treatment necessary
Seborrhea may be seen in newborns and young children up to age 3 years.	None	Scales can become quite thickened and are cosmetically undesirable at times. Associated erythematous papular rash can be noted	N/A	Baby oil-rub on affected area, let sit for 10 min, comb out with fine toothed baby comb Antiseborrheic shampoos Ketoconazole shampoo Topical steroids
Crops last 2–3 weeks Disorder resolves by 2 years of age	None	None	N/A	Topical steroids and antihistamines relieve itch.

OTHER DIAGNOSES TO CONSIDER

The other diagnoses to consider are dependent on the presentation of the infant and lesions seen. Some common important diagnoses to consider are listed below:

- Herpes simplex neonatorum

- Bruises

- Blue nevus

- Staphylococcal skin infection

- Bullous impetigo

- Candidal skin infection

- Infantile atopic dermatitis

- Scabies

WHEN TO CONSIDER FURTHER EVALUATION OR TREATMENT

- Elevated bilirubin levels in the first 24 hrs of life, or above the recommended American Academy of Pediatrics algorithm (http://aappolicy.aappublications.org/cgi/content/full/pediatrics;114/1/297) should be promptly identified and when indicated treated with phototherapy and/or exchange transfusion.

- When neonatal herpes infection is suspected, cultures from multiple sites should be obtained, including any blisters, mucosal surfaces, serum, and CSF (if indicated). Liver function tests should be obtained as well.

- Infants with bullous impetigo or suspected staphylococcal infections should be promptly treated with antibiotics. Strong consideration should be given to obtaining blood cultures and giving parenteral antibiotics pending culture results.

SUGGESTED READINGS

American Academy of Pediatrics, Subcommittee on hyperbilirubinemia. Clinical practice guideline: management of hyperbilirubinemia in the newborn infant 35 or more weeks of gestation. *Pediatrics.* 2004;114:297–316.

Devillers AC, de Waard-van der Spek FB, Oranje AP. Cutis marmorata telangiectatica congenita: clinical features in 35 cases. *Arch Dermatol.* 1999;135(1):34–38.

Fletcher MA. *Physical diagnosis in neonatology.* Philadelphia, PA: Lippincott Williams & Wilkins; 1998:124.

O'Connor, N, McLaughlin M, Ham P. Newborn skin: part I common rashes. *Am Fam Physician.* 2008;77(1):47–52.

Pallor AS, Mancini AJ. Hurwitz clinical pediatric dermatology. *A textbook of skin disorders of childhood and adolescence.* 3rd ed. Philadelphia, PA: WB Saunders; 2006:19, 22–29.

Solomon LM, Esterly NB. Neonatal dermatology. I. The newborn skin. *J Pediatr.* 1970;77(5):888–894.

Treadwell PA. Dermatoses in newborns. *Am Fam Physician.* 1997;56(2):443–450.

Section

TWO

General Appearance

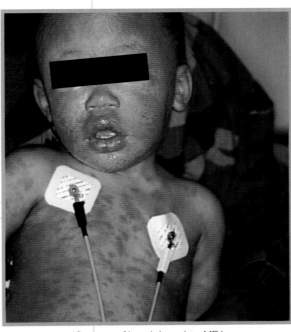

(Courtesy of Joseph Lopreiato, MD.)

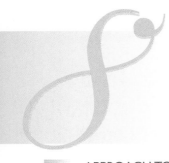

EVAN J. WEINER

General Appearance

APPROACH TO THE PROBLEM

A patient's general appearance is considered one of the most important elements of the physical examination. It represents a subjective impression of the patient's state of being. First and foremost, this impression informs about the patient's overall degree of wellness, distinguishing whether or not the patient is ill-appearing. In addition, one can assess specific aspects of the patient's presentation ranging from the obvious to the more subtle. Specifically, one can examine such patient characteristics as alertness level, nutritional status, facial expression, consolability, developmental ability, respiratory effort, personal interaction, behavior, hygiene, coloring, movement, and gait.

KEY POINTS IN THE HISTORY

- It is essential to ascertain whether the observed general appearance is consistent with that noted by the caregivers.

- Obtaining a patient's baseline status is crucial.

- A changing story, or one inconsistent with physical findings or developmental ability, raises the suspicion of child abuse.

- In the case of a critically ill or injured patient, elicit a SAMPLE history—as described by Pediatric Advanced Life Support—signs and symptoms, allergies, medications, past medical history, last meal, and events leading to presentation.

- When pain is present, assess the patient's subjective degree of pain, or preferably utilize a facial or numerical pain scale.

- When evaluating a febrile child, response to and timing of antipyretics, consolability, and willingness to feed help to distinguish severity of illness. Reevaluation following defervescence is also helpful.

KEY POINTS IN THE PHYSICAL EXAMINATION

- A social smile is rarely present in a child with meningitis or other invasive serious bacterial infections. However, it may be present in occult bacteremia.

- Absent tears, dry mucous membranes, ill general appearance, and delayed capillary refill are reliable external clues of dehydration.

- Tachypnea, nasal flaring, grunting, and accessory muscle use are signs of *respiratory distress*. Depressed sensorium, apnea, bradycardia, and cyanosis are signs of *respiratory failure*.

- Shock can be clinically diagnosed with evidence of poor organ perfusion: for example, altered sensorium, mottled skin, peripheral cyanosis, tachypnea, and decreased peripheral pulses. Septic or "warm" shock may lead to flushing and bounding pulses.

- Elements of a toxic general appearance include grunting, weak or persistent cry, sunken eyes, grey or mottled skin, depressed sensorium, and altered social response.

- Seizure activity may be evidenced by abnormal movements, posturing, extremity jerking, lip smacking, altered mental status, and staring eyes. Seizure activity in neonates may manifest as bicycling movements, chewing, blinking, and/or rigidity.

- A patient with peritoneal irritation lies flat and still. Patients with colicky abdominal conditions appear restless and uncomfortable. Paroxysms of irritability and drawing up of legs may indicate intussusception.

- Children with epiglottitis appear toxic and may be in a "tripod" position. Muffled voice, drooling, and stridor also indicate upper airway obstruction.

PHOTOGRAPHS OF SELECTED DIAGNOSES

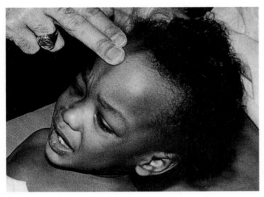

Figure 8-1 Meningitis. (Used with permission from Fleisher GR, Ludwig S, Baskin MN. *Atlas of pediatric emergency medicine*. Philadelphia, PA: Lippincott Williams & Wilkins; 2004:183.)

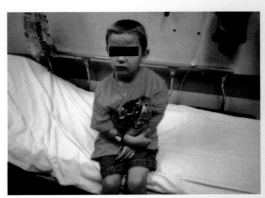

Figure 8-2 Well-appearing child with left supracondylar fracture. This well-appearing, but apprehensive, child's positioning informs of his supracondylar fracture of the left humerus. (Courtesy of Evan J. Weiner, MD, FAAP.)

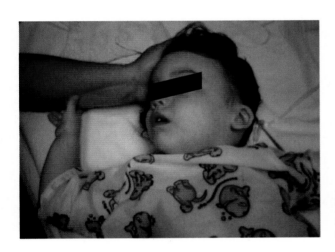

Figure 8-3 Ill-appearing child. This child appears weak and clingy but alert and active. Her ill appearance is the result of a mucocutaneous form of mycoplasma infection. (Courtesy of Evan J. Weiner, MD, FAAP.)

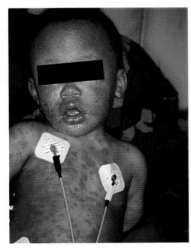

Figure 8-4 Ill-appearing child with Stevens-Johnson syndrome.
(Courtesy of Joseph Lopreiato, MD.)

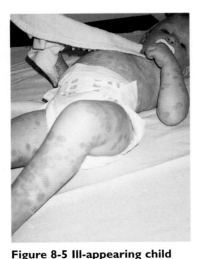

Figure 8-5 Ill-appearing child with urticaria.
(Used with permission from Fleisher GR, Ludwig S, Baskin MN, *Atlas of pediatric emergency medicine*. Philadelphia, PA: Lippincott Williams & Wilkins; 2004:88.)

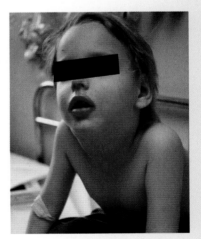

Figure 8-6 Epiglottitis and tripod positioning. This child's "tripod" positioning is indicative of epiglottitis. Note the child's toxic appearance.
(Courtesy of M. Douglas Baker, MD.)

DIFFERENTIAL DIAGNOSIS

DIAGNOSIS	ICD-9	DISTINGUISHING CHARACTERISTICS	DISTRIBUTION	DURATION/ CHRONICITY
Bacterial Meningoencephalitis	320.9	Altered mental status Toxic appearance	Neurologic system	Acute to subacute
Hypovolemia	276.52	Dry mucous membranes Absent tears Sunken eyes Lethargy	Mucosa Skin Eyes Vasculature	Acute to subacute
Congestive Heart Failure	428.0	Orthopnea Jugular venous distension Hepatomegaly Central cyanosis	Cardiac system Lungs Liver Extremities	Subacute
Increased Intracranial Pressure	742.3 Hydrocephalus 959.01 Head Injury	Depressed sensorium Bulging fontanelle Cushing triad	Neurologic system	Acute to subacute
Acute Abdomen	789.0 560.0 (Intussusception)	Abdominal tenderness Irritability	Abdomen	Acute
Respiratory Distress	518.81	Wheezing Stridor Retractions Nasal flaring Tachypnea	Pulmonary system	Acute to subacute
Toxic Ingestion	960–989	Toxidrome Evidence of substance ingested	Multiorgan system	Acute

ASSOCIATED FINDINGS	COMPLICATIONS	PRECIPITATING FACTORS	TREATMENT GUIDELINES
Fever Nuchal rigidity Kernig/Brudzinski signs Seizures Emesis Headache	Sepsis Hearing loss Encephalopathy	Immunocompromise Immunization delay	Broad-spectrum IV antibiotics Steroids prior to the first antibiotic dose
Poor perfusion Decreased urine output Decreased peripheral pulses Cool extremities	Electrolyte derangement Acidosis Renal failure Shock	Vomiting Diarrhea Hemorrhage Anorexia Polyuria	Oral rehydration therapy IV Hydration
Respiratory distress Edema Growth failure Other malformations	Cardiac arrest Renal failure Hypoxia Shock	Congenital heart disease Cardiomyopathy Myocarditis Hypertension	Diuretics Inotropes Afterload reduction Surgery
Emesis Seizures Focal neurologic signs Apnea Sundowning	Cardiopulmonary arrest Traumatic brain injury	Trauma Hydrocephalus Tumor	Hyperventilation Mannitol Surgery Hypertonic saline
Fever Anorexia Vomiting Diarrhea Dehydration Tachypnea Peritoneal signs	Sepsis Bowel perforation	Appendicolith Intestinal obstruction For intussusception: • Meckel diverticulum • Viral illness	Broad-spectrum IV antibiotics Surgery Bowel rest Nasogastric tube For intussusception: • Air contrast enema • Surgery
Apnea Depressed sensorium Grunting Cyanosis	Cardiopulmonary arrest	Infection Bronchospasm Upper airway obstruction Foreign body aspiration	Oxygen IV access Bronchodilators Steroids Airway management Chest radiography
Vomiting Altered sensorium Respiratory distress Apnea Seizures	Arrhythmias Aspiration Brain injury	Lack of childproofing Suicidality	Naloxone Activated charcoal Specific antidotes Cardiac monitoring

OTHER
DIAGNOSES
TO CONSIDER

- Inborn error of metabolism
- Electrolyte derangement
- Hypoglycemia
- Adrenal crisis
- Hepatic encephalopathy
- Uremia
- Autoimmune disease
- HIV (human immunodeficiency virus) infection
- Supraventricular tachycardia
- Failure to thrive
- Child abuse and neglect

WHEN TO
CONSIDER
FURTHER
EVALUATION
OR TREATMENT

- Tachypnea and tachycardia may be subtle clues of a more serious underlying condition and future deterioration. They should prompt urgent evaluation.
- In patients with altered mental status, in addition to pursuing the etiology, one must ensure stability of the airway, even though a primary respiratory process may not be present.
- A shock state may be present, even when a normal blood pressure is maintained due to compensatory mechanisms. Ill general appearance should lead one to consider and treat shock.

SUGGESTED READINGS

Athreya B, Silverman B. Subjective observations. In: *Pediatric physical diagnosis*. Norwalk, CT: Appleton-Century Crofts; 1985:58–70.
Bass JW, Wittler RR, Weisse ME. Social smile and occult bacteremia. *Pediatr Infect Dis J*. 1996;15(6):541.
Gorelick M, Shaw K, Murphy K. Validity and reliability of clinical signs in the diagnosis of dehydration in children. *Pediatrics*. 1997;99(5):E6.
Hsiao AL, Chen L, Baker MD. Incidence and predictors of serious bacterial infections among 57- to 180-day-old infants. *Pediatrics*. 2006;117(5):1695–1701.
Levine DA, Platt SL, Dayan PS, et al. Risk of serious bacterial infection in young febrile infants with respiratory syncytial virus infections. *Pediatrics*. 2004;113(6):1728–1734.
McCarthy P, Sharpe M, Spiesel S, et al. Observation scales to identify serious illness in febrile children. *Pediatrics*. 1982;70(5):802–809.

Section
THREE

Head

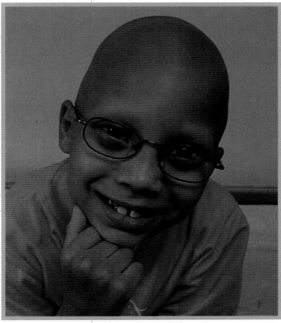

(Courtesy of Paul S. Matz, MD.)

Hair Loss

APPROACH TO THE PROBLEM

Hair loss, or alopecia, may be congenital, hereditary, or acquired. The distribution of hair loss is described as localized, as in alopecia areata, or more diffuse, as in telogen effluvium. Though hair loss often occurs in isolation, it may be a sign of systemic illness. Hair growth cycle disruption in the anagen (active), catagen (regressive), or telogen (resting) phases may cause hair loss. Also, any damage to the follicle or shaft may result in hair loss, as in trichotillomania. Some causes of hair loss, such as tinea capitis, may lead to scalp scarring and permanent hair loss if left untreated, which can be upsetting to the parents and the child.

KEY POINTS IN THE HISTORY

- Hair loss at birth usually occurs with cutis aplasia or sebaceous nevus of Jadassohn.

- Hair loss in younger teens necessitates a search for autoimmune disorders or psychiatric problems.

- Traction alopecia, from tight braiding, is a common cause of hair loss.

- Tinea capitis is the primary cause of alopecia in African American children.

- Home remedies for a child's scaling scalp include hair grease and oils, which may mask the underlying scale of tinea capitis.

- Recent illness may cause the hair to enter the resting (telogen) phase and may manifest as diffuse hair loss (telogen effluvium).

- There may be a family history of hair loss or autoimmune disease, such as in systemic lupus erythematosus.

- Children with systemic symptoms, nail or teeth abnormalities, may have hair loss as a manifestation of a more widespread disease.

- Older children with hair loss need to be assessed for psychological stress, if hair pulling, or trichotillomania, is the cause of their alopecia.

- Hair pulling tends to be biased toward the side of a patient's handedness.

KEY POINTS IN THE PHYSICAL EXAMINATION

- Major hair loss is often related to widespread disease.

- The combination of considerable scalp erythema and hair loss should prompt an investigation into evolving psoriasis or lupus.

- A prepubescent child with a scaly scalp should warrant a scalp culture to check for tinea capitis.

- The breakage of hair shafts close to the scalp in tinea capitis causes the "black dot" sign.

- Intrinsic hair shaft defects, hair pulling, or tight braiding, may cause hair breakage further away from the scalp.

- Kerions and pustules, host inflammatory responses to fungal infections, usually do not represent bacterial superinfection.

- Trichophyton species, accounting for over 90% of tinea capitis in North America, do not fluoresce under a Wood lamp.

PHOTOGRAPHS OF SELECTED DIAGNOSES

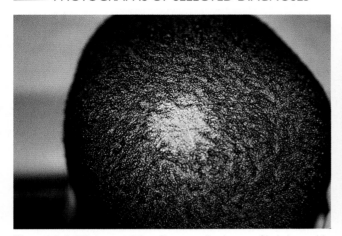

Figure 9-1 Tinea capitis. Circumscribed area of hair loss with scaliness of the scalp.
(Courtesy of George A. Datto, III, MD.)

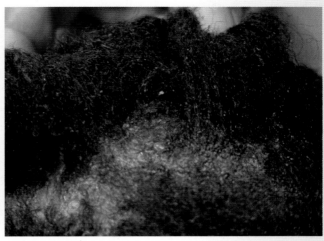

Figure 9-2 Tinea capitis. Diffuse scaling and pustules on the scalp.
(Courtesy of Paul S. Matz, MD.)

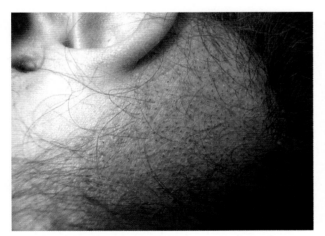

Figure 9-3 "Black dot" sign. Broken hair shafts at the scalp from tinea capitis.
(Courtesy of Paul S. Matz, MD.)

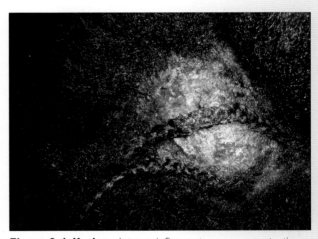

Figure 9-4 Kerion. Intense inflammatory response to tinea capitis.
(Courtesy of Paul S. Matz, MD.)

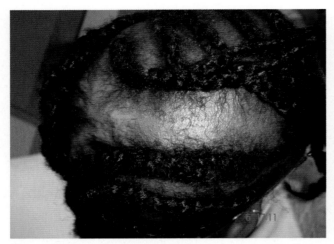

Figure 9-5 Traction alopecia. Alopecia where traction has been applied in association with hair braiding.
(Courtesy of Carrie Ann Cusack, MD.)

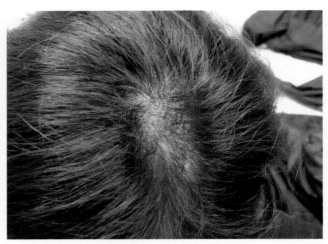

Figure 9-6 Trichotillomania. Broken hair shafts caused by pulling of one's hair.
(Courtesy of George A. Datto, III, MD.)

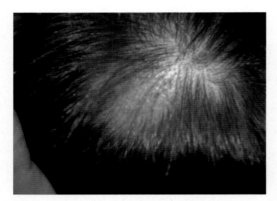

Figure 9-7 Sebaceous nevus of Jadassohn.
Yellowish-orange verrucous plaque on the scalp.
(Courtesy of the Department of Dermatology, Drexel University College of Medicine.)

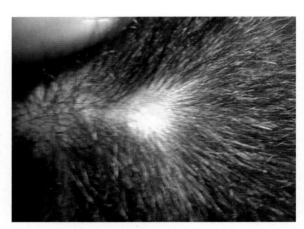

Figure 9-8 Cutis aplasia. Scar on the vertex of the scalp with complete hair loss secondary to cutis aplasia.
(Courtesy of Paul S. Matz, MD.)

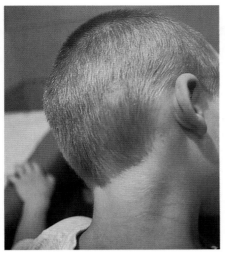

Figure 9-9 Discoid lupus. Oval area of hair loss associated with scalp erythema, scaling, and follicular plugging.
(Courtesy of George A. Datto, III, MD.)

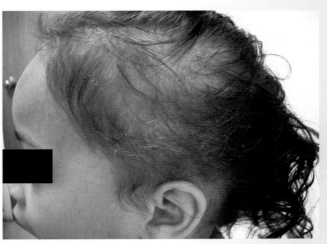

Figure 9-10 Telogen effluvium. Diffuse thinning of hair 3 months after febrile illness.
(Courtesy of Paul S. Matz, MD.)

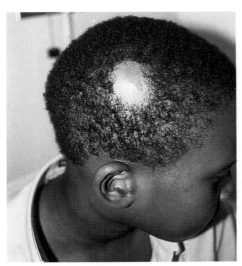

Figure 9-11 Alopecia areata. Localized circular patch of hair loss with normal scalp skin.
(Courtesy of George A. Datto, III, MD.)

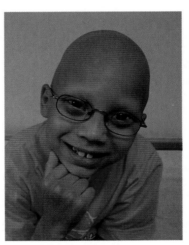

Figure 9-12 Alopecia universalis. Hair loss affecting the scalp, eyebrows, and eyelashes.
(Courtesy of Paul S. Matz, MD.)

DIFFERENTIAL DIAGNOSIS

DIAGNOSIS	ICD-9	DISTINGUISHING CHARACTERISTICS	DISTRIBUTION
Tinea Capitis	110.0	Alopecia, associated with scaling May present as diffuse dryness without alopecia "Black dot" sign	Focal Diffuse
Traction Alopecia	704.0	Hair is thinned at edges of braids	Focal
Trichotillomania	312.39	Broken hair shafts of varying lengths Irregular borders	Crown of head (Friar Tuck sign) Occipital Parietal
Sebaceous Nevus of Jadassohn	706.9	Orange Waxy Congenital	Focal
Cutis Aplasia	709.3	Congenital Oval-shaped alopecia	Midline
Discoid Lupus	695.4	Erythema Scaly	Focal
Telogen Effluvium	704.02	Abrupt hair loss with brushing or washing	Diffuse
Alopecia Areata	704.01	Absence of scaling or erythema in areas of hair loss Sharp borders	Parietal Occipital

ASSOCIATED FINDINGS	COMPLICATIONS	PREDISPOSING FACTORS	TREATMENT GUIDELINES
Occipital and posterior auricular lymphadenopathy Id reaction can occur and worsen with treatment	Kerion	*Trichophyton tonsurans* African American or Hispanic race/ethnicity	Scalp culture Oral antifungals Selenium sulfide shampoo to prevent spread
Small inflammatory papules Regional lymphadenopathy	Scarring of hair follicles	Tight braids or ponytails	Loosen hair braids and/or ponytails Topical antibiotics if infected
Anxious child Obsessive-compulsive disorder	Bezoars due to ingesting pulled hairs	Psychological stress	Cognitive-behavioral therapy Selective serotonin re-uptake inhibitors (SSRIs)
N/A	Potential for basal cell carcinoma after puberty	N/A	Biopsy and removal if worrisome changes
Can be associated with congenital anomalies	Permanent hair loss, due to scarring	N/A	N/A
Similar lesions on sun-exposed skin	Permanent hair loss due to scarring	Autoimmune pathogenesis	Topical immunosuppressants
N/A	Psychological	Acute illness in previous several months	Parental and patient reassurance
Eyebrow hair loss Nail changes Autoimmune diseases	Psychological	Autoimmune pathogenesis Atopy Genetic	Topical corticosteroids Injectible corticosteroids Oral immunosuppressants

OTHER
DIAGNOSES
TO CONSIDER

- Monilethrix

- Pili torti

- Menkes kinky hair syndrome

- Trichorrhexis nodosa

- Progeria

- Ectodermal dysplasia

WHEN TO
CONSIDER
FURTHER
EVALUATION
OR TREATMENT

- Further evaluation and treatment should be considered for areas of intense scalp inflammation.

- Several months of treatment failure for tinea capitis warrants consideration of reinfection or an alternate diagnosis, such as psoriasis.

- Diffuse hair loss warrants a search for a systemic disorder, such as lupus or vitamin D deficiency.

- Consider referral to a psychologist for children with trichotillomania.

SUGGESTED READINGS

Al-Fouzan A, Nanda A. Alopecia in children. *Clin Dermatol.* 2000;18:735–743.

Al Soagir S, Hay JR. Fungal infection in children: tinea capitis. *Clin Dermatol.* 2000;18(6):679–685.

Tay Y, Levy M, Metry D. Trichotillomania in childhood: case series and review. *Pediatrics.* 2004;113(5):e494–e498.

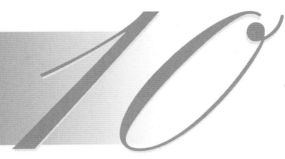

HANS B. KERSTEN

White Specks in the Hair

APPROACH TO THE PROBLEM

White specks in the hair often are a manifestation of diseases involving the scalp, although they may result from infestations in the hair. White specks in the hair do not usually occur in isolation; therefore, it is important to identify the involvement of the disease process on the scalp and other parts of the body. Once properly identified, white specks in the hair can be treated effectively.

KEY POINTS IN THE HISTORY

- Seborrheic dermatitis is common in infants and may also occur in adolescents during puberty.
- Seborrheic dermatitis in infants usually resolves by 7 to 8 months of age and is not typically itchy.
- Children with atopic dermatitis affecting the scalp often complain of itchiness or scratching and commonly have a family history of atopy.
- Tinea capitis is a common cause of white specks in the hair and/or alopecia in children of African descent, but it is uncommon in children of other race/ethnicities.
- Tinea capitis is acquired through personal contact with spores from the lesion.
- Head lice infestation is usually a disease of school-aged children, particularly girls. It is uncommon in children of African descent.
- Head lice and atopic dermatitis cause itching of the scalp.
- Head lice are acquired through close contact with an infested person or contact with infested items such as hats, headsets, combs, brushes, and bed sheets.

KEY POINTS IN THE PHYSICAL EXAMINATION

- Seborrheic dermatitis is characterized by greasy, scaly, yellowish, or salmon-colored lesions on the scalp. Lesions may also appear on the face, eyebrows, neck, shoulders, intertriginous areas, flexural areas of the extremities, or the diaper area.
- Atopic dermatitis may also involve the face and trunk, but the rash usually has popliteal and antecubital involvement that can help distinguish it from seborrheic dermatitis.
- The lesions of seborrheic dermatitis usually are well circumscribed, whereas lesions of atopic dermatitis may be more diffuse.

- With tinea capitis, round patches of inflammation with scale and alopecia are typical.

- Occipital lymphadenopathy is commonly seen with tinea capitis.

- Diffuse tinea capitis may resemble seborrheic dermatitis and present as diffuse scalp dryness without alopecia or erythema.

- Wood lamp examination will produce a yellow-green fluorescence for microsporum dermatophyte species but not for trichophyton species, which account for 90% of tinea capitis cases.

- The nits from head lice are attached firmly to the hair shaft, are difficult to remove by hand, and may be confused with dandruff.

- With head lice, the scalp is normal in appearance. With atopic dermatitis, seborrheic dermatitis, and tinea capitis, there is scaling of the scalp.

- Scales on the scalp may not be appreciated if family members are applying hair grease or other oily hair products to the scalp.

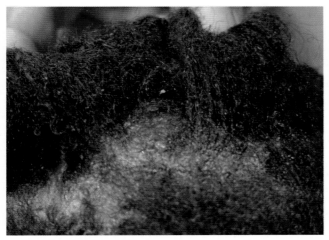

Figure 10-1 Tinea capitis. Note the dry, flaky appearance.
(Courtesy of Paul S. Matz, MD.)

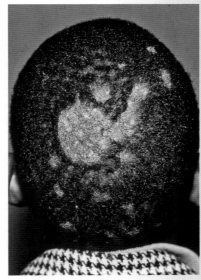

Figure 10-2 Tinea capitis. This photograph shows areas of black-dot alopecia.
(Courtesy of Paul S. Matz, MD.)

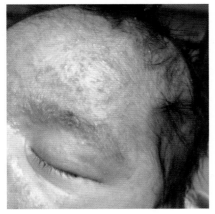

Figure 10-3 Seborrhea. Note the greasy appearance.
(Courtesy of Paul S. Matz, MD.)

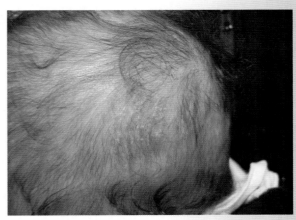

Figure 10-4 Scalp eczema. Note the area of erythema underlying the dry scale.
(Courtesy of Paul S. Matz, MD.)

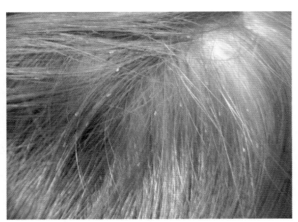

Figure 10-5 Pediculosis capitis. Note the whitish nits found along the hair shafts.
(Courtesy of Hans B. Kersten, MD.)

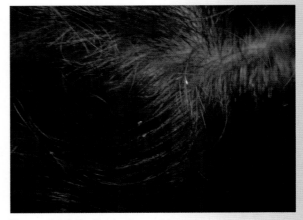

Figure 10-6 Pediculosis capitis.
(Courtesy of Hans B. Kersten, MD.)

DIFFERENTIAL DIAGNOSIS

DIAGNOSIS	ICD-9	DISTINGUISHING CHARACTERISTICS	DISTRIBUTION	ASSOCIATED FINDINGS
Tinea Capitis	110.0	Scaly scalp Black-dot sign	Focal or diffuse	Occipital or cervical adenopathy Id reaction—papulovesicular rash on trunk
Seborrhea	706.3	Greasy, yellowish scale Young infants and adolescents Well-circumscribed lesions Rash on scalp, diaper, or intertriginous areas Generally not itchy Localized cradle cap	Focal or diffuse	Rash involving the face, eyebrows, neck, shoulders, flexural and intertriginous areas of the extremities, and/or diaper area
Eczema	692.9	Always itchy Fluctuating course Rash distribution changes with age Generally worse in the winter time	Diffuse	Diffusely dry skin (xerosis) Lichenification Dermatographism Atopic diseases Hyperaccentuated palmar creases Altered cell-mediated immunity
Head Lice (Pediculosis Capitis)	132.0	Difficult to dislodge nits from the hair shaft Nits right next to the scalp Lice on the scalp Normal scalp	Diffuse nits in the hair Nape of the neck	Lice on the scalp or in the hair Normal scalp

COMPLICATIONS	PREDISPOSING FACTORS	TREATMENT GUIDELINES
Kerion—a boggy, edematous inflammatory reaction to tinea capitis Hair loss	Age—occurs almost exclusively in childhood Gender—boys affected five times more than girls	Systemic antifungals—may need to treat longer because of increased resistance Selenium sulfide shampoo two times per week to reduce spore transmission Oral corticosteroids—may hasten recovery with kerion, but not routinely recommended

Candidal infections in intertriginous areas
 	
Bacterial infections
 	
Intertrigo
 	
Blepharitis
	Age—Infancy (birth–12 months)
	
	Adolescence—at onset of puberty
		Guided by severity and location
		    Attempt to clear scalp lesions.
		    Treat rest of the body with mild-potency corticosteroids.
		Anitseborrheic shampoo (containing sulfur or salicylic acid)
		Mineral oil—loosens thick and adherent scales on the scalp
		Topical corticosteroid lotion to scalp ONLY in difficult-to-treat cases

Secondary infection
 	
Bleeding
 	
Lichenification
 	
Keratosis pilaris
 	
Personality traits—active, restless, irritable, aggressive
 	
Kaposi varicelliform eruption with abrupt vesicular onset
 	
Cataracts—early onset in 4–12% of affected individuals
	Atopy—part of an allergic triad that also includes allergic rhinitis and asthma	Manage itchy dry skin.
		    Moisturizers/lubricants
		    Mild soaps
		    Antihistamines
		    Soft, nonirritating clothing
		    Topical corticosteroids—mainstay of treatment for flares
		    Calcineurin inhibitors as second-line agents (note black box warning and potential risk of malignancies)
		    Systemic corticosteroids—not routinely recommended unless cannot be controlled by other methods

None	Humans—exclusive reservoir for lice Close personal and crowded contact—schools, camps, institutions Rare in blacks; more common among whites	Examination and treatment of all household contacts Permethrin cream rinse 1%—nonprescription Permethrin cream 5%—prescription Pyrethrins and piperonyl butoxide 4% Malathion—effective; treat for 8–12 hr Lindane—occasional neurotoxicity may be seen. High-volume heated air Home products, including olive oil and petroleum jelly, not felt to be as effective

OTHER DIAGNOSES TO CONSIDER

- Acrodermatitis enteropathica
- Wiskott-Aldrich syndrome
- Letterer-Siwe disease
- Psoriasis
- Impetigo

WHEN TO CONSIDER FURTHER EVALUATION OR TREATMENT

- Further evaluation and treatment should be considered for scalp flaking that fails to improve in spite of standard treatment regimens listed in this chapter.
- Severe atopic dermatitis that is unresponsive to the frequent use of emollients and mid-potency topical steroids may require referral to a dermatologist.
- Severe atopic dermatitis that is accompanied by failure to thrive warrants further evaluation and possible referral to a dermatologist.
- Significant hair loss secondary to a kerion found in association with tinea capitis should prompt referral to a dermatologist.
- Tinea capitis recalcitrant to standard medical treatment may require a second treatment course or use of a different antifungal agent.
- Persistent weeping of lesions in seborrhea may signal a secondary candidal infection.
- Recurrent lice is common in school-aged children secondary to poor compliance and repeated exposures at school. Proper treatment technique should be reviewed with parents. Secondary agents should be considered if lice persist.

SUGGESTED READINGS

Ahuja A, Land K, Barnes CJ. Atopic dermatitis. *South Med J.* 2003;96:1068–1072.
Chen BK, Friedlander SF. Tinea capitis update: a continuing conflict with an old adversary. *Curr Opin Pediatr.* 2001;13:331–335.
Goldstein AO, Goldstein BG. Dermatophyte (tinea) infections. In: Rind DM, ed. *Uptodate.* Wellesley, MA: UpToDate; 2008.
Goldstein AO, Goldstein BG. Pediculosis. In: Rind DM, ed. *Uptodate.* Wellesley, MA: UpToDate; 2007.
Gupta AK, Bluhm R. Seborrheic dermatitis. *J Eur Acad Dermatol Venereol.* 2004;18:13–26.
Paller AS, Mancini AJ. *Hurwitz clinical pediatric dermatology: a textbook of skin disorders of childhood and adolescence.* 3rd ed. Philadelphia, PA: Elsevier Saunders; 2006:49–64, 67–69, 451–455, 488–491.

KELLY R. LEITE
AND KATHLEEN CRONAN

Lumps on the Face

APPROACH TO THE PROBLEM

Facial lumps cause concern for parents, but many of these lesions are benign and self-limited. The more common pediatric lesions include dermoid cysts, epidermoid cysts, hemangiomas, buccal cellulitis, panniculitis, fat necrosis, pyogenic granuloma, mumps, and suppurative parotitis. Many of these facial lesions do not require immediate therapy; however, it is important to correctly diagnose and identify those lesions requiring urgent medical attention.

KEY POINTS IN THE HISTORY

- Hemangiomas and dermoid cysts are present at birth or appear during early infancy.

- Epidermoid cysts may appear at any age but more commonly appear after puberty.

- Associated constitutional symptoms, such as fever and malaise, may suggest mumps, suppurative parotitis, or buccal cellulitis.

- Asymptomatic lesions suggest the diagnosis of a dermoid cyst, epidermoid cyst, hemangioma, or fat necrosis.

- Patients with a pyogenic granuloma or fat necrosis may report a history of trauma.

- A lesion that enlarges during the first year of life, and then involutes, supports the diagnosis of hemangioma.

- Recent prolonged exposure to cold objects in the area of swelling suggests (popsicle) panniculitis.

- A history of recurrent parotid swelling or a family history of parotid swelling may indicate juvenile recurrent parotitis, a nonsuppurative, parotid inflammation of unknown etiology.

- The history of an unimmunized child with parotid inflammation strongly suggests mumps.

- Chronic, nonpainful swelling of the parotid gland may be seen in patients with human immunodeficiency virus infection.

KEY POINTS IN THE PHYSICAL EXAMINATION

- Tenderness to palpation is seen with buccal cellulitis, panniculitis, and parotitis/mumps.

- Swelling that obscures the angle of the jaw suggests parotid inflammation or parotitis.

- Children with mumps are rarely extremely ill-appearing.

- Suppurative parotitis, most commonly caused by *Staphylococcus aureus*, is associated with an ill-appearing child who may have purulent discharge from Stensen's duct.

- Nodules or papules with normal overlying skin suggest dermoid cysts, epidermoid cysts, or deep (cavernous) hemangiomas.

- Swelling associated with erythema of the overlying skin suggests buccal cellulitis, panniculitis, fat necrosis, or suppurative parotitis.

- A friable lesion suggests pyogenic granuloma.

PHOTOGRAPHS OF SELECTED DIAGNOSES

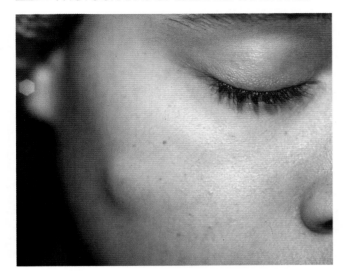

Figure 11-1 Epidermoid cyst. A well-demarcated solitary nodule on the face.
(Used with permission from Goodheart HP. *Goodheart's photoguide of common skin disorders.* Philadelphia, PA: Lippincott Williams & Wilkins; 2003:4.)

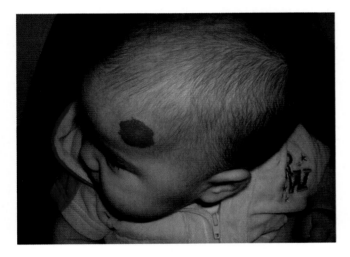

Figure 11-2 Hemangioma. An infant with a rapidly growing vascular mass on the forehead.
(Courtesy of Scott Van Duzer, MD.)

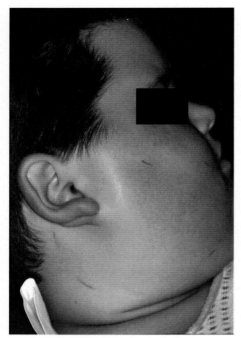

Figure 11-3 Parotitis. Dramatic edema, erythema, and induration of the face overlying the parotid gland.
(Courtesy of Kathleen Cronan, MD.)

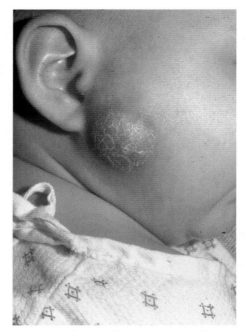

Figure 11-4 Parotid abscess. A well-demarcated fluctuant mass overlying the parotid gland of an infant.
(Courtesy of the late Peter Sol, MD.)

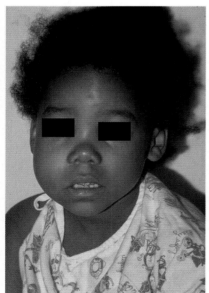

Figure 11-5 Buccal cellulitis secondary to dental abscess. A child with diffuse, unilateral, facial swelling, associated with dental caries.
(Courtesy of the late Peter Sol, MD.)

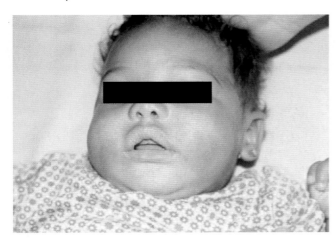

Figure 11-6 Popsicle panniculitis. Bilateral, erythematous firm subcutaneous nodules in the cheeks of an infant.
(Courtesy of Kathleen Cronan, MD.)

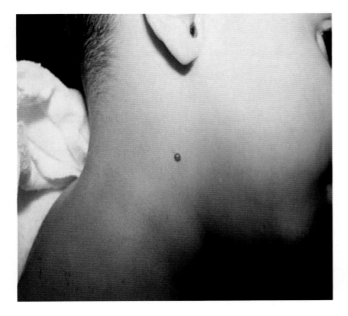

Figure 11-7 Pyogenic granuloma. Isolated erythematous nodule on a child's neck.
(Courtesy of Kathleen Cronan, MD.)

DIFFERENTIAL DIAGNOSIS

DIAGNOSIS	ICD-9	DISTINGUISHING CHARACTERISTICS	DISTRIBUTION
Epidermoid Cyst	706.2	Well-demarcated solitary nodule or papule	Face, scalp, neck, trunk
Dermoid Cyst	709.8	Firm, skin-colored nodule	Often midline, forehead, periorbital area, or lateral eyebrow
Hemangioma	228.01	Superficial or "strawberry" lesion (pink/red) Deep or cavernous lesion (blue/skin colored)	Head and neck, most commonly May occur on trunk, or oral or genital mucosae
Parotitis	072.9 (mumps) 527.2	Painful swelling of the parotid gland that obscures the angle of the mandible	Parotid gland Mumps is usually bilateral. Suppurative type is unilateral.
Buccal Cellulitis	682.0 528.3	Tender to palpation Salmon or violaceous color	Subcutaneous and dermal layers of the cheek Unilateral
Popsicle Panniculitis	729.3	Erythematous nodule Painful to palpation	Perioral Subcutaneous fat Angle of mouth Often bilateral
Fat Necrosis	778.1—newborn 709.3	Multiple or single erythematous, nontender nodule(s)	Cheeks, buttocks, thigh Sites of trauma
Pyogenic Granuloma	686.1	Bright red, exophytic lesion Moist appearance	60% on head/neck Usually solitary

DURATION/CHRONICITY	ASSOCIATED FINDINGS	COMPLICATIONS	TREATMENT GUIDELINES
Slow-growing Persists for life	Normal overlying skin Central dimple	Recurrent inflammation Lesion may rupture	Surgical excision
Congenital	Intracranial extension in midline lesions Spinal cord defects in sacral lesions	Meningitis/infection, particularly if communication with underlying structures	Surgical excision
Rapidly enlarges in the first year of life	Multiple lesions associated with visceral findings Rapidly enlarging lesions seen in Kasabach-Merritt syndrome or PHACE syndrome	Bleeding after trauma Obstruction of airway, vision, or GU tract	Reassurance Dermatology referral for large, obstructing lesions Systemic/intralesional steroids, interferon, pulse dye laser
Viral type in childhood Suppurative type in neonates/older children	Brief prodrome with mumps Increased amylase level in 70% of cases	Rarely: orchitis, encephalitis, pancreatitis, deafness, nephritis, myocarditis	Supportive (mumps) Antistaphylococcal antibiotics for suppurative cases
Acute onset Peak incidence at 9–12 months Resolves with treatment	Acute otitis media commonly seen Ill-appearing child	Bacteremia, meningitis intracranial extension, cavernous sinus thrombosis	Parenteral antibiotics
Lesion persists 2–3 weeks Lesion not apparent immediately	Generally well-appearing child	None	None
Appears between 1–6 weeks of age Heals spontaneously	Associated trauma	Calcification Ulceration Infection	None
Most commonly in childhood Persists unless excised	Associated trauma	Profuse bleeding Infection Recurrence	Curettage and cauterization

OTHER DIAGNOSES TO CONSIDER

- Trichoepithelioma

- Pilomatrixoma

- Idiopathic neuroma

- Mucosal neuromas as seen with multiple endocrine neoplasia IIB

- Lymphocytoma cutis

WHEN TO CONSIDER FURTHER EVALUATION OR TREATMENT

- Epidermoid cysts with recurring inflammation may require surgical excision.

- Enlarging hemangiomas, at risk for obstructing the nose or eye, should be referred to a dermatologist.

- Prompt medical attention is required if parotid or buccal mucosal swelling is accompanied by fever or ill-appearance.

- Pyogenic granulomas with frequent or profuse bleeding require urgent excision by a pediatric dermatologist.

- Dermoid cysts communicating with underlying structures may become infected and require antibiotics.

- A lesion consistent with fat necrosis may require referral to a dermatologist if calcification or ulceration occurs.

SUGGESTED READINGS

Goodheart HP. *Goodheart's photoguide of common skin disorders*. Philadelphia, PA: Lippincott Williams & Wilkins; 2003:4.

McKinzie JP. Clinical pearls: fever and facial swelling—buccal cellulitis. *Acad Emerg Med*. 1998;5(4):347, 368–370.

Miller T, Frieden IJ. Hemangiomas: new insights and classification. *Pediatr Ann*. 2005;34(3):179–190.

Nahlieli O, Shachem R, Shlesinger M, et al. Juvenile recurrent parotitis: a new method of diagnosis and treatment. *Pediatrics*. 2004;114(1):9–12.

Pagliai KA, Cohen BA. Pyogenic granuloma in children. *Pediatr Dermatol*. 2004;21(1):10–13.

Templer J. Acute neonatal suppurative parotitis: case reports and review. *Pediatr Infect Dis J*. 2004;23(1):76–78.

Eyes

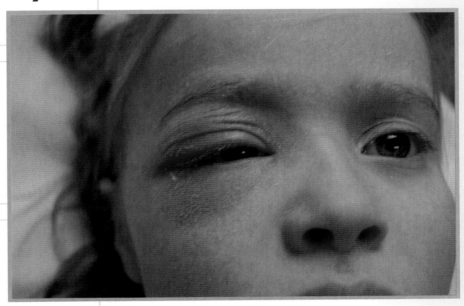

(Courtesy of Parul B. Patel, MD, MPH.)

PARUL B. PATEL
AND STEVEN M. SELBST

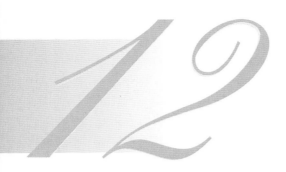

Red Eye

APPROACH TO THE PROBLEM

A red eye is an eye with vascular congestion of the conjunctiva resulting from inflammation, trauma, conjunctivitis, or glaucoma. Redness may also be secondary to eyelid pathology. Conjunctivitis is the most common cause of a red eye, while glaucoma is rare in pediatrics. Conjunctivitis is commonly referred to as "pink eye" when it is caused by a viral or bacterial infection. Conjunctivitis may also have an allergic etiology. Trauma to the eye can cause eye redness in association with corneal abrasions, iritis, and subconjunctival hemorrhage. Red eye may be related to eyelid pathology such as blepharitis and periorbital (preseptal) or orbital (postseptal) cellulitis (see Chapter 13). Red eyes may also be seen in some systemic diseases such as Kawasaki disease (KD).

KEY POINTS IN THE HISTORY

- A history of atopy, allergen exposure, or seasonality will often help distinguish viral from allergic conjunctivitis.

- Pruritus is a common complaint with allergic conjunctivitis.

- While viral and bacterial conjunctivitis may have purulent discharge, early morning lid crusting or gluey eyes usually point to a bacterial etiology.

- The time of presentation is very important in the neonate with conjunctivitis; chemical conjunctivitis usually occurs in the first 24 hours, conjunctivitis secondary to gonococcal infection usually appears within 1 week after birth, and conjunctivitis secondary to chlamydial infection usually appears 1 to 2 weeks after birth.

- Pain after trauma suggests corneal abrasion or iritis, while subconjunctival hemorrhages are usually painless.

- Decreased vision and marked photophobia suggest a more serious diagnosis, such as glaucoma.

- Ocular pain with eye movement distinguishes orbital cellulitis from periorbital cellulitis.

- Consider KD when an irritable child with fever has red eyes but no eye discharge.

- Unilateral conjunctivitis with surrounding vesicular lesions is highly suspicious for keratoconjunctivitis resulting from herpes simplex virus.

- Visual acuity, because it may be impaired, should be tested whenever orbital cellulitis is suspected.

- Fluorescein examination is extremely helpful in diagnosing a corneal abrasion. Holding the fluorescein strip near the outer canthus, while having the patient blink, allows the dye to taint the tears. To further limit discomfort, fluorescein dye may be applied to the conjunctiva following the application of an ocular anesthetic.

- Signs of orbital cellulitis, such as limited eye movement and decreased vision, may mimic those of orbital pseudotumor and neoplasm.

- A palpable, preauricular lymph node in association with conjunctivitis is suspicious for viral conjunctivitis.

- Forty percent to fifty percent of those who have conjunctivitis in association with acute otitis media (formerly described as the otitis media-conjunctivitis syndrome) may have infection due to nontypeable *Haemophilus influenzae*.

- Consider other diagnoses, such as keratitis, iritis, or uveitis, when the limbus (the sclerocorneal junction) is involved.

- Conjunctivitis associated with pharyngitis is often caused by adenovirus.

- A history of gluey or sticky eyelids and physical findings of mucoid or purulent discharge are highly predictive of bacterial infection.

- Chemosis is swelling of the conjunctiva due to allergy or irritation.

PHOTOGRAPHS OF SELECTED DIAGNOSES

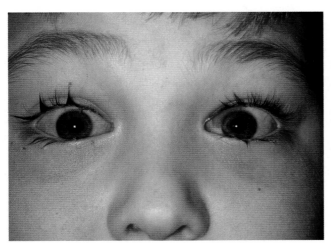

Figure 12-1 Conjunctivitis with a subconjunctival hemorrhage. Note the subconjunctival hemorrhage on the left. (Courtesy of Steven M. Selbst, MD, FAAP.)

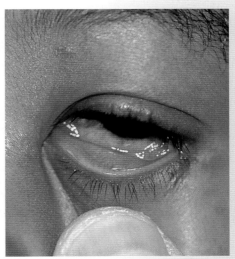

Figure 12-2 Allergic conjunctivitis with lid edema and conjunctival injection. (Used with permission from Fleisher GR, Ludwig S, Baskin MN. *Atlas of pediatric emergency medicine.* Philadelphia, PA: Lippincott Williams & Wilkins; 2004:271.)

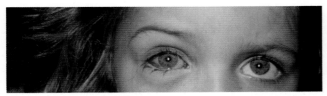

Figure 12-3 Viral conjunctivitis. Note the classic appearance of the red eye, absence of thick eye discharge. (Courtesy of Parul B. Patel, MD, MPH.)

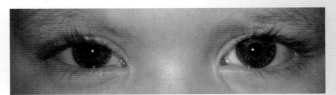

Figure 12-4 Bacterial conjunctivitis. The early-morning eyelid gluing and/or crusting may be absent on examination. (Courtesy of Steven M. Selbst, MD, FAAP.)

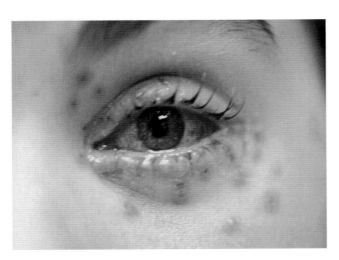

Figure 12-5 Herpes keratoconjunctivitis. Note the classic vesicular lesions around the eye. (Courtesy of Steven M. Selbst, MD, FAAP.)

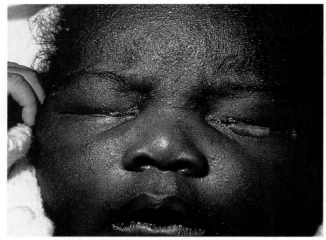

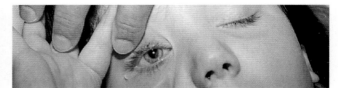

Figure 12-7 Corneal abrasion. Note the prominence of fluorescein medially.
(Courtesy of Kathleen Cronan, MD.)

Figure 12-6 Gonococcal ophthalmia neonatorum.
(Used with permission from Ostler HB, Maibach HI, Hoke AW, et al. *Diseases of the eye and skin: a color atlas.* Philadelphia, PA: Lippincott Williams & Wilkins; 2004:269.)

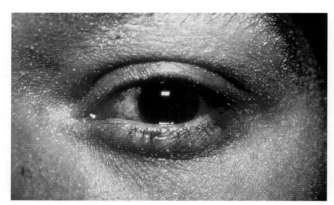

Figure 12-8 Conjunctivitis seen with KD.
(Used with permission from Goodheart HP. *Goodheart's photoguide to common skin disorders.* 2nd ed. Philadelphia, PA: Lippincott Williams & Wilkins; 2003:198.)

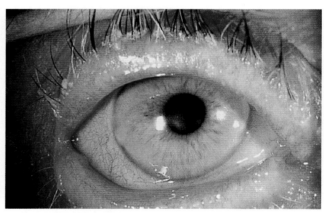

Figure 12-9 Blepharitis. Note the irritation of the eyelid margins.
(Used with permission from Weber J, Kelley J. *Health assessment in nursing.* 2nd ed. Philadelphia, PA: Lippincott Williams & Wilkins; 2003:196.)

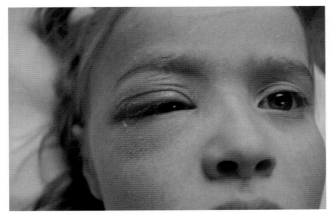

Figure 12-10 Periorbital cellulitis. Note the erythema and swelling of the eyelids.
(Courtesy of Parul B. Patel, MD, MPH.)

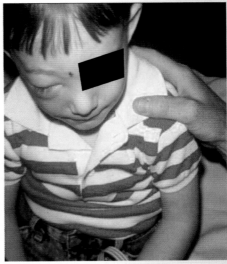

Figure 12-11 Orbital cellulitis. Note swelling and proptosis of the right.
(Courtesy of Steven M. Selbst, MD, FAAP.)

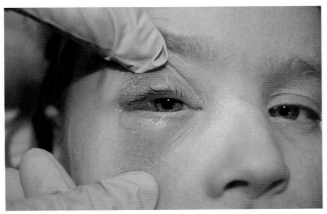

Figure 12-12 Chemosis. Note the impressive swelling of the conjunctiva.
(Courtesy of Parul B. Patel, MD, MPH.)

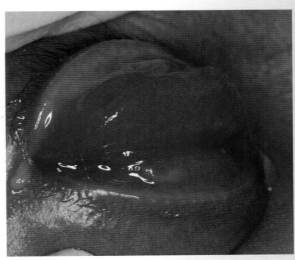

Figure 12-13 Chlamydia conjunctivitis. Note the severe chemosis and purulent discharge.
(Courtesy of Parul B. Patel, MD, MPH.)

DIAGNOSIS	ICD-9	DISTINGUISHING CHARACTERISTICS	DISTRIBUTION	DURATION/ CHRONICITY
Subconjunctival Hemorrhage	372.72	Painless Benign Spontaneous resolution	Localized rupture of small subconjunctival vessels	Resolves in 2–3 weeks
Allergic Conjunctivitis	372.14	Seasonal Pruritic Conjunctival edema (chemosis) Usually watery discharge Bilateral	Diffuse (involves whole conjunctiva and sclera)	Resolves with allergen removal and/or treatment Recurs every season
Viral Conjunctivitis	077.99	History of exposure Ocular discomfort Watery discharge Tender preauricular lymph node Follicular aggregates	Diffuse (involves whole conjunctiva and sclera)	3–7 days Self-limited
Bacterial Conjunctivitis	372.30	Usually mucopurulent discharge Early-morning crusty or "gluey" eye	Diffuse marked erythema	7–10 days Generally self-limited in infants and older children
	098.4	*Gonococcal conjunctivitis* Profuse purulent discharge Lids often swollen High risk in neonates usually less than 2 weeks old and sexually active adolescents	Diffuse hyperacute conjunctival injection	Variable, depends on treatment
Herpes Keratoconjunctivitis	370.40	Lid often swollen Watery discharge Painful Unilateral Photophobia Foreign body sensation Periorbital vesicles Dendritic (tree-like) pattern with fluorescent stain seen with slit lamp	Diffuse	Variable, depends on treatment May be recurrent
Corneal Abrasion	918.1	Intense pain Tearing (+/–) photophobia	Localized	Improves within 24–48 hrs
Conjunctivitis with KD	446.1	Nonpurulent Nonulcerative Bilateral	Bulbar conjunctivitis (spares limbus)	1–2 weeks if untreated
Blepharitis	373.00	Redness and swelling of eyelid margins Scaly, flaky debris on lid margins Gritty, burning sensation Matting upon awakening	Eyelid margins	Chronic/recurrent
Periorbital (Preseptal) Cellulitis	373.13	Infection of the space anterior to the orbital septum Lid warmth, edema, erythema, and tenderness More common in children <5 years Usually unilateral	Eyelids, upper and lower	7–10 days with oral antibiotic treatment
Orbital (Postseptal) Cellulitis	376.10	Infection involving the orbital structures posterior to the orbital septum Lid warmth, edema, erythema, and tenderness Chemosis Proptosis Decreased extraocular movement Periocular pain Usually unilateral	Eyelids, upper and lower Mild, diffuse conjunctival injection	10–14 days with IV and oral antibiotic treatment
Glaucoma	365.9	Cloudy or hazy cornea (because of corneal edema) Tearing but discharge is unusual Photophobia, blurred vision Irregular corneal reflex Rare in children except congenital variety The eye may appear large.	Circumcorneal injection (ciliary flush)	Variable

ASSOCIATED FINDINGS	COMPLICATIONS	PREDISPOSING FACTORS	TREATMENT GUIDELINES
Periorbital trauma	None	Direct trauma Spontaneous Childbirth or birth trauma Increased intrathoracic pressure (as seen with coughing, vomiting)	Self-resolving
Atopy Teary eyes Photophobia	Usually none	Allergens including pollen, ragweed, dust, animal dander (usually airborne)	Oral or topical antihistamines
Viral syndrome (fever, pharyngitis, adenopathy) Ocular discomfort Eyelid swelling	Infectious to others	Exposure from direct contact or from fomites	Self-resolving Emphasis on hand washing
Sometimes occurs with acute otitis media (usually because of nontypeable *H. influenzae*) Ocular discomfort	Infectious to others	Exposure from direct contact with other infected individuals	Ocular antibiotics Add oral antibiotics if suspecting *H. influenzae* Consult ophthalmologist if contact lens wearer
Sepsis-like picture in neonates May be associated with disseminated gonococcal disease (arthritis, rash) or urethral discharge in adolescents	Loss of eye from abscess, corneal ulceration, and perforation when untreated Infectious to others	Vertical transmission (mother to baby) Sexually active adolescents Victims of sexual abuse Exposure to (direct contact) infected person	Consider full sepsis workup in neonates and admission for IV antibiotics Consult ophthalmologist
Mucocutaneous or predominantly periorbital vesicles Corneal ulceration Systemic involvement Sepsis-like picture or seizures in neonates	Systemic infection in neonates Infectious to others	Neonates of infected mothers are at risk Sexually active adolescents	Consult ophthalmologist
Facial trauma Other eye injury	Infection Ulceration (contact lens wearers)	Direct trauma Rubbing eyes Foreign body Insertion/removal of contact lenses	Ocular antibiotics Follow-up with ophthalmology if no improvement in 2 days or promptly if contact lens wearer Discontinue use of contact lenses
Signs and symptoms of acute phase of KD (fever, irritability, rash, lymphadenopathy, mucous membrane and extremities changes) Acute iridocyclitis Punctate keratitis Subconjunctival hemorrhage	Coronary artery aneurysms, myocardial infarction, and/or death when KD is left untreated	Uncertain	Admission for IVIG, aspirin, Echocardiogram, cardiology consultation
Rosacea or seborrheic dermatitis	Hordeolum	Usually none	Consider ocular antibiotics
Fever and pain	Orbital cellulitis Bacteremia/sepsis Meningitis	Minor trauma or insect bite Localized lid infections Bacteremia because of *H. influenzae* type B	Oral antibiotics, IV antibiotics if ill appearing, not improving
Fever Associated URI (upper respiratory tract infection) symptoms Decreased visual acuity Malaise	Blindness Brain abscess Meningitis Cavernous sinus thrombosis	Sinusitis Minor trauma Dental abscess Periorbital cellulitis	CT scan of the orbits Ophthalmology consult Otolaryngology consult if sinus infection, abscess found IV antibiotics
Increased intraocular pressure Acute periocular pain Nausea and vomiting with acute angle glaucoma	Blindness	Trauma Congenital Other ocular diseases	Consult ophthalmologist

OTHER
DIAGNOSES
TO CONSIDER

- Keratitis
- Episcleritis/scleritis
- Chemical or toxin conjunctivitis
- Iritis (anterior uveitis or iridocyclitis)
- Dacryocystitis

WHEN TO
CONSIDER
FURTHER
EVALUATION
OR TREATMENT

- Consider full sepsis workup and admission of neonates suspected to have gonoccocal conjunctivitis.
- All patients suspected to be infected with herpes keratitis should follow up with an ophthalmologist.
- For patients with corneal abrasions, prescribe an ocular antibiotic such as erythromycin for prophylaxis against conjunctivitis.
- Corneal abrasions usually heal within 24 to 48 hours. Consultation with an ophthalmologist and a slit lamp examination may be necessary if symptoms persist. Prompt consultation is mandatory if the patient wears contact lenses.
- Do not prescribe steroids to treat patients with red eye without an ophthalmology consultation.
- Patients with orbital cellulitis should be admitted for IV antibiotics, ophthalmology evaluation, and CT scan of the orbits to rule out abscess formation.

SUGGESTED READINGS

Alessandrini EA. The case of the red eye. *Pediatr Ann.* 2000;29(2):112–116.

Coote MA. Sticky eye, tricky diagnosis. *Aust Fam Physician.* 2002;31(3):225–231.

Pasternak A, Irish B. Ophthalmologic infection in primary care. *Clin Fam Pract.* 2004;6(1):19–25.

Patel PB, Diaz MCG, Bennett JE, et al. Clinical features of bacterial conjunctivitis in children. *Acad EM.* 2007;14(1):1–5.

Rietveld RP, van Weert HCPM, ter Riet G, et al. Predicting bacterial cause in infectious conjunctivitis: cohort study on informativeness of combinations of signs and symptoms *BMJ.* 2004;329:206–210.

Teoh DL, Reynolds S. Diagnosis and management of pediatric conjunctivitis. *Pediatr Emerg Care.* 2003;19(1):48–55.

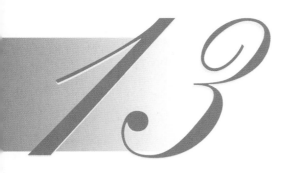

Swelling of/Around the Eye

APPROACH TO THE PROBLEM

The causes of swelling of/around the eye range from temporary irritations to ophthalmological emergencies. The causes can be broadly divided into two categories, conditions with diffuse swelling and conditions with discrete masses. Diffuse swelling around the eye results from edema. Edema results from a localized extravasation of the capillary fluid as with allergies or infection, from hypoalbuminemia as in a renal disease or from a reduced cardiac output state such as heart failure. Discrete masses usually result from growths like hemangiomas, the occlusion of the nasolacrimal duct system, or the inflammation/infection of the eyelid glands as seen with a hordeolum.

KEY POINTS IN THE HISTORY

- Preseptal cellulitis often occurs after an insult to skin integrity as seen with an insect bite. Timing of the swelling in relationship to timing of the bite will help distinguish between a superimposed infection and a simple bite. Generally, bacterial infections do not set in until 2 to 3 days after the initial bite.

- Preseptal cellulitis is often preceded by a history of a bacterial infection such as acute otitis media or sinusitis.

- In cases of IgE-mediated allergic reactions, consider not only airborne allergens but also contact irritants from substances rubbed into the eye. Food allergies are unlikely to cause isolated periorbital swelling.

- A history of pruritus suggests allergy; however, allergy-induced swelling can be deceivingly nonpruritic.

- Cardiac failure patients may report dyspnea or diaphoresis on exertion (infants during feeding, older children during exercise), poor growth, orthopnea, nocturnal dyspnea, cyanosis, or respiratory distress.

- A history of abdominal pain may be associated with both Henoch-Schönlein purpura (HSP) and hereditary angioedema.

- An intermittent history of swelling may be associated with hereditary angioedema (plasma protein C1 inhibitor deficiency). Tingling in the area may precede swelling.

- Hemangiomas and lymphangiomas often appear the same on physical examination. However, hemangiomas are not present at birth and tend to be more rapidly growing than lymphangiomas. Approximately half of all lymphangiomas are present at birth.

- Sudden appearance of a tender eyelid mass suggests a hordeolum.

- Chalazia are generally painless and can be present for weeks prior to presentation.

KEY POINTS IN THE PHYSICAL EXAMINATION

- The presence of fever or tenderness (subjective or on examination) points toward infection. This is particularly important to note when differentiating between an insect bite and periorbital cellulitis (also see Chapter 14). In periorbital cellulitis, look for the presence of other bacterial infections such as acute otitis media or sinusitis.

- Signs of orbital infection include proptosis, the restriction of extraocular movements (usually inability to look up), visual changes, and pain with eye movement. Systemic symptoms such as fever, drowsiness, vomiting, or headache may be present and should raise the suspicion for bacteremia, meningitis, or brain abscess.

- In hypoalbuminemia and cardiac failure states, other areas of dependent edema should be present. In infants, look for sacral edema, and in children who can stand, look for ankle edema. In cardiac failure, hepatosplenomegaly or crackles on auscultation of the lung fields may be present. Tachycardia may be a sign of cardiomyopathy.

- Unilateral diffuse swelling results from a localized extravasation of the capillary fluid into the periorbital area.

- Bilateral diffuse swelling usually represents edema from hypoalbuminemia or low cardiac output states. Although less common, allergic reactions can sometimes present as bilateral diffuse swelling.

- In ocular trauma, look for decreased visual acuity, tearing, and pain. The presence of an orbital-rim step-off signals a fracture. Crepitus over the eyelids may be evident if there is a fracture in the paranasal sinuses. The presence of hyphema (blood in the anterior chamber) may result after blunt trauma. Photophobia can be a sign of traumatic iritis. Restricted eye movement and double vision are ominous signs for globe rupture.

- A purpuric lower extremity rash is associated with HSP.

- Dermoids tend to be firm masses, while hemangiomas and lymphangiomas are soft.

- Deep hemangiomas often have a bluish hue. Superficial hemangiomas may be bluish but are more often "strawberry" red. Hemangiomas blanch with pressure.

- Congenital nasolacrimal duct obstruction (dacryostenosis), which manifests as tear overflow with mild palpebral erythema, predisposes infants to dacryocystitis.

- Most chalazia point toward the conjunctival surface, while hordeola may point either way. When looking for hordeola or chalazia, palpate the eyelid for nodules and visualize beneath the eyelid.

PHOTOGRAPHS OF SELECTED DIAGNOSES

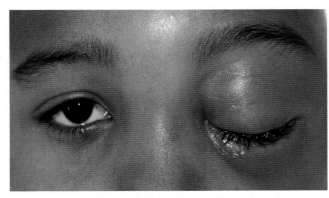

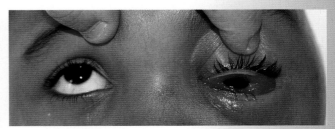

Figure 13-2 Orbital cellulitis. This is the same patient as in the previous photograph. Note the presence of chemosis and ophthalmoplegia.
(Courtesy of Scott Goldstein, MD.)

Figure 13-1 Orbital cellulitis. The swelling and erythema seen externally with orbital cellulitis may be similar to that seen with periorbital cellulitis.
(Courtesy of Scott Goldstein, MD.)

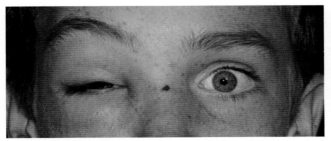

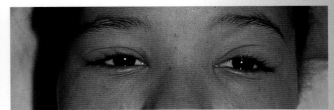

Figure 13-4 Eyelid edema. Bilateral eyelid edema from nephrotic syndrome.
(Courtesy of George A. Datto, III, MD.)

Figure 13-3 Insect bite. This patient was stung by an insect at dusk but did not notice any swelling until the next morning.
(Courtesy of Naline Lai, MD.)

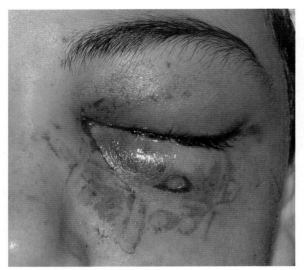

Figure 13-5 Trauma. This child was hit by a baseball.
(Courtesy of Scott Goldstein, MD.)

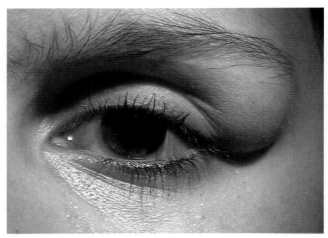

Figure 13-6 Dermoid. Note the swelling in the upper eyelid.
(Courtesy of Barry Oppenheim, MD.)

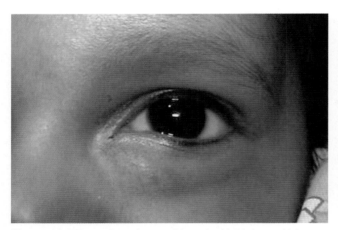

Figure 13-7 Lymphangioma. Note the bluish hue, which can also be seen in deep hemangiomas.
(Courtesy of Barry Oppenheim, MD.)

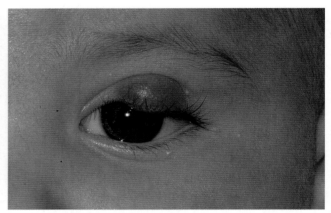

Figure 13-8 Hemangioma. This hemangioma is beginning to obscure this child's vision.
(Courtesy of Scott Goldstein, MD.)

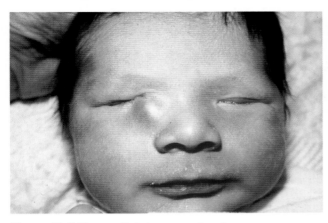

Figure 13-9 Congenital dacryocystocele.
(Courtesy of Terri L. Young, MD.)

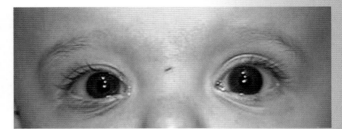

Figure 13-10 Positive dye test for nasolacrimal duct obstruction. Poor drainage leading to pooling of dye.
(Courtesy of Barry Oppenheim, MD.)

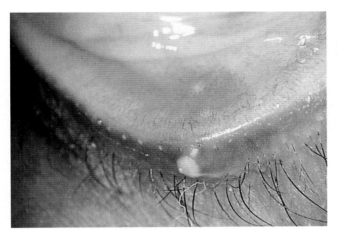

Figure 13-11 Hordeolum. This tender lesion points toward the conjunctival surface in this patient.
(Used with permission from Weber J, Kelley J. *Health assessment in nursing.* 2nd ed. Philadelphia, PA: Lippincott Williams & Wilkins; 2003:196.)

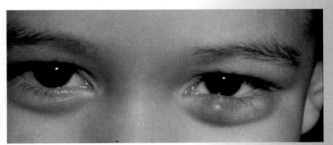

Figure 13-12. Chalazion. This is a relatively painless lesion.
(Courtesy of Terri L. Young, MD.)

DIAGNOSIS	ICD-9	DISTINGUISHING CHARACTERISTICS	DISTRIBUTION	DURATION/ CHRONICITY
Diffuse Swelling				
Periorbital (Preseptal) and Orbital Cellulitis	373.13 (abscess of eyelid) 376.01 (orbital cellulitis)	Either: warm, tender, erythematous, nonpruritic Orbital cellulitis: proptosis, ophthalmoplegia, decreased visual acuity	Unilateral Upper and/or lower palpebrae	Acute
Allergic Reaction	372.05	Warm, nontender, ±erythematous, ±pruritic, diffuse swelling	Bilateral Periorbital	Acute Often appears on awakening after night time exposure
Insect Bite	918.0	Warm, nontender, nondurated erythematous, pruritic, ±punctation, diffuse swelling	Unilateral	Acute Often appears on awakening after night time exposure
Edema from Nephrotic Syndrome	581.9	Not warm, nontender, nonerythematous, nonpruritic, diffuse swelling	Bilateral	Acute or chronic
Edema from Cardiovascular Causes	428.0 (heart failure)	Not warm, nontender, nonerythematous, nonpruritic, diffuse swelling	Bilateral	Acute
Trauma	921.1 (contusion of eyelids and periocular area) 374.82 (edema of the eyelid) 216.3 (edema of the eyebrow) 870.0 (laceration of the skin of the eyelid and periocular area)	Not warm, tender, ecchymosis/erythema, diffuse swelling	Unilateral	Acute
Hereditary Angioedema	277.6 (hereditary angioneurotic edema)	Not warm, nontender, nonerythematous, nonpruritic, diffuse swelling	Unilateral or bilateral	Intermittent, usually presents in adolescence
Discrete Masses				
Dermoid	216.1 (neoplasm benign, eyelid)	Nontender, smooth, discrete mass, firm, usually fixed	Unilateral Usually over the brow or upper eyelid	Congenital: may increase in size with age, usually recognized by age 16
Lymphangioma	228.1	Nontender, smooth, discrete mass, soft	Unilateral	May be present at birth (approx. 50%) Slow growth Often stabilizes in adulthood
Hemangioma	228.01	Nontender, discrete mass, soft or firm Bright red "strawberry" Deeper lesions have a bluish hue Blanches with pressure	Unilateral	Usually not present at birth, appears shortly thereafter Grows quickly in the first year of life, often involutes by age 6
Lacrimal System Infections (Dacryocystitis, Canaliculitis)	375.3 (dacryocystitis) 771.6 (neonatal conjunctivitis)	Tender, discrete mass, soft or firm, erythematous	Unilateral, nasolacrimal area	Acute
Congenital Dacryocystocele (Mucocele)	375.42 (lacrimal mucocele)	Bluish hue, discrete mass, firm	Unilateral, nasolacrimal area	At birth or shortly after
Hordeolum (common name, sty)	373.11	Tender, discrete mass, firm May point toward or away from the conjunctival surface	Infection of eyelid glands (Meibomian gland in internal hordeolum or Zeis in external hordeolum)	Acute
Chalazion	373.2	Nontender, discrete mass, firm Usually points toward the conjunctival surface	Meibomian gland dysfunction	Chronic

ASSOCIATED FINDINGS	COMPLICATIONS	PRECIPITATING FACTORS	TREATMENT GUIDELINES
Prior insult to skin integrity Concomitant bacterial infection	Venous sinus thrombosis Meningitis	Bacterial infection, such as sinusitis, acute otitis media, or conjunctivitis Trauma	Second generation oral antibiotics are still the mainstay of uncomplicated periorbital cellulitis Consider coverage for CA-MRSA. Admit if suspicion of orbital cellulitis, fever, not improving.
Chemosis (gelatinous-appearing reaction to allergen)	Bacterial superinfection	Exposure to environmental allergens Allergens often carried on hands and rubbed into eyes	Irrigate area well Cool compresses Oral antihistamines Oral steroid Antihistamine and/or mast stabilizer ophthalmic drops
Other bites present on body	Bacterial superinfection	N/A	Oral antihistamines Cool compresses Over-the-counter pain management Consider oral steroids
Edema over other dependent areas, bilateral ankles after standing or sacral edema after lying down Urine with 3–4+ proteinuria	Renal failure	N/A	Manage underlying renal disease.
Edema over other dependent areas, bilateral ankles after standing or sacral edema after lying down Signs of heart failure including hepatosplenomegaly, dyspnea or diaphoresis on exertion poor growth, orthopnea, nocturnal dyspnea, cyanosis, respiratory distress	Heart failure	N/A	Manage underlying cardiac disease.
N/A	Lens dislocation, retinal detachment, uveal hemorrhage, retinal artery occlusion with sudden increases in intraocular pressure, optic nerve compression	N/A	If suspicion of a ruptured globe, no further examination to be attempted except by ophthalmologist, protect the eye with a shield (paper or foam cup can be substituted). If there is visual impairment, an inability to fully examine an eye or any suspicion of anything beyond mild soft-tissue injury and corneal abrasion, an ophthalmologist should be consulted.
May be associated with autonomic instability Usually one area involved but may have several including face, hands, arms, legs, genitalia, and buttocks Vomiting and/or abdominal pain may mimic a surgical emergency. Upper airway obstruction may occur from laryngeal edema.	Airway obstruction, autonomic instability	N/A	Prophylaxis with androgens During attack may require respiratory support and intravenous fluids for maintenance of autonomic stability
Eyelid, iris colobomas, microphthalmos, retinal and choroidal defects, first brachial arch defects Common in Goldenhar syndrome	Occlusion of vision with resulting amblyopia, cosmetic issues Risk of cyst rupture which can produce secondary granulomatous inflammation	N/A	Complete surgical excision
Other facial lymphangiomas may be present.	Occlusion of vision with resulting amblyopia, cosmetic issues	N/A	Surgical excision often must be repeated because lymphangiomas are difficult to remove in a single surgical procedure.
N/A	Amblyopia if vision is occluded	N/A	Referral to ophthalmologist if occluding vision
Congenital nasolacrimal duct obstruction (dacryostenosis) predisposes to dacryocystitis.	Periorbital cellulitis Orbital cellulitis	N/A	Massage nasolacrimal area four times per day. Massage bilaterally in case there is a subtle contralateral dacryocystitis.
If bilateral, assess breathing for possibility of nasal obstruction.	Infection/abscess	Blocked nasolacrimal duct	Warm compresses, massage, antibiotic ointment, may need surgical intervention if recurring infection or abscess develops If bilateral, assess breathing for any associated nasal obstruction.
N/A	Periorbital cellulitis	Bacterial blepharitis	Usually caused by infection with *S. aureus* Warm compresses QID, gently wash with baby shampoo If infection suspected, use topical antibiotic
N/A	Corneal abrasions Astigmatism from mass effect causing pressure on the globe	N/A	May need surgical intervention Intervene after 3–4 weeks or if mass effects present.

OTHER
DIAGNOSES
TO CONSIDER

- Xanthomata (also xanthomas; yellowish fleshy masses resulting from cholesterol deposition, rare in children)

- Langerhans cell histocytosis

- Dermatomyositis

- Graves disease

- Infarction of orbital bones seen with sickle cell disease

WHEN TO
CONSIDER
FURTHER
EVALUATION
OR TREATMENT

- When there is minimal eyelid swelling with preseptal cellulitis in an afebrile, well-appearing, older child with reliable follow-up and no suspicion of orbital cellulitis, outpatient treatment with oral antibiotics is recommended. While pneumococcus and hemophilus remain the most common causes of periorbital cellulitis, increasing consideration must be given to the role of community-acquired methicillin-resistant *Staphylococcus aureus* (CA-MRSA).

- In any case where there is visual impairment or an inability to fully examine the eye, consult an ophthalmologist. Even if benign, mass lesions that are large enough to obstruct vision may lead to amblyopia or induce astigmatism and should, therefore, be evaluated by a pediatric ophthalmologist. Dermoids are at high risk for cyst rupture. Therefore, the treatment for dermoids is complete surgical excision.

- If dacryocystitis is recurrent or if nasolacrimal duct obstruction continues beyond age 1, probing is indicated.

- If a hordeolum has not resolved in 48 hours of medical treatment, drainage is indicated.

- Chalazia need surgical intervention after 3 to 4 weeks or if mass effects are present.

SUGGESTED READINGS

Klein BR, Sears ML. Pediatric ocular injuries. *Peds Rev.* 1992;13;422–428.

Kunimoto DY, Kanitkar KD, Makar MS, et al., eds. *The Wills Eye Manual. Office and emergency room diagnosis and treatment of eye disease.* 4th ed. Philadelphia, PA: Lippincott Williams & Wilkins; 2004:14–39, 126–127.

Rafailidis PL, Falagas ME. Fever and periorbital edema: a review. *Surv Ophthalmol.* 2007;52(4):422–433.

Riordan-Eva P, Whitcher J, eds. *Vaughan and Asbury's general ophthalmology.* 17th ed. New York, NY: McGraw-Hill; 2008.

Wald ER. Periorbital and orbital infections. *Peds Rev.* 2004;25;312–320.

Yanoff M, Duker J, eds. *Ophthalmology.* 2nd ed. St. Louis: Mosby; 2004:708–709, 740–741, 763–765.

14

**KATHRYN R. CROWELL,
DEAN JOHN BONSALL,
AND MARYELLEN E. GUSIC**

Discoloration of/Around the Eye

**APPROACH TO
THE PROBLEM**

Pediatricians often see children with ocular complaints, whether in the scope of routine well-child care or under more emergent situations. Visual inspection of the eye may reveal a change in color of the bulbar conjunctivae or discoloration of the lids and tissues around the eye. Discoloration of the sclera related to pigmentary changes may be seen. Children and adults with increased skin pigmentation may have increased pigmentation in the basal layer of the bulbar conjunctivae. This normal discoloration is usually bilateral and most evident in the interpalpebral area. Icterus is a yellow discoloration of the sclerae that is more uniform in distribution and occurs as a result of bilirubin binding to the bulbar conjunctivae. Icterus is an indicator of hemolytic disorders or liver dysfunction. In disorders such as Ehlers-Danlos syndrome, Marfan syndrome, and osteogenesis imperfecta, the sclerae appear blue because the underlying brown uvea shows through abnormally thin sclerae. Bluish sclerae are seen with congenital glaucoma and aniridia.

Discoloration around the eyes may be seen with "allergic shiners," which refers to discoloration below the eyes that results from venous congestion due to nasal and paranasal sinus mucosal edema. The conjunctivae may appear injected if allergic conjunctivitis is present. Blunt trauma to the eye or forehead may lead to the extravasation of blood into the surrounding tissues. Bilateral periorbital ecchymoses are seen with a basilar skull fracture. Neuroblastoma, a tumor of embryonic sympathetic neuroblasts, may metastasize to involve the orbit. The unilateral or bilateral discoloration associated with the spread of the tumor to the eye, and subsequent obstruction of palpebral blood vessels, appears similar to the ecchymosis following trauma. In periorbital (or preseptal) cellulitis, the entire eyelid may appear erythematous, swollen, and feel warm to the touch. Infection is limited to the skin and subcutaneous tissues of the eyelid that lie anterior to the orbital septum. In orbital (postseptal) cellulitis, infection extends into the orbital fat and tissues around the eye, commonly in association with concurrent sinusitis. In both conditions, the bulbar conjunctivae may appear injected.

- A family history of atopic disease including allergic rhinitis, eczema, and asthma may be elicited in patients with allergic shiners. Patients with allergic rhinitis often report nasal itching, sneezing, congestion, and rhinorrhea.

- Scleral epithelial melanosis, seen as a result of pigmentation of the conjunctivae, does not change in appearance or location. It is more commonly seen in people of African, Hispanic, or Asian descent. Lesions may contain more pigment following sun exposure or when the conjunctivae are inflamed.

- A nevus of Ota is congenital hyperpigmentation of the tissues of the eye (melanosis oculi) in association with the pigmentation of the surrounding skin. A nevus of Ota is present at birth in 50% of cases.

- The sclera will appear uniformly yellow with icterus from hyperbilirubinemia. This can be distinguished from the brownish discoloration of muddy sclera (a normal variant) by having the patient look up. With muddy sclera, the inferior portion of the sclera will appear white.

- In traumatic injuries, the timing of the injury determines the discoloration observed— bruising that is initially purple or deep blue may later change to a yellowish color as the bruising resolves.

- Visual complaints may occur with concomitant trauma to the eye and its surrounding tissues.

- Poor visual acuity or double vision may occur with infiltrative disease of the orbit and extraocular muscles.

- In children, orbital cellulitis most commonly results from the spread of a sinus infection.

- Periorbital cellulitis may be a complication of superficial eyelid trauma, dacryocystitis, a stye, or a chalazion.

KEY POINTS IN
THE PHYSICAL
EXAMINATION

- The lesions of scleral epithelial melanosis are flat and are not inflamed or vascularized. They are usually brown/gray in appearance.

- The increased pigmentation of a nevus of Ota is usually unilateral and located below the conjunctiva. The affected part of the sclera is gray or blue in appearance.

- Blue sclerae and joint hyperextensibility should raise suspicion for Ehlers-Danlos and Marfan syndromes.

- Jaundice in an otherwise healthy child should raise suspicion for hemolytic or hepatic disease. Careful attention should be placed on the abdominal examination, noting any hepatosplenomegaly.

- Proptosis found in association with eye discoloration may also be seen with an infiltrative disease of the orbit, such as neuroblastoma or retinoblastoma.

- The ecchymotic discoloration seen with metastatic neuroblastoma may precede diagnosis of the primary tumor, which is typically found in the abdomen or thorax.

- In orbital cellulitis, but not periorbital cellulitis, proptosis and/or painful decreased extraocular movements are often found on physical examination. One way to assess proptosis is to look for asymmetry when standing over the seated patient and looking at the top of his/her head.

PHOTOGRAPHS OF SELECTED DIAGNOSES

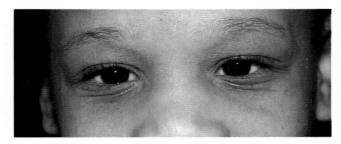

Figure 14-1 Allergic shiners. Note the darkening of the periorbital areas, the lichenification, and the characteristic double fold (Dennie-Morgan fold) that extends from the inner to the outer canthus of the lower eyelid.
(Used with permission from Goodheart HP. Goodheart's photoguide of common skin disorders. 2nd ed. Philadelphia, PA: Lippincott Williams & Wilkins; 2003:48.)

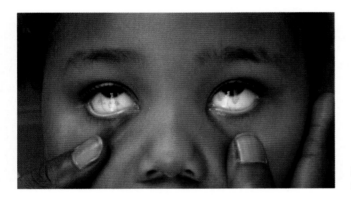

Figure 14-2 Scleral epithelial melanosis.
(Courtesy of Julie A. Boom, MD.)

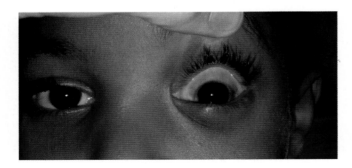

Figure 14-3 Nevus of ota.
(Courtesy of Brian Forbes, MD.)

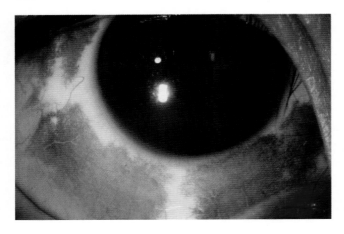

Figure 14-4 Nevus of ota.
(Courtesy of Dean John Bonsall, MD, MS, FACS.)

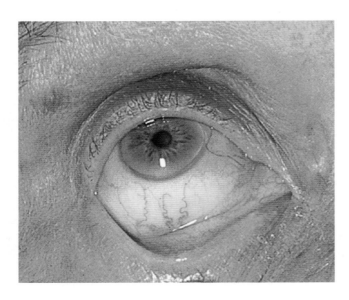

Figure 14-5 Scleral icterus.
(Used with permission from Bickley LS, Szilagyi P. Bates' guide to physical examination and history taking. 8th ed. Philadelphia, PA: Lippincott Williams & Wilkins; 2003:147.)

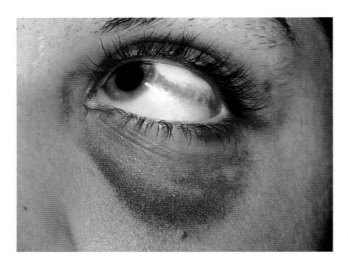

Figure 14-6 Black eye from trauma.
(Courtesy of Dean John Bonsall, MD, MS, FACS.)

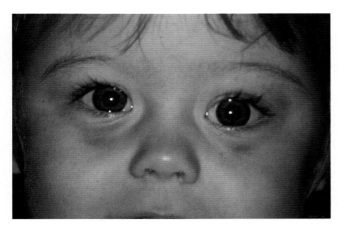

Figure 14-7 Metastatic neuroblastoma.
(Courtesy of Julia L. Stevens, MD, University of Kentucky.)

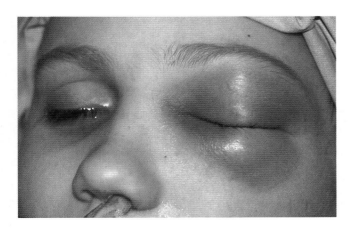

Figure 14-8 Orbital cellulitis.
(Courtesy of the Penn State Hershey Eye Center.)

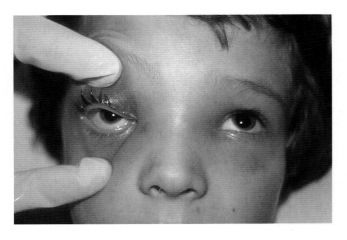

Figure 14-9 Periorbital cellulitis. Note the absence of proptosis and symmetric upward gaze.
(Courtesy of James W. McManaway, III, MD, Hershey Pediatric Ophthalmology Associates.)

DIFFERENTIAL DIAGNOSIS

DIAGNOSIS	ICD-9	DISTINGUISHING CHARACTERISTICS	DISTRIBUTION	DURATION/ CHRONICITY
Allergic Shiners	477.9 (allergic rhinitis)	Bilateral darkening of the skin below the orbits Symptoms and signs of allergic rhinitis	Skin below eyelids	Concurrent with symptoms of rhinitis
Scleral Epithelial Melanosis	743.49	Flat, patchy pigmentation of conjunctivae Moves with conjunctivae	Bilateral, although not necessarily symmetric Limbal area	Congenital
Nevus of Ota	216.1	Blue or gray macules located on the forehead, temple, or periorbital skin as well as the sclera and cornea	Most cases are unilateral, although pigmentation may be present bilaterally in up to 10% of cases.	Congenital
Scleral Icterus	782.4	Yellow discoloration of the scleral conjunctivae Jaundice of skin	Sclerae Conjunctivae	Associated with serum hyper-bilirubinemia May persist for a short time after serum bilirubin level reaches normal levels
Raccoon Eyes seen with Basilar Skull Fracture	Basilar skull Fracture 801.00	History of trauma Bilateral periorbital ecchymoses (raccoon eyes) Bruising behind auricle (Battle sign)	Periorbital	Raccoon eyes resolve over several weeks.
Metastatic Neuroblastoma	198.4	Unilateral or bilateral ecchymoses Proptosis Periorbital swelling Palpable abdominal mass	Periorbital	Precedes, follows, or is concurrent with primary tumor
Orbital Cellulitis	376.01	Erythema and swelling of the eyelid Proptosis Decreased and/or painful extraocular movements	Periorbital	Concurrent or following sinus infection, dental infection, or orbital trauma
Periorbital Cellulitis	373.13	Erythema and swelling of the eyelid Normal extraocular movements No proptosis	Periorbital	Acute

ASSOCIATED FINDINGS	COMPLICATIONS	PREDISPOSING FACTORS	TREATMENT GUIDELINES
Dennie-Morgan lines Allergic salute Deepened nasolabial folds Mouth breathing	Of rhinitis: • Epistaxis • Infection • Change in the bony structure of the face and palate • Malocclusion	Inhaled allergens	Treatment should be targeted at underlying allergic condition. Consider systemic antihistamine and/or inhaled corticosteroid use
Pigmentation of the skin	Not a risk factor for ocular melanoma	More common in children of African, Hispanic, and Asian descent May be induced by UV-light exposure or inflammation of the conjunctivae	N/A
Pigmentation of oral mucosa	Ocular melanoma can arise from nevus of Ota, and up to 10% of patients may develop glaucoma.	More common in females	Infrequent association with glaucoma and ocular melanoma; therefore, symptomatic patients should be referred to an ophthalmologist.
Yellow discoloration of skin and mucous membranes May be associated with hepatomegaly May be associated with signs of anemia	Icterus does not cause long-term consequences, but the underlying conditions are associated with their own complications.	Hemolytic disease Increased bilirubin production Impaired uptake or conjugation of bilirubin Biliary obstruction Hepatocellular injury	Serum total and direct bilirubin levels and determination of cause for hyperbilirubinemia
CSF otorrhea and/or rhinorrhea	Of basilar skull fracture: • Intracranial infection • Intracranial air collections • Cerebral injury/bleed • Increased intracranial pressure • Seizures	Trauma	Cranial CT imaging Treatment depends on the patient's neurologic status. May require surgical intervention as well as cardiopulmonary support
Proptosis Palpable abdominal mass Fever Opsoclonus myoclonus Ataxia Bone pain Anemia	Of associated tumor: • Flushing • Hypertension • Tachycardia • Urinary obstruction • Airway obstruction • Superior vena cava syndrome	Unknown	Requires consultation with oncology and extensive workup including the measurement of urinary catecholamines, CT scanning/magnetic resonance imaging of chest and abdomen, bone marrow biopsy, bone scan, and histological assessment of tumor type/grade. Treatment based upon tumor grade/type
Proptosis Decreased and/or painful extraocular movements Fever	Orbital abscess Permanent vision loss Decreased ocular motility Meningitis Cavernous sinus thrombosis Intracranial, epidural, or subdural abscess	Sinus infection due to staphylococcal or streptococcal infection Ascending dental infections Orbital trauma	Orbital CT scan to determine the extent of tissue involvement Consultation with ophthalmology and/or otolaryngology Systemic antibiotics to cover both S. aureus and S. pyogenes. S. pneumonia and H. flu should also be considered. May require surgical intervention
Fever	Orbital involvement	Local trauma, infection of contiguous structures (hordeolum, conjunctiva, lacrimal duct), and nasopharyngeal infections	Systemic antibiotics to cover most common organisms and close follow-up

- Conjunctival nevus

- Phlyctenule—a vesicle or ulcer on the cornea or conjunctivae with localized vascular injection

- Episcleritis/scleritis

- Uveitis

- Vernal conjunctivitis—severe conjunctivitis occurring in warm seasons as a result of exposure to allergens

- Ruptured globe

- Orbital tumors, including metastatic neuroblastoma and retinoblastoma

- Children with suspected allergic conjunctivitis who are unresponsive to first-line topical antihistamines should be evaluated to rule out vernal conjunctivitis.

- Scleral icterus should initially be evaluated with serum total and direct bilirubin levels.

- Children with suspected infiltrative disease of the orbit, or tumor, should be evaluated with an orbital computed tomography (CT) scan. Further imaging may be necessary to identify the primary tumor site. As neuroblastoma is the most common metastatic orbital tumor, measuring urinary catecholamines (homovanillic acid and vanillylmandelic acid) may be useful. Imaging is required to identify the primary tumor site.

- Periorbital bruising suggestive of basilar skull fracture warrants an urgent cranial CT scan.

- Children with suspected orbital cellulitis should have an orbital CT scan and be treated with systemic antibiotics. Ophthalmology and/or otolaryngology should be consulted without delay.

- Children with periorbital cellulitis may be treated with oral antibiotics and close follow-up required.

SUGGESTED READINGS

Bickley LS, Szilagyi P. Bates' guide to physical examination and history taking. 8th ed. Philadelphia, PA: Lippincott Williams & Wilkins; 2003:147.

Goodheart HP. Goodheart's photoguide of common skin disorders. 2nd ed. Philadelphia, PA: Lippincott Williams & Wilkins; 2003:48.

Kanski JJ. Clinical ophthalmology: a systemic approach. 5th ed. Edinburgh: Butterworth-Heinemann; 2003.

Liesegang TJ. Pigmented conjunctival and scleral lesions. Mayo Clin Proc. 1994;69:151–161.

Oski FA, DeAngelis CD, Feigin RD, et al. Metastatic neuroblastoma. In: Principles and practice of pediatrics. 2nd ed. Philadelphia, PA: JB Lippincott Co.; 1994:892.

Wright KW. Eyelid, orbital masses, and ocular pigmentation abnormalities. In: Pediatric ophthalmology for pediatricians. Baltimore, MD: Williams & Wilkins; 1999:229–247, 283–286.

RENEE M. TURCHI
AND ESTHER K. CHUNG

Pupil, Iris, and Lens Abnormalities

APPROACH TO THE PROBLEM

There are various abnormalities of the pupils, iris, and lens in children. In most cases, timely diagnosis and management are critical. The assessment of visual acuity is the most integral facet of the ophthalmologic examination. More than half of the visual abnormalities in children are first discerned by their primary care physician. Many diagnoses, such as leukocoria, require prompt referral to an ophthalmologist. When in doubt, referral is a prudent approach in managing many of these diagnoses.

KEY POINTS IN THE HISTORY

- Congenital cataracts are associated with intrauterine infections (such as congenital rubella and congenital varicella syndrome) and metabolic disorders, and they may be associated with Down, Edward, and Turner syndromes.

- One third of cataracts are hereditary, and nearly one third of cataracts in children have no identifiable etiology.

- Brushfield spots occur in up to 85% to 90% of children with Down syndrome, but they may be seen in normal children as well.

- Colobomas may occur in normal children or as part of genetic syndromes (such as CHARGE syndrome).

- Iritis and uveitis raise suspicion for conditions associated with systemic inflammation as in juvenile rheumatoid arthritis (JRA).

- Hyphemas are often the result of blunt trauma to the globe.

KEY POINTS IN THE PHYSICAL EXAMINATION

- Small, centrally located cataracts are often clinically stable without an impact on vision.

- Leukocoria, or a white pupillary reflex, is an important clinical sign of intraocular tumors, such as retinoblastoma. Retinoblastoma is the leading malignant ocular tumor in children.

- Leukocoria is bilateral in 30% to 40% of cases.

- It is important to rule out scleral rupture or the presence of a foreign body when chemosis is present.

- Kaiser-Fleischer rings are rims of brown-green pigment in the cornea. Although occasionally visible to the naked eye, slit lamp examination is sometimes necessary to visualize these rings.

- Iritis is characterized by pain, tearing, photophobia, and decreased visual acuity. Symptoms may be acute and develop rapidly over 1 to 2 days. Iritis may be asymptomatic in children with rheumatologic disease such as JRA.

- Blunt traumatic injuries to the eye warrant an inspection of the anterior chamber (space between cornea and iris) for hyphemas.

- Small hyphemas require slit lamp examination, while larger ones may be visible to the naked eye.

- When blood pools in the inferior portion of the eye from a hyphema, it often causes elevated intraocular pressure and decreased visual acuity.

PHOTOGRAPHS OF SELECTED DIAGNOSES

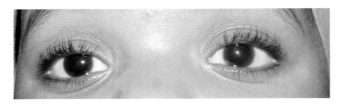

Figure 15-1   Aniridia. This photograph shows a child with bilateral aniridia.
(Courtesy of Brian Forbes, MD.)

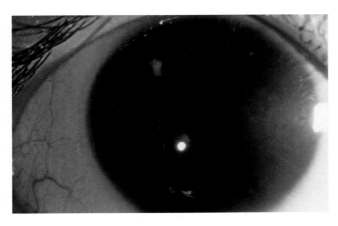

Figure 15-2   Aniridia.
(Courtesy of Sophia M. Chung, MD.)

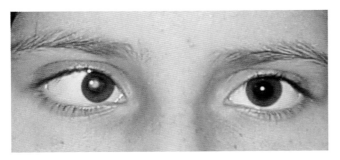

Figure 15-3   Cataract. Note the central haze in the right eye of this patient.
(Courtesy of Brian Forbes, MD.)

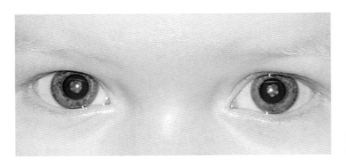

Figure 15-4   Bilateral central cataracts.
(Courtesy of Brian Forbes, MD.)

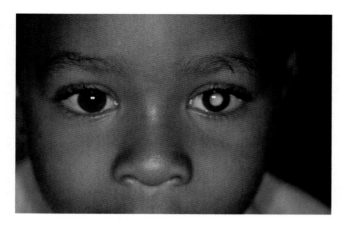

Figure 15-5 Leukocoria.
(Used with permission from Rubin E, Farber JL. *Pathology*. 3rd ed.
Philadelphia, PA: Lippincott Williams & Wilkins; 1999:765.)

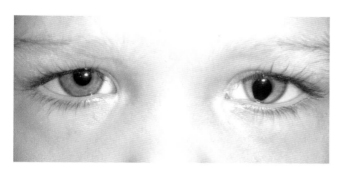

Figure 15-6 Coloboma in the left eye.
(Courtesy of Brian Forbes, MD.)

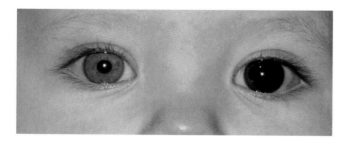

Figure 15-7 Heterochromia iridium.
(Courtesy of Brian Forbes, MD.)

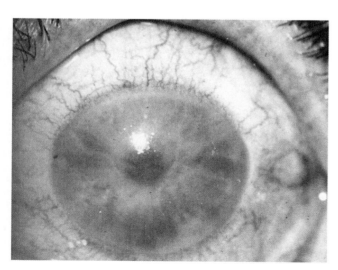

Figure 15-8 Iritis.
(Used with permission from Harwood-Nuns A, Wolfson, et al. *The clinical
practice of emergency medicine*. 3rd ed. Philadelphia, PA: Lippincott Williams
& Wilkins; 2001:66.)

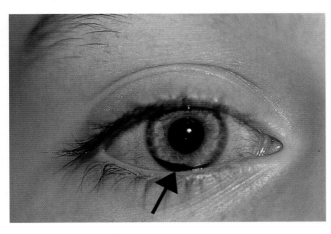

Figure 15-9 Hyphema. This 7-year-old girl was struck by a hard rubber ball and presented with blurred vision. The 1-mm hyphema was only visible when she was upright.
(Used with permission from Fleisher GR, Ludwig S, Baskin MN. *Atlas of pediatric emergency medicine.* Philadelphia, PA: Lippincott Williams & Wilkins; 2004:403.)

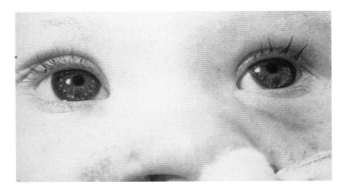

Figure 15-10 Brushfield spots.
(Used with permission from Bickley LS, Szilagyi P. *Bates' guide to physical examination and history taking.* 8th ed. Philadelphia, PA: Lippincott Williams & Wilkins; 2003:771.)

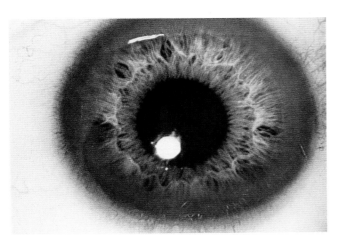

Figure 15-11 Kaiser-Fleischer ring.
(Used with permission from Tasman W, Jaeger E. *The Wills Eye Hospital atlas of clinical ophthalmology.* 2nd ed. Philadelphia, PA: Lippincott Williams & Wilkins; 2001:466.)

DIAGNOSIS	ICD-9	DISTINGUISHING CHARACTERISTICS	DISTRIBUTION	DURATION/ CHRONICITY
Aniridia	743.45	Iris hypoplasia Pupil is same size as cornea. Edge of lens visible Incidence 1:64,000–1:96,000	Usually bilateral Some cases asymmetrical	May employ pigmented contact lens to ameliorate symptoms.
Anisocoria	379.41 (pupil) 743.46 (congenital)	Unequal pupil size Change in light reactivity	N/A	Related to etiology
Cataract	366.9	Haze over eyes Apparent with red reflex testing	Location and density of cataract determine visual effects	Dense bilateral cataracts require urgent surgery. Partial cataracts removed after visual assessment
Leukocoria	360.44	White pupillary reflex	May be unilateral or bilateral, depending on etiology (up to 40% of time bilateral in retinoblastoma)	Related to diagnosis and ability to treat
Coloboma	743.49	Notch, hole, or defect in iris or choroids	Defect often located inferior and nasal May be unilateral or bilateral	Visual loss related to affected area
Heterochromia Iridium	364.53 Acquired hetero-chromia of the iris	Rare May be isolated finding	Iridium—different colors between irises Iridis—different colors within one iris	N/A
Iritis	364.3	Pain, redness, and photophobia In severe cases, may have vision disturbances and hypotonia of the eye.	Inflammation of the iris	Pain, redness, and photophobia may last weeks in acute cases. Chronic cases may have milder symptoms for months to years. Blurred vision Poor pupillary light response
Hyphema	364.41 921.3 (traumatic)	Collection of blood in anterior chamber of the eye	Superior located meniscus in ante-rior chamber	Clot often gone in 3–5 days Rebleeding can occur if there is inadequate rest, unstable intraocular pressure; and is more prevalent in sickle-cell disease
Brushfield Spots	743.800	White and yellow spots evenly arranged around pupil in iris Iris looks speckled	Often bilateral	N/A
Kaiser-Fleischer Rings	275.1	Corneal staining from copper that is brown to orange-green in color	Staining more common at upper pole or cornea	Often present after systemic disease treated

ASSOCIATED FINDINGS	COMPLICATIONS	PRECIPITATING FACTORS	TREATMENT GUIDELINES
Photophobia Nystagmus Cataracts Glaucoma Part of WAGR and Gillespie syndromes	Poor vision	May be genetically inherited (usually autosomal dominant—sporadic in one third)	• Depends on features present • Correct vision (glasses) • Surgery (rarely) • Regular follow-up
Horner syndrome Drugs Lesion of parasympathetic system (including CN III)	Changes in vision with severe cases	Physiological (20%) Horner syndrome Drugs Tonic pupil Lesion of parasympathetic system (including CN III) Trauma to pupil	• Treatment related to etiology • Nerve palsy, trauma or mydriasis may require surgical intervention.
Decrease in visual acuity	Blindness Amblyopia Glaucoma Strabismus	Intrauterine infections Metabolic disorders (i.e., hypoglycemia, hypocalcemia) Genetic disorders (Trisomy 21)	• Medical management if no visual impairment • Surgery (often when >3mm in diameter, nystagmus, strabismus or any visual impairment)
Orbital tumors Also may find: proptosis, pain, diplopia, conjunctival edema	Blindness Myopia Cataracts	Retinoblastoma is most serious etiology. Other etiologies: • Congenital cataracts (most common) • Retinopathy of prematurity (ROP) • Retinal detachment • Persistent hyperplastic primary vitreous • Coat disease • Toxocariasis	• Dilating drops for better examination may require imaging if suspect retinoblastoma. • Treatment of underlying condition—intraocular tumor, cataract, ROP, retinal detachment, infection
Small eye Glaucoma Retinal detachment Disc degeneration Cataracts	Poor vision	Dominant inheritance when present without systemic manifestations Syndromes associated: • Trisomy 13 and 18 • Cat eye syndrome • Wolf-Hirschhorn • Rieger syndrome • CHARGE association	• Usually no treatment • Cosmetic contact lenses and sunglasses may be used. • Vision correction if impaired
Irises two different colors	Glaucoma (rare)	Trauma Congenital pigmented nevi Waardenburg syndrome Piebald trait Horner syndrome	• Treat underlying cause/disease if applicable. • Cosmetic contact lenses if desired
Cataract Glaucoma	Amblyopia Corneal changes and blurry vision Band keratopathy Macular edema Red eye Light sensitivity	JRA (most common) Trauma Kawasaki disease Infections (measles, mumps, varicella, Epstein-Barr virus, leprosy, Lyme) Spondyloarthropathies Sarcoidosis	• Mitigate cause of inflammation if known. • Topical steroid drops
Occasional blood staining of the cornea	Glaucoma (10%) Increased intraocular pressure Rebleeding	Trauma (most common) Herpes zoster Iritis Orbital tumors Juvenile xanthogranulomatosis	• Topical corticosteroids • Antifibrinolytic agents • Usually outpatient management • Risk for re-bleeding and increased intraocular pressure
Most often seen in children with Trisomy 21 (90%)	N/A	Trisomy 21 (most often)	• Typically no intervention necessary
Liver disease, neurological impairment, and cognitive deficits in Wilson disease	No visual impairment Often fade with treatment	Wilson disease (defect in copper metabolism) Liver failure Carotenemia Multiple myeloma	• Treatment aims to manage copper metabolism as part of treatment for Wilson Disease • Correct visual impairment.

<table>
<tr><td>

OTHER
DIAGNOSES
TO CONSIDER

</td><td>

Pupil abnormalities:

- Horner syndrome

- Adie syndrome

- Third cranial nerve palsy

- Persistent pupillary membrane

Lens abnormalities:

- Lens subluxation

- Dystrophy

- Cystinosis

- Lenticular myopia

Iris abnormalities:

- Ocular albinism

- Iridodialysis

- Cyclodialysis

</td></tr>
</table>

WHEN TO
CONSIDER
FURTHER
EVALUATION
OR TREATMENT

- Leukocoria is a diagnosis warranting immediate attention and referral as it may result in visual impairment and may be life threatening.

- Retinoblastoma, the most common intraocular tumor in childhood, typically presents with leukocoria. Mean age at diagnosis is 12 months for bilateral and 24 months for unilateral tumors.

- Iritis and uveitis require prompt attention and a slit lamp examination. In addition, patients should be evaluated for other systemic diseases to determine the cause of inflammation.

SUGGESTED READINGS

Halder S, Oureshia W, Ali A. Leukocoria in children. *J Pediatr Ophthalmol Strabismus.* 2008;45(3):179–180.

Krishnamurthy R, VanderVeen DK. Infantile cataracts. *Inter Ophthalmol Clin.* 2008;48(2):175–192.

Lai JC, Ferkat S, Barron Y, et al. Traumatic hyphema in children: risk factors for complications. *Arch Ophthalmol.* 2001;119(1):64–70.

Melamud A, Palekar R, Singh A. Retinoblastoma. *Am Fam Physcian.* 2006;73(6):1039–1044.

Patel H. Pediatric uveitis. *Pediatr Clin North Am.* 2003;50:125–136.

Tasman W, Jaeger E. *The Wills Eye hospital atlas of clinical ophthalmology.* 2nd ed. Philadelphia, PA: Lippincott Williams & Wilkins; 2001:466.

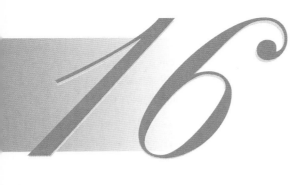

MARY ELIZABETH WROBLEWSKI
AND DAVID M. KROL

Misalignment of the Eyes

APPROACH TO THE PROBLEM

Misalignment of the eyes is collectively termed strabismus. The direction of deviation of the nonfixating eye determines the type of strabismus. Esotropia is a medial or nasal deviation of the nonfixating eye, exotropia is a lateral or temporal deviation, and hypertropia is an upward deviation of either eye. A misalignment, which is associated with ocular muscle restriction or nerve palsy, may be the same in all fields of gaze (comitant strabismus) or may differ depending on the field of gaze (incomitant strabismus). Failure to recognize and address strabismus during visual development may lead to amblyopia, a decrease or loss of vision in the misaligned eye. Though neonatal strabismus may be a normal finding, pediatricians should be able to recognize it and address any strabismus that persists or develops beyond 3 months of age. Examining the eyes is an important part of routine examinations, beginning at birth.

KEY POINTS IN THE HISTORY

- Parents are often the first to bring concerns about their child's eyes to the attention of a physician; many children do not realize when they are having difficulty seeing.

- Family photographs can help pinpoint the onset of the misalignment and may show abnormalities in the red reflex.

- Misalignment may be present constantly, limited to when the child is tired, or present only when the child looks in certain directions.

- Some forms of strabismus may be hereditary, and the family may know of a relative with a "lazy eye."

- Strabismus may occur in association with migraine headaches.

- Strabismus following head trauma warrants emergent evaluation and treatment.

- Misalignment may recur years after surgical correction.

- A child with a cranial nerve palsy may turn or tilt the head in order to maintain binocular vision.

- An older child with strabismus may cover one eye or squint one eye when focusing on the television or another object to eliminate bothersome double vision.

KEY POINTS IN THE PHYSICAL EXAMINATION

- The earliest visual screening tool is the simultaneous red reflex test (Brückner test), which may be performed from birth onward. If there is any difference in the size, color, or brightness of red reflexes between the eyes, it could be a sign of misalignment, accommodative error, retinal pathology such as retinoblastoma, or a lens opacity such as a cataract.

- The corneal light reflex, or Hirschberg, test should show symmetric reflection of a light source centered approximately 2 ft from the patient. If the reflection is not symmetric, suspect misalignment. The reflection will be symmetric in children with broad nasal bridges or wide epicanthal folds if they have pseudostrabismus.

- In the cover test, the child fixates on a target and one eye is covered. If the opposite eye (not covered) moves to refixate on the target, strabismus is present. This should be done on both eyes.

- In the cover-uncover test, one eye is again covered for a few seconds and then the cover is rapidly removed. If the eye that was under the cover moves laterally, suspect an accommodative strabismus.

- By 2 months of age, when a child is old enough to track a moving target, extraocular movements may be examined for the presence of cranial nerve palsies, including sixth nerve (abducens), third nerve (oculomotor), and fourth nerve (trochlear) palsies.

- Visual acuity testing should be performed starting as young as 3 years of age using a tumbling E chart, Snellen chart, HOTV chart, or Allen card/chart to screen for possible amblyopia. If there is a greater than two-line difference between eyes, long-standing strabismus may be present. Poor vision in the misaligned eye is due to the suppression of the visual cortex to prevent diplopia.

PHOTOGRAPHS OF SELECTED DIAGNOSES

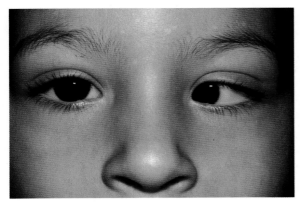

Figure 16-1 Esotropia.
(Courtesy of Dean John Bonsall, MD, MS, FACS.)

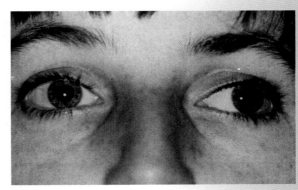

Figure 16-2 Exotropia.
(Used with permission Wright KW. *Pediatric ophthalmology for pediatricians*. Baltimore, MD: Williams and Wilkins; 1999:41.)

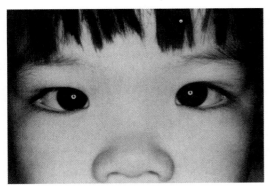

Figure 16-3 Pseudostrabismus.
(Used with permission from Wright KW. *Pediatric ophthalmology for pediatricians*. Baltimore, MD: Williams and Wilkins; 1999:49.)

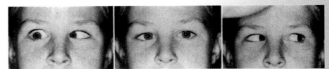

Figure 16-4 Right sixth nerve palsy.
(Used with permission from Wright KW. *Pediatric ophthalmology for pediatricians*. Baltimore, MD: Williams and Wilkins; 1999:59.)

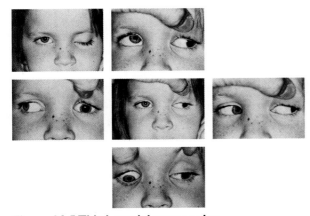

Figure 16-5 Third cranial nerve palsy.
(Used with permission from Wright KW. *Pediatric ophthalmology for pediatricians*. Baltimore, MD: Williams and Wilkins; 1999:63.)

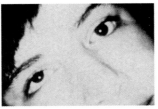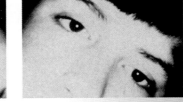

Figure 16-6 Fourth cranial nerve palsy.
(Used with permission from Wright KW. *Pediatric ophthalmology for pediatricians*. Baltimore, MD: Williams and Wilkins; 1999:57, 58.)

DIFFERENTIAL DIAGNOSIS

DIAGNOSIS	ICD-9	DISTINGUISING CHARACTERISTICS	DISTRIBUTION	DURATION/ CHRONICITY
Infantile Strabismus	378	Onset <6 months of age	Monocular/ binocular	May be present at birth.
Pseudostrabismus	743.63	Appearance of eyes deviating inward due to wide nasal bridge	N/A	Present until nose narrows with facial development
Accommodative Esotropia	378.35	Age >2 months Typically 1–5 years of age Inward turning of one eye when focusing on a near object	Monocular	Chronic
Sensory Esotropia/ Exotropia	378 369	<2 years: esotropia >2 years: exotropia	Monocular	Chronic
Intermittent Exotropia	378.23	Ages 2–8 years Exotropia when the child is tired	Monocular/binocular	Chronic
Convergence Insufficiency	378.83	Intermittent exotropia with near vision, but aligned with distance vision	Monocular/binocular	Chronic
Sixth Cranial Nerve Palsy	378.54	Inability to abduct affected eye Esotropia	Monocular	Chronic
Third Cranial Nerve Palsy	378.51	Eye does not move up or down and is exotropic.	Monocular	Chronic
Fourth Cranial Nerve Palsy	378.53	Vertical deviation of eye due to paralysis of superior oblique muscle	Monocular	Chronic
Duane Syndrome	378.71	Congenital absence of cranial nerve VI with aberrant innervation of lateral rectus muscle by cranial nerve III	Monocular/binocular	Chronic

ASSOCIATED FINDINGS	COMPLICATIONS	PRECIPITATING FACTORS	TREATMENT GUIDELINES
Vertical strabismus Latent nystagmus when one eye is covered	Visual loss Lack of binocular fusion	N/A	Surgical weakening of bilateral medial rectus muscles between 6 months and 2 years of age Eyeglasses are prescribed if there is significant farsightedness.
Centered corneal light reflex Negative cover-uncover test Asian descent	N/A	N/A	Reassurance
Farsightedness	Amblyopia	Farsightedness	Eyeglasses to treat accommodative error Sometimes miotic drops are used. Surgical correction may be needed if eyes are still misaligned with eyeglasses.
Blindness in one eye	N/A	Monocular blindness	Surgical correction of the muscles of the blind eye
Covering one eye causes it to become exotropic.	Significant amblyopia is rare.	Fatigue	Surgical correction if the deviation is not controlled
Reading fatigue	Diplopia when reading	Ocular muscle fatigue	Eye exercises to strengthen extraocular muscles
Diplopia	Amblyopia	Congenital Closed head injury Infratentorial neoplasms Post-viral infection Following lumbar puncture	Varies depending on underlying condition
Ptosis Dilated, unresponsive pupil	Amblyopia	Congenital Closed head injury Migraine	Surgical correction
Compensatory head tilt to the strong side Deviation worsens with head tilt to the weak side Subtle facial asymmetry	Amblyopia Chronic head tilt	Congenital Closed head injury	Surgical correction to reduce head tilt
Head turn to keep eyes aligned Narrowing of the fissure (affected eye) with adduction Widening of the fissure with abduction	Amblyopia	Congenital	Surgical correction to reduce head turn

OTHER
DIAGNOSES
TO CONSIDER

- Migraine headaches

- Intracranial mass

- Hydrocephalus

- Möbius syndrome (palsies of the cranial nerves VI and VII; limb and craniofacial anomalies)

- Brown syndrome (also known as superior oblique tendon sheath syndrome)

- Myasthenia gravis

WHEN TO
CONSIDER
FURTHER
EVALUATION
OR TREATMENT

- If a parent reports seeing misalignment of a child's eye at any time even if the eye examination appears normal, intermittent strabismus should be considered and the child should be referred to an ophthalmologist.

- If esotropia is constant or persists after 4 months of age, refer to an ophthalmologist.

- If the corneal light reflex is not symmetric for both eyes, the simultaneous red-reflex test shows asymmetric red reflexes or the cover-uncover test elicits even slight movement of one eye, strabismus should be suspected and the child should be referred to ophthalmology.

- If there is a visual acuity difference of greater than two lines between eyes on a Snellen, HOTV, tumbling E or Allen chart, the child may have amblyopia and should be further evaluated.

- If torticollis is present but not due to a musculoskeletal etiology, refer to an ophthalmologist for further evaluation.

SUGGESTED READINGS

Aronson S, Bridge C, Brunner RT, et al, eds. *Preschool vision screening for healthcare professionals.* Chicago, IL: Prevent Blindness America; 2005.

Committee on Practice and Ambulatory Medicine, Section on Ophthalmology. American Association of Certified Orthoptists, American Association for Pediatric Ophthalmology and Strabismus, American Academy of Ophthalmology. Eye examination in infants, children, and young adults by pediatricians. *Pediatrics.* 2003;111(4 Pt 1):902–907.

Donahue SP. Pediatric strabismus. *N Engl J Med.* 2007;356(10):1040–1047.

Doshi NR, Rodriguez MLF. Amblyopia. *Am Fam Physician.* 2007;75(3):361–367.

Magramm I. Amblyopia: etiology, detection, and treatment. *Pediatr Rev.* 1992;13:7–14.

Wright K. *Pediatric ophthalmology for pediatricians.* Baltimore, MD: Williams and Wilkins; 1999:21–69.

Section
FIVE

EARS

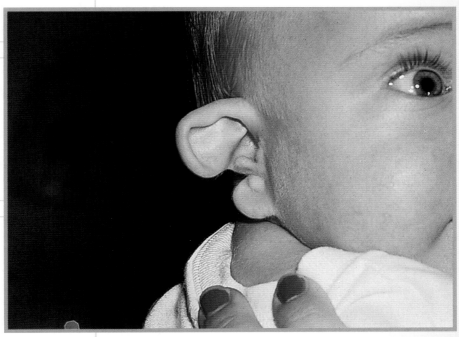

(Courtesy of Steven D. Handler, MD, MBE.)

17

CHARLES A. POHL

Abnormalities in Ear Shape and Position

APPROACH TO THE PROBLEM

Normally, there is a wide variation of shapes, sizes, and positions of ears in children. Most auricular growth (85%) is completed by 3 years of age, cartilaginous formation by 5 to 6 years, and ear width and its distance from the scalp by 10 years. Abnormalities in ear shape or position may occur as isolated findings or as part of a complex of congenital anomalies. Congenital malformations of the external ear, which occur in 1:10,000 to 1:20,000 live births, include problems with ear size (e.g., micro-ear), position (e.g., posteriorly rotated, low-set ears), maldevelopment (e.g., anotia, microtia, cleft earlobe, lobular attachment), and protrusion (e.g., prominent, lopped, cupped).

Malformed or underdeveloped auricles are frequently seen with genetic problems such as Beckwith-Wiedemann syndrome (creased lobes), CHARGE association (lopped or cupped ears), facio-auriculo-vertebral spectrum (Goldenhar syndrome; microtia), Levy-Hollister (cupped ears), or Trisomy 21 (small ears). Low-set ears commonly occur in syndromes such as Noonan, Smith-Lemli-Opitz, Treacher Collins, and Trisomy 18. Several studies have found an association between renal anomalies and various ear abnormalities. Although the underlying etiology is unclear, the anomalies usually are not found as isolated findings, but rather as components of more complex congenital syndromes, such as Beckwith-Wiedemann or Trisomy 18.

When inspecting the external ear, it is important to evaluate its position, size, shape, and symmetry compared with the other ear. The protrusion angle of the ear should not exceed 15 degrees in children. Fifteen percent of the auricle (the superior attachment of the pinna) should be above the horizontal line (an imaginary line drawn from the inner canthus through the outer canthus). The angle between the vertical axis (the line perpendicular to the horizontal line) and the longitudinal axis of the ear (superior aspect of the outer helix to the inferior border of the earlobe) is normally between 10 degrees and 30 degrees. In addition, the length of an ear can be roughly estimated by measuring the distance between the arch of the eyebrow and the base of the ala nasi.

- Because hearing impairment is associated with microtia, lopped, or cupped ears, and with meatal atresia, it is essential to ask about hearing and language development.

- Underlying renal anomalies should be considered when children with ear abnormalities have a history of deafness or a maternal history of gestational diabetes.

- Children with microtia often have hearing loss on the side of their normal-appearing auricle.

- Familial inheritance patterns are seen with abnormal earlobe attachments and cupped ears; therefore, asking about a family history of ear abnormalities may be helpful.

KEY POINTS IN
THE PHYSICAL
EXAMINATION

- Children with posteriorly rotated, low-set ears should be inspected carefully for other congenital abnormalities.

- When a child has protruding ears, normal auricular architecture distinguishes prominent ears from lopped or cupped ears.

- Micro-ears, unlike maldeveloped auricles such as microtia, are small but normally formed.

- Marked skull molding can make normal auricles appear protruded.

- Abnormal facial features including small chin, midfacial or nose hypoplasia, and highly arched eyebrows, can give the false impression of low-set, posteriorly rotated ears.

- Normally developed helices distinguish intrauterine compression abnormalities from the array of helix deformities. Also, intrauterine positioning effects do not generally result in symmetric abnormalities.

- Evaluation for renal anomalies should be considered when a patient with an auricular abnormality has other dysmorphic features, including facial asymmetry, choanal atresia, micrognathia, colobomas of the eye, branchial cysts, cardiac abnormalities, imperforate anus, and/or distal limb abnormalities.

PHOTOGRAPHS OF SELECTED DIAGNOSES

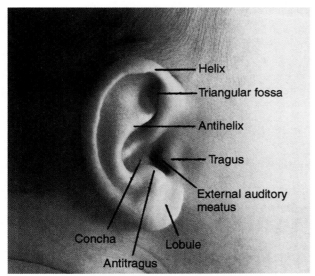

Figure 17-1 Normal anatomy of external ear.
(Used with permission from Fletcher MA, ed. *Physical diagnosis in neonatology*. Philadelphia, PA: Lippincott–Raven Publishers; 1998:285.)

Helix
Triangular fossa
Antihelix
Tragus
External auditory meatus
Concha
Lobule
Antitragus

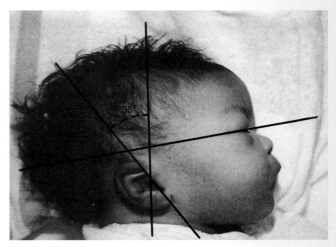

Figure 17-2 Posteriorly rotated, low-set ears.
(Used with permission from Fletcher MA, ed. *Physical diagnosis in neonatology*. Philadelphia, PA: Lippincott–Raven Publishers; 1998:287.)

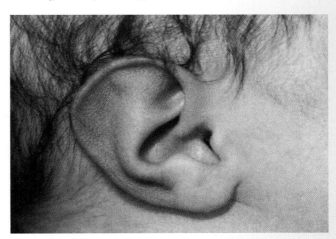

Figure 17-4 Helix deformity.
(Used with permission from Fletcher MA, ed. *Physical diagnosis in neonatology*. Philadelphia, PA: Lippincott–Raven Publishers; 1998:288.)

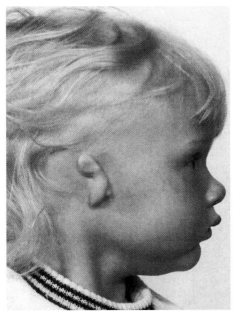

Figure 17-3 Microtia.
(Used with permission from Cotton RT, Myer CM III, eds. *Practical pediatric otolaryngology*. Philadelphia, PA: Lippincott–Raven Publishers; 1999:345.)

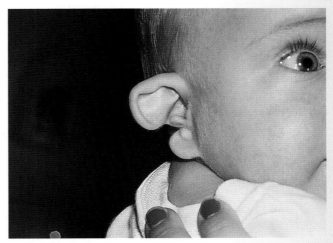

Figure 17-5 Cleft ear.
(Courtesy of Steven D. Handler, MD, MBE.)

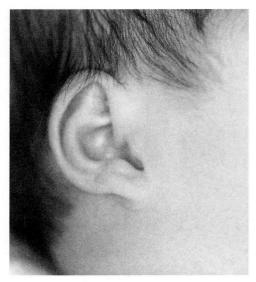

Figure 17-6 Adherent lobule/lobular attachment.
(Used with permission from Fletcher MA, ed. *Physical diagnosis in neonatology*. Philadelphia, PA: Lippincott–Raven Publishers; 1998:289.)

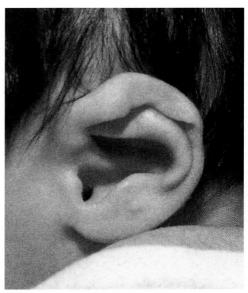

Figure 17-7 Lopped ear.
(Used with permission from Fletcher MA, ed. *Physical diagnosis in neonatology*. Philadelphia, PA: Lippincott–Raven Publishers; 1998:297.)

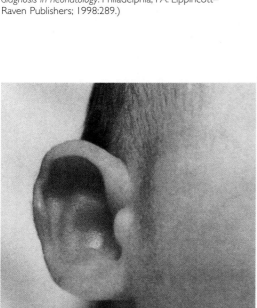

Figure 17-8 Cupped ear.
(Used with permission from Fletcher MA, ed. *Physical diagnosis in neonatology*. Philadelphia, PA: Lippincott–Raven Publishers; 1998:298.)

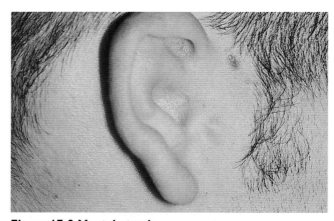

Figure 17-9 Meatal atresia.
(Courtesy of Steven D. Handler, MD, MBE.)

DIFFERENTIAL DIAGNOSIS

CATEGORY	DIAGNOSIS	ICD-9	DISTINGUISHING CHARACTERISTICS	ASSOCIATED FINDINGS	OTHER FEATURES	TREATMENT GUIDELINES
Ear Size	Micro-ear	872.11	Normal auricular architecture, but smaller size	Usually none	N/A	Cosmetic reconstructive surgery if severe
Ear Position	Posteriorly rotated, low-set ears	744.2	External ear located inferior to normal location and rotated posteriorly	Isolated or component of complex syndrome, often involving the renal system	N/A	N/A
Maldeveloped Auricles	Microtia	744.23	Dysplastic or disorganized external ear Variable presentation—from a small deformed auricular appendage to gross hypoplasia with a blind or absent external canal	Hearing loss (even in normal appearing ear) Other auditory malformations common (e.g., external auditory meatus, middle ear abnormality, ossicular abnormality)	1.7/10,000 live births 2:1 male-to-female ratio Autosomal dominant or recessive	Cosmetic reconstructive surgery if severe Hearing augmentation
	Helix deformity	744.29	Partial abnormality of auricle	Usually isolated	N/A	Cosmetic reconstructive surgery if severe
	Cleft ear (bifid lobule)	744.2	Isolated maldevelopment of earlobe	N/A	N/A	Cosmetic reconstructive surgery if severe
	Adherent lobule/lobular attachment	744.21	Earlobe attached anteriorly	Usually isolated	Familial	N/A
Protrusion	Prominent	744.29	Helix of ear is normally shaped and attached to the skull, but protrudes forward	N/A	N/A	Cosmetic reconstructive surgery if severe
	Lopped ear	744.29	Ear's helix and scapula fold downward because of inadequate development of antihelix; absence of antihelical fold	Hearing loss Similar to microtia Associated with anencephaly, microencephaly, severe congenital neuromotor deficiency; ossicular malformation	N/A	Cosmetic reconstructive surgery if severe
	Cupped ear	744.29	Ear malformation causes anterior protrusion of pinna and an exaggerated concave concha	Similar to lopped ear	Familial or sporadic	Cosmetic reconstructive surgery if severe
Maldevelopment of Ear Canal	Meatal atresia (aural atresia)	872	Atresia of auditory canal with or without pinna abnormality	Microtia Hearing impairment Craniofacial abnormality	1.5/20,000 live births Sporadic, autosomal dominant or recessive, chromosomal syndrome (e.g., Goldenhar syndrome)	Cosmetic reconstructive surgery if severe Early bone surgery if bilateral hearing impairment

OTHER
DIAGNOSES
TO CONSIDER

- Intrauterine compression, such as folded helix

- Marked skull molding (appears "protruded")

- Craniofacial disproportion forms such as severe microcephaly (ear appears large)

- Appearance of "low-set" or "posteriorly rotated" ears when abnormal facial features are present, such as a small chin, midface hypoplasia, or highly arched eyebrows

- Epidermal nevus on ear

- Arteriovenous malformation

WHEN TO
CONSIDER
FURTHER
EVALUATION
OR TREATMENT

- Malformed or underdeveloped auricles, as well as low-set ears, are often associated with more complex congenital syndromes or part of genetic disorders. Maldeveloped ears should be evaluated by otolaryngology and/or plastic surgery particularly when considering cosmetic, reconstructive surgery.

- Closely monitor hearing, with periodic hearing evaluation, and language development in children with microtia, lopped, and cupped ears, as well as meatal atresia.

- Renal anomalies, often diagnosed by renal ultrasound, should be considered if a child with an ear abnormality has a history of deafness, a maternal history of gestational diabetes, or other dysmorphic features.

SUGGESTED READINGS

Bellucci RJ. Congenital aural malformation: diagnosis and treatment. *Otolaryngol Clin North Am.* 1981;14:95–124.

Bordley JE, Brookhouser PE, Tucker GK, eds. *Ear, nose and throat disorders in children.* New York: Raven Press; 1986.

Cotton RT, Myer CM III, eds. *Practical pediatric otolaryngology.* Philadelphia, PA: Lippincott–Raven Publishers; 1999:345.

Fletcher MA, ed. *Physical diagnosis in neonatology.* Philadelphia, PA: Lippincott–Raven Publishers; 1998:285, 287–289, 297, 298.

Jones KL. *Smith's recognizable patterns of human malformation.* 5th ed. Philadelphia, PA: WB Saunders; 1997.

Wang RY, Earl DL, Ruder RO, et al. Syndromic ear anomalies and renal ultrasounds. *Pediatrics.* 2001;108(2):E32.

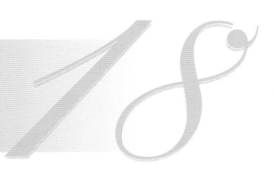

KATHLEEN CRONAN

Ear Swelling

APPROACH TO THE PROBLEM

Swelling of the external ear may be a concerning symptom to parents. Most causes of ear swelling are benign. Insect bites, for example, are a common cause of ear swelling in pediatric patients. However, the swelling seen with insect bites and other benign entities may mimic other diseases, such as cellulitis, bacterial chondritis, and mastoiditis, all of which require immediate attention. Otitis externa can become diffuse and cause external ear swelling with an appearance similar to cellulitis. Blunt trauma to the ear results in swelling and discoloration of the auricle, pinna, or both. Mastoiditis, an uncommon bacterial infection, causes swelling and erythema of the pinna in addition to posterior auricular swelling and tenderness.

KEY POINTS IN THE HISTORY

- Pruritus, associated with swelling and erythema, is the typical presentation of an insect bite to the ear.

- A previous history of ear piercing or laceration to the ear lobe should raise the suspicion for a keloid. Patients with keloids will often have a history of keloids on other parts of their body.

- Recent ear pain with or without drainage in conjunction with posterior auricular swelling, fever, or both may indicate mastoiditis.

- The duration of symptoms often helps to distinguish an insect bite from cellulitis. Swelling and erythema resulting from an insect bite occur suddenly; whereas, the swelling, tenderness, and redness of cellulitis may gradually develop.

- A history of active or recent, localized otitis externa may result in cellulitis of the auricle or diffuse otitis externa.

- A history of paroxysmal ear burning, redness, and swelling may indicate otomelalgia (red ear syndrome).

| KEY POINTS IN THE PHYSICAL EXAMINATION | • Trauma, which may present as an auricular hematoma, and cellulitis typically present as a swelling of the pinna and auricle; whereas, mastoiditis presents as swelling and redness of the posterior auricular (e.g., in the area of the mastoid) and auricular areas. |

KEY POINTS IN THE PHYSICAL EXAMINATION

- Trauma, which may present as an auricular hematoma, and cellulitis typically present as a swelling of the pinna and auricle; whereas, mastoiditis presents as swelling and redness of the posterior auricular (e.g., in the area of the mastoid) and auricular areas.

- Forward displacement of the pinna usually indicates mastoiditis, although diffuse external otitis or a posterior auricular insect bite may cause ear displacement when significant associated swelling is present.

- A rubbery, fleshy mass that extends beyond the wound margins indicates keloid formation.

- Erythema, swelling, warmth, and tenderness of the auricle usually indicate cellulitis. If there is no tenderness in association with the swelling and redness, an insect bite is more likely than cellulitis.

- Pain elicited with traction on the pinna and/or pressure on the tragus is associated with otitis externa.

- A bluish discoloration of the auricle accompanied by swelling suggests trauma. Petechial lesions on top of or inside the pinna are highly suspicious for an intentional injury that may be the result of pinching and pulling the pinna as seen with boxing or child physical abuse.

- Erythema and tenderness of the overlying skin and perichondrium suggest perichondritis.

PHOTOGRAPHS OF SELECTED DIAGNOSES

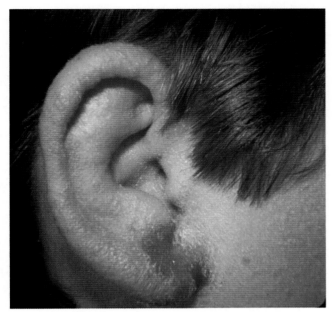

Figure 18-1 Cellulitis. Note the erythema and swelling.
(Courtesy of Kathleen Cronan, MD.)

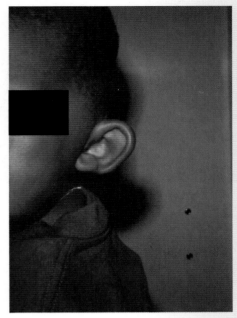

Figure 18-2 Insect bite. Ear protrusion and swelling in a well child with a papule on the posterior ear demonstrating an insect bite to ear.
(Courtesy of Kathleen Cronan, MD.)

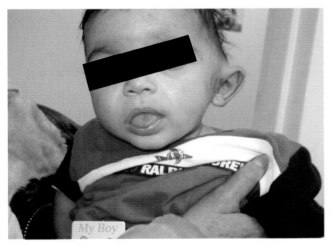

Figure 18-3 Mastoiditis. A protruding ear with evidence of acute otitis media, indicating mastoiditis. Frontal view.
(Courtesy of Paul S. Matz, MD.)

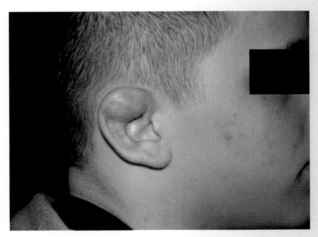

Figure 18-4 Auricular hematoma. This resulted from a direct blow to the ear.
(Courtesy of Kathleen Cronan, MD.)

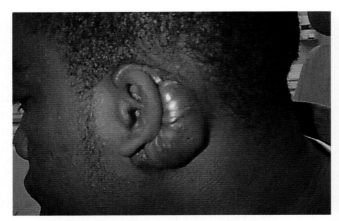

Figure 18-5 Keloid. Rubbery mass at the site of ear piercing is compatible with a keloid.
(Courtesy of Steven P. Cook, MD.)

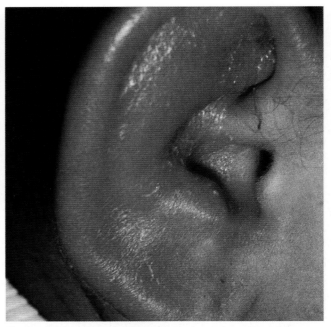

Figure 18-6 Perichondritis. Erythema and swelling of the pinna are consistent with perichondritis.
(Used with permission from Handler SD, Myer CM. *Atlas of ear, nose and throat disorders in children.* Ontario, Canada: BC Decker; 1998:12.)

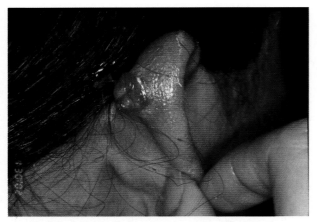

Figure 18-7 Infected ear-piercing site. Pustule with drainage at ear piercing site, indicating infection.
(Courtesy of Ellen Deutsch, MD.)

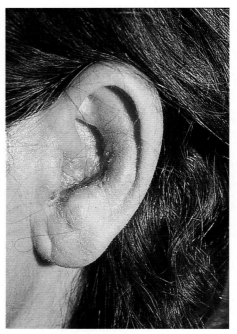

Figure 18-8 Ramsay Hunt syndrome. Vesicles in external auditory canal demonstrating Ramsay Hunt syndrome.
(Courtesy of Steven D. Handler, MD, MBE.)

DIFFERENTIAL DIAGNOSIS

DIAGNOSIS	ICD-9	DISTINGUISHING CHARACTERISTICS	DISTRIBUTION	ASSOCIATED FINDINGS	PREDISPOSING FACTORS	TREATMENT GUIDELINES
Cellulitis	380.1	Erythema Warmth Tenderness Originating from a wound Edema	Pinna Earlobe Preauricular and postauricular spaces	Fever Red streaking Wound	Insect bites Laceration Earring related Ear piercing	Oral antibiotics; IV antibiotics if infection is spreading or no response to oral antibiotics If there is concurrent otitis externa, antibiotic drops are required.
Diffuse Otitis Externa	380.10	Swelling Erythema Warmth Pain with manipulation of the pinna and pressure on the tragus Drainage from external auditory canal	External auditory canal Auricle Posterior auricular area	Forward displacement of auricle Fever Thick otorrhea	Swimming Excoriation of external auditory canal	Antibiotic ear drops
Otomelalgia (Red Ear Syndrome)	388.8	Erythema Swelling Burning Unilateral Episodic	Entire ear, including earlobe	Migraine type headache	Migraine headache	Application of ice
Insect Bite	910.8	Erythema Swelling of sudden onset Nontender Papule or punctum at site of bite Pruritus	Pinna Posterior auricular space	Other papules on skin surface	Insect bite Sting	Oral antihistamines Cold packs
Mastoiditis	383.00	Edema of pinna and skin overlying mastoid Erythema of pinna/skin over mastoid process Tenderness of mastoid process Displacement of pinna inferiorly and anteriorly	Postauricular area Mastoid periosteum Pinna	Acute otitis media Purulent otorrhea Fever Toxicity	Acute otitis media	Urgent evaluation IV antibiotics Drainage of abscess Referral to otolaryngology
Trauma	959.09	Discoloration with ecchymoses Hematoma between the perichondrium and the cartilage Pallor of area	Pinna Earlobe Auricle	Hemotympanum Perforated tympanic membrane	Direct blow to the ear Frost bite	Surgical evaluation for possible hematoma drainage If intentional injury from child abuse suspected, contact the local department of human services
Keloid	701.4	Flesh colored mass May be tender and pruritic initially Rubbery Extends beyond margins of wound	Ear lobe Site of wound or ear piercings	Other sites of keloid formation	Pierced ear Ear laceration Insect bites Burn Race/ethnicity of African descent	Intralesional steroid injections Surgical excision by plastic surgery, followed by steroid injections Topical gel sheeting for several hours per day
Perichondritis	380.00 (pinna, auricle) 380.01 (acute, of pinna) 380.02 (chronic, of pinna)	Erythema Tenderness Swelling	Pinna Auricular cartilage Site of wound	Puncture from earring Laceration Nodule Fever, chills Nausea	Trauma Ear piercing through the cartilage Laceration through cartilage	IV antibiotics Surgical drainage if abscess present

OTHER
DIAGNOSES
TO CONSIDER

- Malignant otitis externa

- Xanthomatosis

- Relapsing polychondritis

- Henoch-Schönlein purpura involving the ear lobe and pinna

- Ramsay Hunt syndrome or herpes zoster oticus

- Frostbite after rewarming

WHEN TO
CONSIDER
FURTHER
EVALUATION
OR TREATMENT

- Medical evaluation should be sought if ear swelling is accompanied by fever or ill appearance.

- Suspected cellulitis requires oral antibiotic treatment.

- Swelling from insect bites usually resolves with antihistamines and local treatment, such as ice or cold compresses.

- Mastoiditis requires urgent evaluation by an otolaryngologist.

- If the external ear is pale or ecchymotic following trauma and there is suspicion for an underlying hematoma, surgical evaluation is required to determine the need for emergent evacuation of the hematoma.

- Keloids may improve after monthly, intralesional injection of triamcinolone suspension by a dermatologist or plastic surgeon.

- Perichondritis requires systemic antibiotics and removal of all ear jewelry. Cartilage is susceptible to rapid destruction by bacterial infection; therefore, prompt treatment is essential.

- Otomelalgia resolves with the application of ice.

SUGGESTED READINGS

Arnett AM. Pain-earache. In: Fleisher GR, Ludwig S, Henretig FM, eds. Textbook of pediatric emergency medicine. 5th ed. Philadelphia, PA: Lippincott Williams & Wilkins; 2006:505–510.

Feigin RD, Alexander JJ. Otitis externa. In: Feigin RD, Cherry JD, Demmler GJ, Kaplan SL, eds. Textbook of pediatric infectious diseases. 5th ed. Philadelphia, PA: WB Saunders; 2004:212–213.

Handler SD, Myer CM. Atlas of ear, nose and throat disorders in children. Ontario, Canada: B.C. Decker, Inc.; 1998:12.

Lewis K, Shapiro NL, Cherry JD. Mastoiditis. In: Feigin RD, Cherry JD, Demmler GJ, Kaplan SL, eds. Textbook of pediatric infectious diseases. 5th ed. Philadelphia, PA: WB Saunders; 2004:235–240.

Maffei FA, Davis HW. Minor lesions and injuries. In: Feigin RD, Cherry JD, Demmler GJ, Kaplan SL, eds. Textbook of pediatric infectious diseases. 4th ed. Philadelphia, PA: WB Saunders; 2000:1509.

Paller A, Mancini A. Collagen vascular disorders. In: Hurwitz Clinical Pediatric Dermatology: A Textbook of Skin Disorders of Childhood and Adolescence, 3rd edition, Paller, AS, Mancini, AJ, (Eds). 3rd ed. Philadelphia, PA: Elsevier Saunders; 2006:602–603.

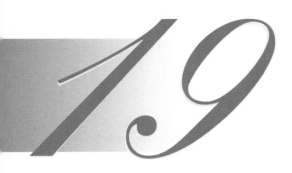

VALARIE STRICKLEN
AND DAVID M. KROL

Ear Pits and Tags

APPROACH TO THE PROBLEM

The discovery of pits and tags on or around a child's ear often raises the question of whether further evaluation is needed. Ear pits and tags occur equally in both sexes and occur in all races, with an increased incidence in children of African and Asian descent. Overall, the incidence is approximately 0.3% to 0.9% in the general population. Ear pits are typically located in front of the ear (preauricular) and mark a sinus tract lined with epithelium that travels beneath the skin. Most are superficial, but some may connect to a cystic structure. Ear tags, fleshy mounds of skin that are often pedunculated, are also typically located near the tragus and anterior to the ear. These anomalies arise during the sixth week of gestation when the fetal auricle develops.

The inner and outer ear structures develop during the same time period, and it is important that audiological screening be performed on all newborns with outer ear anomalies since these children have a slightly higher incidence of sensorineural hearing loss. Many studies have shown an association between ear and renal abnormalities. Based on recent studies, routine ultrasonography of the renal system is not recommended for ear pits and tags in the absence of other congenital anomalies.

KEY POINTS IN THE HISTORY

- Ear pits and tags are usually asymptomatic and can be unilateral or bilateral.

- Often, ear pits are present in other family members.

- Most ear pits and tags are isolated deformities; however, they may be associated with several craniofacial syndromes listed below.

- Preauricular pits and cysts should not be confused with first branchial cleft cysts, which are closely linked to the external auditory canal, tympanic membrane, the angle of the mandible and the facial nerve.

- Branchiootorenal (BOR) syndrome should be ruled out with a renal ultrasound if both a preauricular pit and first branchial cleft cyst are present.

KEY POINTS IN THE PHYSICAL EXAMINATION

- Ear tags are fleshy, nontender, skin-colored anomalies located anterior to the tragus and are most commonly unilateral although they may be bilateral.

- Ear tags are typically cosmetic deformities without any underlying structural abnormalities.

- Ear tags may be solitary or found in clusters; ear pits are generally solitary lesions.

- Ear pits are pinpoint holes located in front of the ear and above the tragus.

- Branchial cleft cysts and sinuses are in close approximation to the facial nerve and should not be confused with simple preauricular anomalies.

- Additional congenital malformations should prompt further investigation into craniofacial syndromes listed below.

PHOTOGRAPHS OF SELECTED DIAGNOSES

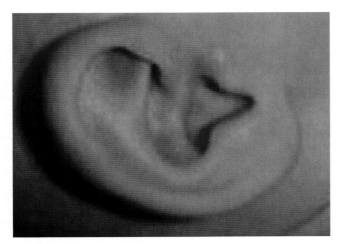

Figure 19-1 Preauricular ear tag.
(Courtesy of Valarie Stricklen, MD, FAAP.)

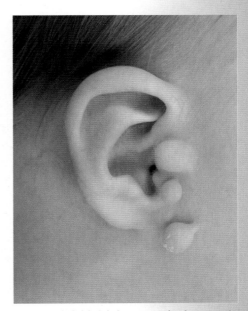

Figure 19-2 Multiple preauricular tags in a child with oculoauriculovertebral spectrum disorder.
(Courtesy of David Tunkel, MD.)

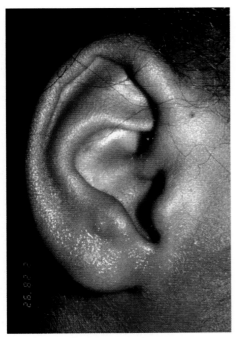

Figure 19-3 Preauricular pit. Note how visualization can be obscured by hairline.
(Courtesy of David Tunkel, MD.)

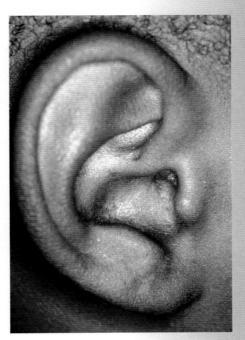

Figure 19-4 Auricular sinus on the inferior crus area of the pinna.
(Courtesy of David Tunkel, MD.)

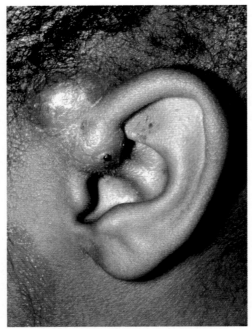

Figure 19-5 Infected preauricular sinus.
The swelling nearly obscures identification of the
offending sinus tract opening.
(Courtesy of David Tunkel, MD.)

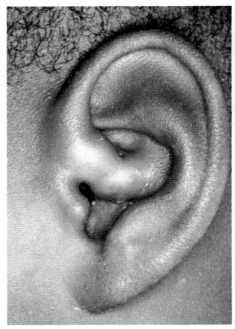

**Figure 19-6 Infected auricular pit on
the inferior crus.** Note erythema and
edema.
(Courtesy of David Tunkel, MD.)

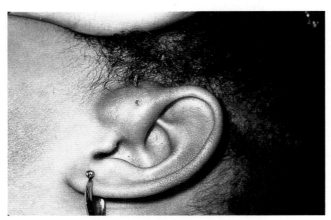

Figure 19-7 Preauricular abscess.
(Courtesy of Steven D. Handler, MD, MBE.)

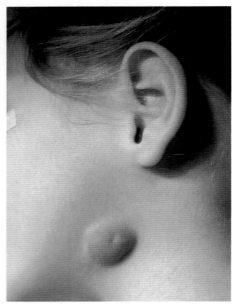

Figure 19-8 First branchial cleft sinus.
While not a true a preauricular sinus, this
lesion must be considered in the differential
diagnosis.
(Courtesy of David Tunkel, MD.)

DIFFERENTIAL DIAGNOSIS

DIAGNOSIS	ICD-9	DISTINGUISHING CHARACTERISTICS	DISTRIBUTION	ASSOCIATED FINDINGS	COMPLICATIONS	TREATMENT GUIDELINES
Preauricular Tags	744.1	Fleshy, skin-colored Painless Unilateral or bilateral	Anterior to the tragus Attached to the cheek, tragus, or ear lobe	Craniofacial syndromes with related renal anomalies	Cosmetic Rarely hearing loss may accompany the lesion.	Surgical excision for cosmetic reasons
Preauricular Pits, Sinuses/Cysts	744.46 744.47	Pinpoint holes that mark a tract that travels beneath the skin	Typically, anterior to the tragus and in front of the ear	Found in different syndromes and craniofacial sequences	Infection of the pit, sinus, and/or tract with common skin bacteria, such as staphylococcus and streptococcus Rarely hearing loss may accompany the lesion.	Surgical excision for cosmetic reasons
Preauricular Pit Infection	682.9 (cellulitis, unspecified site)	Erythema Swelling Tenderness Possible drainage	N/A	Swelling Erythema Drainage	Recurrent infections	Antibiotic therapy Surgical excision with repeated infections
First Branchial Cleft Sinus/ Cyst	744.41 (sinus) 744.42 (cyst)	Associated with the external auditory canal and angle of the mandible	Lateral and superior to the facial nerve and the external auditory canal	Associated ear pit usually found in close approximation with the cyst	May become infected Involvement of the facial nerve makes surgical removal difficult.	Antibiotic treatment Consultation with otolaryngology and/or plastic surgery

OTHER
DIAGNOSES
TO CONSIDER

- Duplication of the ear canal

- Body piercing/secondary trauma from piercing

- Associated craniofacial or chromosomal syndromes, such as:

  - BOR syndrome

  - Beckwith-Wiedemann syndrome

  - Oculoauriculovertebral spectrum

  - Chromosome 11q duplication

  - Chromosome 4p deletion

WHEN TO
CONSIDER
FURTHER
EVALUATION
OR TREATMENT

- Ear pits that consistently drain or are frequently infected require antibiotic therapy and possible excision by a skilled surgeon.

- Antibiotic therapy directed at staphylococcal and streptococcal species should be started if swelling, erythema, tenderness, and associated drainage ensue.

- Excision of large ear tags for cosmetic reasons requires expertise and knowledge of Langer lines. Smaller ear tags may be ligated with suture material; however, for optimal cosmetic outcomes and to avoid complications, removal and ligation of ear tags should be done by otolarygologists or plastic surgeons.

- Multiple preauricular anomalies should prompt further investigation into other congenital malformations. If multiple anomalies are found, a renal ultrasound should be considered to rule out renal anomalies.

- Branchial cleft anomalies, which often involve the facial nerve, should not be confused with simple preauricular anomalies.

SUGGESTED READINGS
Bianca S, Ingegnosi C, Ettore G. Preauricular tags and associated anomalies: considerations for genetic counseling. *Genet Couns.* 2003;14(3):321–324.
Deshpande SA. Renal ultrasonography not required in babies with isolated minor ear anomalies. *Arch Dis Child Fetal Neonatal Ed.* 2006;91(1):F29–F30.
Huang XY, Tay GS, Wansaicheong GKL, et al. Preauricular sinus: clinical course and associations. *Arch Otolaryngol Head Neck Surg.* 2007;133:65–68.
Kohelet D, Arbel E. A prospective search for urinary tract abnormalities in infants with isolated preauricular tags. *Pediatrics.* 2000;105(5):E61.
Kugelman A, Hadad B, Ben-David J, et al. Preauricular tags and pits in the newborn: the role of hearing tests. *Acta Paediatr.* 1997;86:170–172.
Wang RY, Earl DL, Ruder RO, et al. Syndromic ear anomalies and renal ultrasounds. *Pediatrics.* 2001;108(2):E32.

LEE R. ATKINSON-McEVOY AND ESTHER K. CHUNG

20 Ear Canal Findings

APPROACH TO THE PROBLEM

Physicians caring for children frequently see patients who have complaints about the ear, including pain, itching, drainage, and decreased hearing. Often, the initial concern is focused on middle ear abnormalities, but external auditory canal (EAC) abnormalities may cause complaints that are similar to those caused by middle ear pathology. Common diseases of the EAC include otitis externa (affecting up to 10% of the population), impacted cerumen, trauma, and foreign bodies in the ear.

There are many variations in cerumen, and canal size and shape. Flaky, dry cerumen may be found in East Asian patients. In some cases, as in Down syndrome, the canals may be narrowed, making it difficult for the examiner to evaluate the tympanic membrane on routine otoscopy.

KEY POINTS IN THE HISTORY

- School-aged children may be exceptionally precise in their description of pain. Therefore, it is important to ask them to describe what they are feeling. Often, when parents report pain, the child instead reports ringing or fullness. For example, one child with water in his ear reported, "It sounds like I am under water."

- The use of cotton swabs or other objects to clean the ear may result in trauma to the EAC and tympanic membrane, and retained pieces of cotton may cause irritation or subsequent inflammation.

- The placement of a foreign body in the ear may lead to trauma and most often presents with pain. If the foreign body is not promptly removed, the EAC may become infected.

- Tinnitus and bleeding, in addition to pain, may be symptoms that occur from trauma to the external ear canal.

- Decreased hearing often occurs with cerumen impaction, fluid in the external canal, or otitis externa, but it may also be seen in trauma, particularly when perforation of the tympanic membrane exists.

- Drainage from the EAC may occur in acute otitis media with perforation, otitis externa, and external fluid in the canal (residual from swimming or bathing).

- The drainage seen with acute otitis media with perforation is often described as brownish and sticky, but at other times may be whitish and creamy.

- Pseudomonal and fungal infections should be considered in children with chronic symptoms of otitis externa.

- History of frequent swimming or submersion of ears while in the bathtub is suggestive of otitis externa (also known as *swimmer's ear*). Water from the pool or tub is believed to cause alterations in the normal flora of the EAC.

- Patients with eczema, seborrhea, or psoriasis may have the involvement of the epidermis of the EAC and may complain of pruritus.

- The use of medication or topical substances to the ear may result in an eczematous dermatitis.

- Earrings, particularly those made of alloy metals, may cause inflammation at the earring site and an eczematous dermatitis of the surrounding tissues.

KEY POINTS IN THE PHYSICAL EXAMINATION

- It is important to note that there may be variations in the amount, color, and consistency of cerumen.

- If blood is present, suspect trauma and carefully inspect the tympanic membrane for perforation or other injury.

- Pain elicited from pressure on the tragus and/or outward traction on the pinna is suggestive of otitis externa.

- Edema and inflammation of the ear canal are typically seen with otitis externa.

- When a significant amount of discharge is present, it may be difficult to differentiate acute otitis media with perforation from otitis externa.

- Greasy scales, dry or flaky skin, excoriation, and crusting of the external ear canal and pinna may be seen with eczematous or psoriatic dermatitis and seborrhea.

- Pustules on the outer portion of the EAC suggest furunculosis.

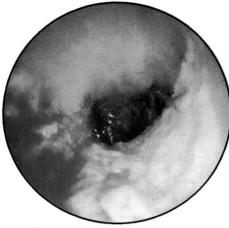

Figure 20-1 Cockroach in external canal.
Note the visible body and legs from the cockroach. There is also surrounding edema and
hyperemia.
(Courtesy of Ellen Deutsch, MD.)

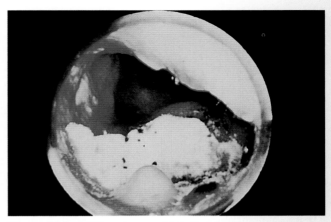

Figure 20-2 Otitis externa. Note that the EAC is edematous
with narrowing. There is also discharge present.
(Courtesy of Steven D. Handler, MD, MBE.)

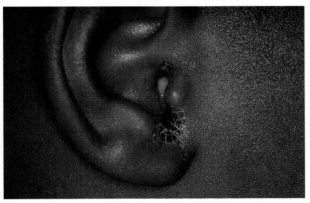

**Figure 20-3 Otorrhea associated with a
cholesteatoma.** Note the white-colored discharge visible at
the os of the EAC, as well as crust on the antitragus.
(Courtesy of Ellen Deutsch, MD.)

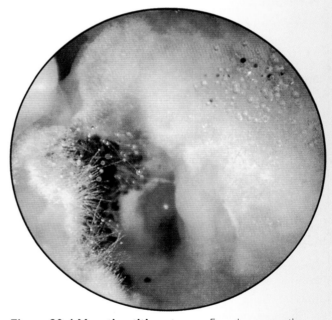

Figure 20-4 Mycotic otitis externa. Fungal overgrowth
produces a moist appearing, whitish-colored plaque.
(Used with permission from Handler SD, Myer CM. *Atlas of ear, nose and
throat disorders in children.* Hamilton: BC Decker; 1998:24.)

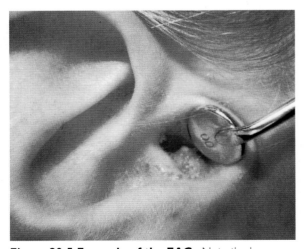

Figure 20-5 Furuncle of the EAC. Note the large
erythematous papule with a pustular tip.
(Used with permission from Handler SD, Myer CM. *Atlas of ear,
nose and throat disorders in children.* Hamilton: BC Decker; 1998:24.)

DIAGNOSIS	ICD-9	DISTINGUISHING CHARACTERISTICS	DISTRIBUTION	DURATION/ CHRONICITY
Foreign Body in EAC	385.83	Foreign bodies—most commonly seen in younger children	N/A	May present acutely or chronically
Trauma/Superficial Injury to EAC	910.8	Bleeding or pain of the ear	N/A	Acute onset of symptoms
Acute Otitis Media with Perforation	382.01	Mucoid, whitish, grayish or brownish discharge in canal Canal walls, when visualized, are not irritated or red.	N/A	Acute
Otitis Externa	380.10	Tenderness with pressure on the tragus and outward traction on the pinna	N/A	Acute or chronic
Seborrheic Otitis Externa	690.10	Greasy appearing scales that may involve the auricle	N/A	Often chronic
Eczematous Otitis Externa	380.22	Dry, flaky skin that may be pruritic	N/A	Often chronic
Psoriatic Otitis Externa	696.1	Dry scaly plaques with a silvery quality	N/A	Often chronic
Chronic Mycotic Otitis Externa	380.15	Intense itching, but usually painless Moist-appearing, white-colored plaque	N/A	Often chronic
Furunculosis	680.0	Erythematous pustules in the anterior portion of the external ear canal	N/A	Acute or recurrent

ASSOCIATED FINDINGS	COMPLICATIONS	PRECIPITATING FACTORS	TREATMENT GUIDELINES
Acute setting—possibly pain or decreased hearing Chronic setting—foul odor or discharge	Hearing loss Infection	Cleaning ears with cotton swabs Young age, particularly in the toddler years	Removal of foreign body relieves symptoms. Can be removed directly with forceps or with irrigation If inflammation of the EAC is present, combination antibiotic and steroid topical treatments can be used.
Bloody discharge Decreased hearing whenever the tympanic membrane is affected	Hearing loss	Foreign body in ear Aggressive cleaning with an object of EAC	Careful exploration to evaluate for presence of concomitant perforation of the tympanic membrane Combination of antibiotic and steroid topical treatment can be used to treat symptoms of inflammation of EAC in the absence of perforated tympanic membrane If the tympanic membrane is perforated, refer to otolaryngologist.
May be associated with systemic symptoms, such as fever	Hearing loss Speech delays if recurrent	Associated with preceding upper respiratory infection	Treatment with topical antibiotics or systemic antibiotics, if warranted based on age and severity of infection
Edema of the external ear canal with seropurulent discharge or whitish to grayish exudate Generally no fever	Rarely, acute otitis media from invasion through the tympanic membrane Cellulitis	Trauma to external ear canal or exposure to water	Combination of antibiotic and steroid topical treatment can be used to treat symptoms of inflammation of EAC. For swimmers, prophylactic use of earplugs can help prevent otitis externa. Also installation of 1 teaspoon of a solution of equal parts of white vinegar and rubbing alcohol can prevent bacterial and fungal overgrowth
Patient may have seborrheic dermatitis in other areas, especially the scalp.	Scarring and narrowing of external ear canal	Family history of seborrheic dermatitis	Treatment with topical steroids can eliminate symptoms.
History of diffuse eczema	Scarring and narrowing of external ear canal	Use of topical medications or exposure to metals (earrings) or cosmetics	Treatment with emollients and topical steroids can eliminate symptoms.
History of psoriasis	Scarring and narrowing of external ear canal	History of psoriasis	Treatment with topical steroids can eliminate symptoms.
May form an exudate that may have a musty odor	Untreated infections can lead to bacterial superinfection.	Recurrent or chronic otitis externa	Treatment with topical antifungal agents can eliminate symptoms. In patients who are immunocompromised, systemic treatment may be warranted.
Point tenderness at the site of the furuncle	Scarring and narrowing of external ear canal	Infection of hair follicle	Heat, analgesics, and oral antistaphylococcal antibiotics are mainstays of treatment.

OTHER
DIAGNOSES
TO CONSIDER

- Osteomyelitis

- Acne

- Cholesteatoma

- EAC exostosis

- Malignant otitis externa

WHEN TO
CONSIDER
FURTHER
EVALUATION
OR TREATMENT

- In immunocompromised patients, consider parenteral treatment for EAC infections and consider less common organisms as possible etiologic agents.

- If penetrating injury is suspected, consider imaging and consultation with subspecialists from trauma surgery, neurosurgery, and/or otolaryngology to evaluate for further injury.

- If acute otitis media with perforation is suspected, treat with oral antibiotics and consider the use of topical antibiotic drops to the EAC.

- If symptoms do not improve within 48 to 72 hours of initiating treatment, consider other etiologies and referral to an otolaryngologist.

SUGGESTED READINGS

Beers SL, Abramo TJ. Otitis externa review. *Pediatr Emerg Care.* 2004;20(4):250–253.

Dohar JE. Evolution of management approaches for otitis externa. *Pediatr Infect Dis J.* 2003;22(4):299–308.

Ely JW, Hansen MR, Clark EC. Diagnosis of ear pain. *Am Fam Physician.* 2008;77(5):621–628.

Handler SD, Myer CM. *Atlas of ear, nose, and throat disorders in children.* Hamilton: B.C. Decker; 1998:22–27.

McCoy SI, Zell ER, Besser RE. Antimicrobial prescribing for otitis externa in children. *Pediatr Infect Dis J.* 2004;23(2):181–183.

Osguthorpe JD, Nielsen DR. Otitis externa: review and clinical update. *Am Fam Physician.* 2006;74(9):1510–1516.

Roland PS, Stroman DW. Microbiology of acute otitis externa. *Laryngoscope.* 2002;112:1166–1177.

Tympanic Membrane Abnormalities

APPROACH TO THE PROBLEM

Acute otitis media (AOM) is one of the most common diagnoses and reasons for antibiotic prescriptions in children. With more than five million cases diagnosed annually, it is associated with individual discomfort, family disruption, financial costs, serious sequelae, and antimicrobial resistance. For these reasons, it is important to make the correct diagnosis when evaluating the tympanic membrane (TM).

Pneumatic otoscopy allows the visualization of TM characteristics: color, contour, position (normal, retracted, full, bulging), and mobility. A normal TM is described as translucent, pearly gray, and mobile. A light reflex and boney landmarks, such as the arm of the malleus, are generally easily viewed. The examination, though, requires the child to be restrained or held still and to have a clean ear canal. Also, a pneumatic otoscope with a good seal and light source must be available.

KEY POINTS IN THE HISTORY

- Acute onset, hyperpyrexia, and otalgia are features of AOM and not otitis media with effusion (OME).

- Concomitant or recent upper respiratory tract infections or allergies are commonly seen with AOM and OME.

- Hearing loss is a nonspecific finding that may be caused by middle ear fluid (AOM, OME), as well as by structural damage of the TM or ossicles (severe tympanosclerosis, TM perforation, or cholesteotoma).

- Refer children to a pediatric otolaryngologist whenever TM perforation is accompanied by either hearing loss or vertigo, or when middle ear fluid is chronic and associated with hearing loss and/or speech delay.

- Suspect cholesteatoma if persistent middle ear effusion (MEE) or hearing impairment, greasy and/or whitish mass, or no clinical response is present when treating another suspected TM problem.

- When a cholesteatoma is associated with ataxia or headaches, neuroimaging should be considered to evaluate for the presence of a brain abscess.

KEY POINTS IN THE PHYSICAL EXAMINATION

- One must immobilize the head carefully and firmly when evaluating the TM and ear canal, while using a snug-fitting ear speculum. The small (2.5 mm diameter) ear speculum should be used in infants and preschool children, while the large (4 mm diameter) ear speculum should be used in school-aged children and adolescents.

- The light reflex may be absent in some normal children.

- Mobility, assessed by pneumatic otoscopy, should be measured especially when the history and/or physical examination suggest a problem. Poor TM mobility is associated with AOM, MEE, TM perforation, or TM structural damage as with tympanosclerosis.

- Mild TM erythema can occur in association with fever, crying, upper respiratory viral infections, or irritation from cerumen or foreign objects.

- AOM should have evidence of MEE and acute inflammation, including TM bulging or fullness, marked erythema, otorrhea, or yellow or cloudy fluid.

- Air bubbles and amber TM discoloration are associated with serous middle ear fluid or OME.

- Blood in the ME causes a bluish, deep red, or brown ("chocolate") appearance of the TM.

- Chalky white plaques on TM (tympanosclerosis) are seen with healed inflammation.

- TM mobility is absent or decreased with TM perforation.

- Manipulation of the ear pinna to ensure proper visualization of TM varies with age. As in adults, the pinna should be lifted posterosuperiorly in older children. The pinna should be pulled horizontally backward in infants and younger children.

- Localized TM atelectasis, especially in the posterosuperior quadrant of the pars tensa, is seen with retraction pockets.

- Excessive localized mobility reflects a healed perforation or TM thinning.

- OME is evidenced by fluid bubbles and air-fluid levels or by at least two of the following TM changes: abnormal color including white, yellow, amber, or blue; opacification; decreased mobility.

PHOTOGRAPHS OF SELECTED DIAGNOSES

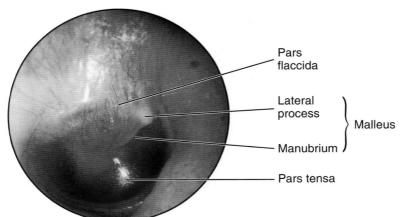

Pars flaccida
Lateral process
Manubrium
Malleus
Pars tensa

Figure 21-1 Normal tympanic membrane.
(Photo used with permission from Handler SD, Myer CM. *Atlas of ear, nose and throat disorders in children*. Ontario, Canada: BC Decker; 1998:28.)

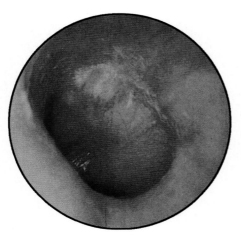

Figure 21-2 Acute otitis media.
(Courtesy of Steven D. Handler, MD, MBE.)

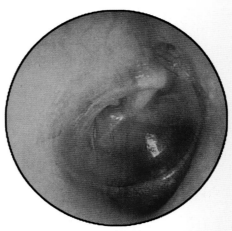

Figure 21-3 Otitis media with effusion.
(Courtesy of Glenn Isaacson, MD.)

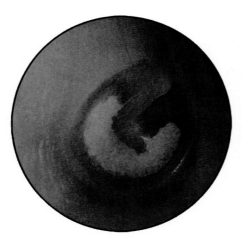

Figure 21-4 Tympanosclerosis.
(Courtesy of Steven D. Handler, MD, MBE.)

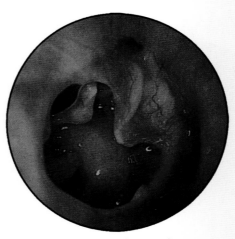

Figure 21-5 Tympanic membrane perforation.
(Courtesy of Steven D. Handler, MD, MBE.)

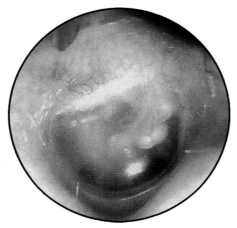

Figure 21-6 Cholesteatoma.
(Used with permission from Handler SD, Myer CM.
Atlas of ear, nose and throat disorders in children.
Ontario, Canada: BC Decker; 1998:30.)

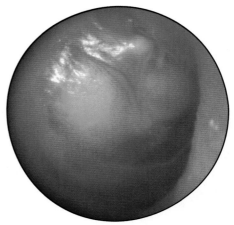

Figure 21-7 Cholesteatoma. Note the
white, pearly lesion seen behind the tympanic
membrane in the anterior and posterior
superior quadrants.
(Courtesy of John A. Germiller, MD, PhD.)

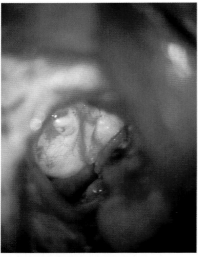

Figure 21-8 Cholesteatoma.
Intraoperative view of the lesion that
corresponds with the previous figure.
(Courtesy of John A. Germiller, MD, PhD.)

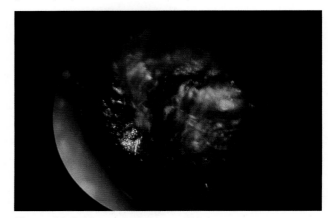

Figure 21-9 Hemotympanum. This hemotympanum was
seen in association with a left temporal bone fracture.
(Courtesy of Ellen Deutsch, MD.)

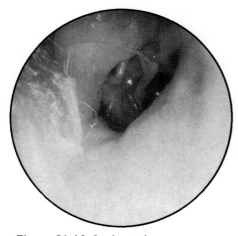

Figure 21-10 Atelectasis, severe.
(Courtesy of Ellen Deutsch, MD.)

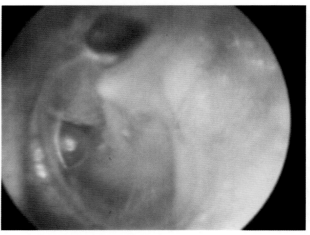

Figure 21-11 Retraction pocket.
(Courtesy of Steven D. Handler, MD, MBE.)

DIAGNOSIS	ICD-9	DISTINGUISHING CHARACTERISTICS	ASSOCIATED FINDINGS	COMPLICATIONS	PRECIPITATING FACTORS	TREATMENT GUIDELINES
Acute Otitis Media	382.0	Usually under the age of 6 years MEE and features of acute inflammation: otalgia, fullness or bulging TM, marked TM erythema, otorrhea, yellow or cloudy fluid Malleus may be obscured TM will have poor mobility Acute onset	Fever Otalgia Dizziness Unsteady gait	Structural damage of TM or ear bones (ossicles) Hearing impairment Mastoiditis Facial paralysis Persistent perforation Intracranial infection (rare) Cholesteatoma formation	Upper respiratory tract infection Allergies Environmental tobacco smoke	Antimicrobial therapy covering *Streptococcus pneumoniae, Haemophilus influenzae, Moraxella catarrhalis, Streptococcus pyogenes*
Otitis Media with Effusion	381.4	Absence of pain or fever Nonerythematous, nonmobile TM with serous or mucoid fluid Bubbles or air-fluid interface noted on otoscopy TM discoloration (white, yellow, or amber) TM atelectasis common (prominence of the short process of the malleus) Usually indolent course	Ear popping Feeling of fullness or pressure Hearing loss Vertigo	Hearing loss Speech/language delay TM atelectasis Developmental/learning impairment Cholesteatoma Usually spontaneously resolves (50% to 60% resolve 2 weeks after AOM treated, 80% after 4 weeks treatment, 90% after 8 weeks treatment)	Concomitant resolving AOM Allergies Upper respiratory tract infection	Supportive care Decongestants and steroids have not been shown to have long-term benefits.
Tympanosclerosis (Myringosclerosis)	385.0	"Chalky white plaque" in fibrous layer of TM Reddish or yellowish, localized deposit early Poor mobility when severe	Conductive hearing loss when AOM is present Asymptomatic if small patch	Conductive hearing loss	Ear infections (severe AOM) Ventilation tube insertion	Supportive care
TM Perforation	384.2 382.01	Hole in TM Everted, ragged edges resulting from sudden pressure changes; bloody when resulting from direct TM trauma Anteroinferior quadrant when resulting from sudden pressure changes; posteriorly when resulting directly from trauma	Hearing loss Bleeding Pain Tinnitus	Marginal perforation less likely to heal than central ones and more likely to lead to cholesteatoma or intracranial infection Residual perforation Water entering middle ear Ear infections Ossicular damage (more likely when resulting from direct TM trauma)	Direct TM trauma (e.g., from cotton swab, hairpins) Ear trauma Sudden ear pressure changes in ear canal (e.g., gunfire or violent slap) AOM Chronic OME	Usually heals spontaneously Refer if vertigo, persistent hearing loss, or when perforation does not heal Surgical repair if persistent hearing loss
Cholesteatoma	385.32	Greasy, whitish mass of keratin debris	Dizziness Ataxia and headaches (suggests brain abscess) Hearing loss Chronic otorrhea	Bony structure erosion Hearing loss Facial nerve paralysis Intracranial process (e.g., brain abscess, meningitis)	Congenital Recurrent AOM Persistent MEE	Referral to otolaryngology Surgical resection
Hemotympanum	385.89	Extravasated blood or blood stained fluid in ME space Bright red or dark red, blue, or brown ("chocolate" ear drum) TM	Hearing loss Pain Feeling of pressure or fullness	Usually resolves spontaneously Hearing loss TM perforation	Head injury Barotrauma (e.g., flying, diving) Basilar skull, including temporal bone, fracture Severe AOM Middle ear surgery	Consider CT to rule-out basilar skull fracture from accidental or nonaccidental trauma. Referral to otolaryngology Surgical evacuation if associated with significant pain or persistent hearing loss
Atelectasis	384.9	Retracted and atrophic TM Golden-yellow serous effusion TM thinning and transparent over time (may resemble perforation)	Often asymptomatic Muffled sounds; feeling of pressure or fullness	Fluctuating conductive hearing loss	Untreated OME (prolonged negative pressure)	Supportive care Refer if persistent hearing loss or persistent symptoms
Retraction Pockets	384.9	Localized atelectasis Usually on posterosuperior quadrants of pars tensa	Usually asymptomatic	Cholesteatoma Hearing loss	Atrophic TM from recurrent OM, atelectasis, chronic eustachian tube dysfunction Trauma	Supportive care Refer if you suspect a cholesteatoma or if persistent hearing loss

- Bullous myringitis

- Improper technique (e.g., inadequate light resource, poor speculum seal)

- Cerumen

- Mastoiditis

- Trauma to temporal bone

- Foreign body in ear canal

- Bleeding disorder

- Glomus tympanicum or glomus jugulare tumor

- Otosclerosis (Schwartze's sign)

- Consider antibiotic treatment when MEE is associated with acute inflammation, as evidenced by TM bulging or fullness, marked erythema, otorrhea, or yellow or cloudy fluid.

- Chronic MEE associated with hearing loss and/or speech delay should be referred to a pediatric otolaryngologist.

- Children with a TM perforation associated with hearing loss or vertigo should be referred to an otolaryngologist.

- Investigate for a cholesteatoma if MEE persists or AOM does not respond to antibiotic therapy.

- Suspect a brain abscess when a cholesteatoma is associated with ataxia or headaches.

- Consider an atypical or resistant organism in a child who is immunocompromised or has been exposed to frequent or recent antimicrobial therapy.

- Persistent TM perforation should be referred to an otolaryngologist especially if associated with hearing loss.

SUGGESTED READINGS

American Academy of Family Physicians, American Academy of Otolaryngology—Head and Neck Surgery, American Academy of Pediatrics Subcommittee on Otitis Media With Effusion. Otitis media with effusion. Pediatrics. 2004;113:1412–1429.

American Academy of Pediatrics Subcommittee on Management of Acute Otitis Media. Diagnosis and management of acute otitis media. Pediatrics. 2004;113:1451–1465.

Handler SD, Myer CM. Atlas of ear, nose and throat disorders in children. Ontario, Canada: B.C. Decker, Inc.; 1998:28, 30.

Pichichero ME. Acute otitis media: improving diagnostic accuracy—Part I. AFP. 2000;61:2051–2056.

Stool SE, Berg AO, Berman S, et al. Otitis Media with Effusion in Young Children. Clinical Practice Guideline, Number 12. AHCPR Publication No. 94-0622. Rockville, MD: Agency for Health Care Policy and Research, Public Health Service, US Department of Health and Human Services. July 1994.

Section

SIX

Nose

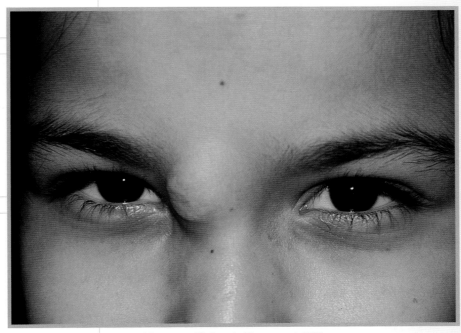

(Courtesy of E. Douglas Thompson, Jr, MD.)

Nasal Bridge Swelling

APPROACH TO THE PROBLEM

Swelling of the nasal bridge is an uncommon problem that may present a diagnostic dilemma to the practitioner. Lesions resulting in swelling may be divided into congenital and acquired etiologies. Congenital lesions of the nose occur in 1 in 20,000 to 40,000 live births. The most common congenital lesions to consider in the differential diagnosis of nasal bridge swelling include dermoid cysts, dacryocystoceles, gliomas, encephaloceles, and hemangiomas. Teratomas, lymphangiomas, lipomas, and angiofibromas are less frequently encountered. Acquired lesions may occur secondary to trauma or infection.

KEY POINTS IN THE HISTORY

- Increased size when crying or straining raises the possibility of a connection to the central nervous system consistent with an encephalocele.

- Intermittent discharge of sebaceous materials may occur with nasal dermoid cysts.

- A history of trauma is associated with a nasal fracture or contusion.

- Fever can be evidence of abscess or cellulitis, infection of a congenital cystic lesion, or meningitis complicating lesions that extend to the central nervous system.

- Rapid growth of the lesion in the first weeks to months of life is suggestive of a hemangioma.

KEY POINTS IN THE PHYSICAL EXAMINATION

- Dermoid cysts are midline lesions.

- Hair protruding from a midline mass most likely represents a dermoid cyst.

- Cystic lesions located on the lateral aspect of the nose just under the medial canthus indicate the presence of a dacryocystocele.

- New deformity of the nasal bridge along with edema and contusions suggests nasal bridge fracture.

- Transillumination may be evident in encephaloceles.

- A positive Furstenberg sign, represented by enlargement of the mass with compression of the jugular veins, makes the diagnosis of an encephalocele probable.

- Compressible lesions suggest encephaloceles and hemangiomas.

- Reddish or bluish discoloration and telangiectasias are most consistent with hemangiomas, but may be seen in gliomas.

PHOTOGRAPHS OF SELECTED DIAGNOSES

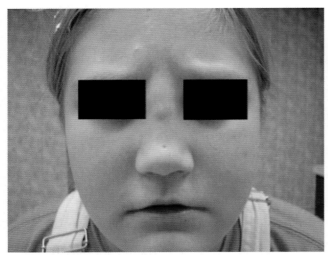

Figure 22-1 Dermoid cyst. A midline mass on the upper nasal bridge.
(Courtesy of Kathleen Cronan, MD.)

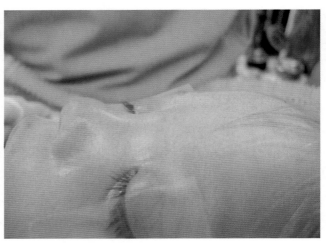

Figure 22-2 Dermoid cyst. Preoperative view.
(Courtesy of John A. Germiller, MD, PhD.)

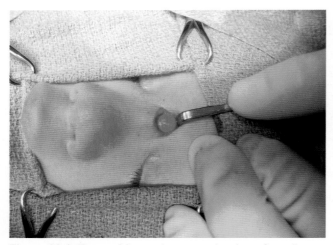

Figure 22-3 Dermoid cyst. Intraoperative view of a well-circumscribed dermoid cyst that corresponds with the previous figure.
(Courtesy of John A. Germiller, MD, PhD.)

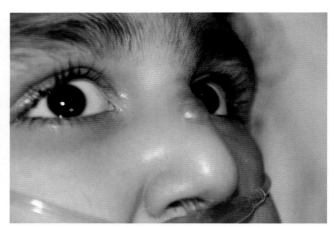

Figure 22-4 Hypertrophic scar. Nasal bridge scarring due to use of a continuous positive airway pressure machine.
(Courtesy of E. Douglas Thompson, Jr, MD.)

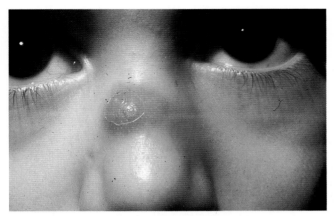

Figure 22-5 Nasal bridge abscess. Painful, erythematous lesion with purulent center on a child's nasal bridge.
(Courtesy of the late Peter Sol, MD.)

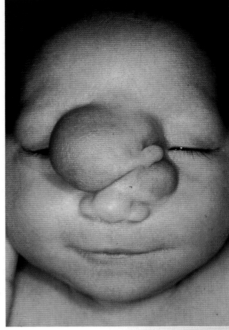

Figure 22-6 Nasal bridge encephalocele. Large nasal bridge mass in a neonate.
(Courtesy of Joseph Piatt, MD.)

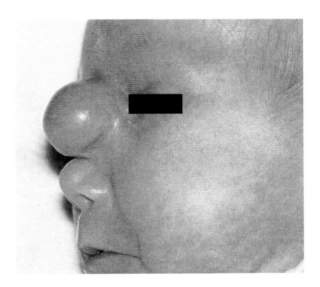

Figure 22-7 Large frontal encephalocele. A midline nasal protrusion in a newborn.
(Used with permission from Handler SD, Myer CM. *Atlas of ear, nose, and throat disorders in children.* Ontario, Canada: BC Decker; 1998:48.)

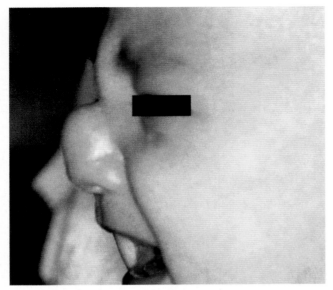

Figure 22-8 Large glioma under the nasal dorsum.
Deformity of the nasal bridge in a newborn.
(Used with permission from Handler SD, Myer CM. *Atlas of ear, nose, and throat disorders in children.* Ontario, Canada: BC Decker; 1998:48.)

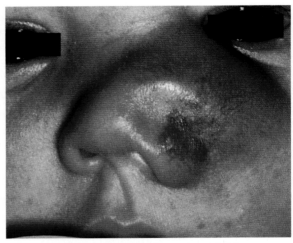

Figure 22-9 Nasal hemangioma in a child 6 months of age. Note the vascularity of this nasal mass.
(Used with permission from Handler SD, Myer CM. *Atlas of ear, nose, and throat disorders in children.* Ontario, Canada: BC Decker; 1998:55.)

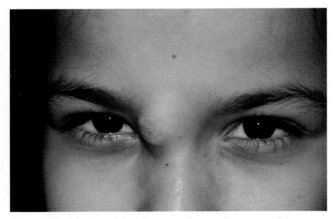

Figure 22–10 Resolving hemangioma. A compressible mass without obvious vascularity on the nasal bridge of a child.
(Courtesy of E. Douglas Thompson, Jr, MD.)

DIFFERENTIAL DIAGNOSIS

DIAGNOSIS	ICD-9	DISTINGUISHING CHARACTERISTICS	ASSOCIATED FINDINGS	COMPLICATIONS	TREATMENT GUIDELINES
Dermoid Cyst	216.3	Midline mass Variable presence of a pit Hair may protrude from mass	Drainage of sebaceous material	Abscess Bony erosion CNS infection Recurrence, if not completely resected	CNS imaging (generally MRI) to rule out intracranial extension Surgical resection
Dacryocystocele	375.43	Cystic mass Lateral aspect of nose below medial canthus of eye	Eye drainage and tearing	Dacryocystitis Nasal obstruction Recurrence after drainage	May drain spontaneously Digital massage Lacrimal duct probing under anesthesia by an ophthalmologist
Nasal Trauma	959.09	Swelling Deformity Ecchymosis Lacerations Epistaxis	Facial trauma or fracture	Nasal fracture Septal hematoma Septal abscess Nasal obstruction Facial asymmetry Cerebrospinal fluid (CSF) leak	Pain control Brain CT if CSF leak is suspected Closed reduction, if possible, otherwise open reduction under anesthesia
Encephaloceles	742.0	Compressible mass Demonstrates transillumination Positive Furstenberg sign	CSF leak Cleft palate	Meningitis Brain abscess Nasal obstruction Displacement of the globe	Neurosurgical evaluation Brain MRI Surgical resection
Gliomas	748.1	Firm mass lateral to the midline that is unaffected by crying, straining, or compression of the jugular veins	Tearing	Nasal obstruction	CNS imaging (generally MRI) to rule out intracranial extension Surgical resection
Hemangiomas	228.00	Soft, compressible mass Red or blue discoloration	Other cutaneous hemangiomas Hemangiomatosis	Bleeding Ulceration Scarring Airway obstruction Visual axis obstruction Amblyopia	Observation only for most lesions Referral to dermatology and/or surgery for corticosteroids, laser therapy, or surgical excision when airway or visual axis obstruction occurs

OTHER
DIAGNOSES
TO CONSIDER

- Diffuse neonatal hemangiomatosis

- Teratoma and other tumors

- Complex craniofacial anomalies

- Neurofibroma/plexiform neurofibroma (seen in neurofibromatosis I)

- Keloid or other scarring

WHEN TO
CONSIDER
FURTHER
EVALUATION
OR TREATMENT

- MRI and neurosurgical referral are indicated if a dermoid cyst, glioma, or encephalocele is suspected.

- Routine imaging is not necessary in most cases of nasal trauma, but CT should be considered if other facial fractures or a cerebrospinal fluid leak is suspected.

- Nasal hemangiomas resulting in the obstruction of the airway or visual axis should be referred to the appropriate specialists.

- Corticosteroids may be used to slow the growth of a hemangioma but, due to the attendant side effects, should only be used when lesions obstruct the airway or visual axis.

SUGGESTED READINGS

Dasgupta NR, Bentz ML. Nasal gliomas: identification and differentiation from hemangiomas. *J Craniofac Surg.* 2003;14(5):736–738.

Lee WT, Koltai PJ. Nasal deformity in neonates and young children. *Pediatr Clin North Am.* 2003;50(2):459–467.

Mahapatra AK, Suri A. Anterior encephaloceles: a study of 92 cases. *Pediatr Neurosurg.* 2002; 36(3):113–118.

Smolinski KN, Yan AC. Hemangiomas of infancy: clinical and biological characteristics. *Clin Pediatr.* 2005;44:747–766.

Wong RK, VanderVeen DK. Presentation and management of congenital dacryocystocele. *Pediatrics.* 2008;122(5):e1108–e1112.

Zapata S, Kearns DB. Nasal dermoids. *Curr Opin Otolaryngol Head Neck Surg.* 2006;14(6):406–411.

SHAREEN F. KELLY

23 Nasal Swelling, Discharge, and Crusting

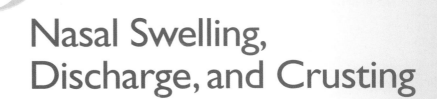

APPROACH TO THE PROBLEM

Investigating the causes of nasal swelling and discharge involves acquiring a careful history that includes the duration and timing of symptoms, the environment in which the symptoms occurred, whether anything has relieved the symptoms, and to what extent the problem has disrupted the child's daily functioning. Radiological studies may be useful in select cases. Noting the age of the patient is important because the sinus and nasopharyngeal complex changes with age. Asking about sick contacts will help in identifying infectious causes of rhinorrhea that may vary with age.

KEY POINTS IN THE HISTORY

- Rhinorrhea accompanying viral infections may be associated with fever, cough, and/or lymphadenopathy.

- Most rhinorrhea from viral upper respiratory tract infections resolves in 6 to 10 days.

- Prolonged purulent rhinorrhea (>10 days) or acute symptoms including headache, facial pain, and/or fever are suggestive of bacterial rhinosinusitis.

- Seasonal allergic rhinitis is generally accompanied by sneezing and intense nasal pruritus (and is often associated with ocular pruritus).

- Children with allergic rhinitis often have family members with atopic diseases.

- Fits of sneezing, which occur soon after rising from sleep and nasal symptoms in the presence of specific allergens, such as dust or animals, are characteristic of seasonal allergic rhinitis.

- Nasal drainage resulting from a foreign body, typically occurring in younger children, is usually acute, unilateral, and often associated with a foul odor.

- Children with impetigo generally do not complain of pain at the affected site.

- Recurrent nasal infections or persistent inflammation may contribute to the development of nasal polyps.

- Direct trauma to the nose may result in a septal hematoma.

- Viral rhinorrhea may be of varied color, thickness, and amount.

- Tenderness over the facial bones and increased headache and/or facial pain on forward bending of the neck are signs of sinusitis.

- Difficulty with nasal breathing in the absence of swollen turbinates is usually indicative of enlarged adenoids.

- Rhinorrhea from allergic rhinitis is generally thin, profuse, and clear.

- Examination of the nares in a child with allergic rhinitis usually reveals enlarged nasal turbinates with pale boggy mucosa.

- Children with allergic rhinitis often have associated Dennie-Morgan lines and allergic shiners.

- Nasal drainage from a foreign body is unilateral, thick, purulent, and sometimes bloody or foul smelling.

- Impetigo may occur as a single "honey-crusted" lesion of the nares. Because of autoinoculation, it often presents with multiple lesions in close proximity to the original lesion.

- Nasal polyps are painless, lucent-gray, yellow, or erythematous nasal masses that are most often solitary.

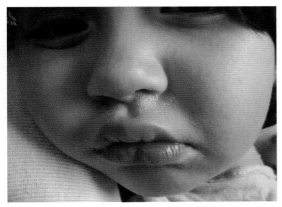

Figure 23-1 Viral rhinorrhea. Scant mucoid rhinorrhea in a child with an upper respiratory tract infection.
(Courtesy of Paul S. Matz, MD.)

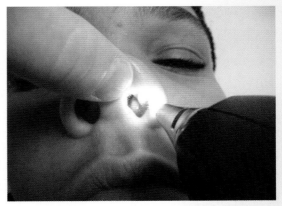

Figure 23-2 Allergic rhinitis. Pale boggy inferior turbinates are visible.
(Courtesy of Paul S. Matz, MD.)

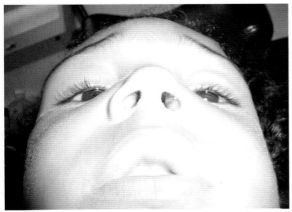

Figure 23-3 Nasal discharge/crusting because of a foreign body. This child had persistent unilateral, foul-smelling discharge until paper was removed from the left side by an otolaryngologist.
(Courtesy of Paul S. Matz, MD.)

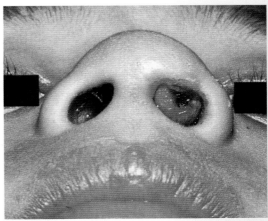

Figure 23-4 Nasal polyp. Erythematous mass visible in the left nare.
(Used with permission from Handler SD, Myer CM. *Atlas of ear, nose and throat disorders in children*. Ontario, Canada: BC Decker; 1998:59.)

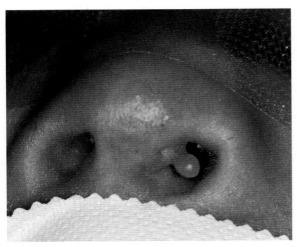

Figure 23-5 Skin tag at nasal vestibule. Small protuberant nodule at entrance to left nare.
(Used with permission from Handler SD, Myer CM. *Atlas of ear, nose and throat disorders in children*. Ontario, Canada: BC Decker; 1998:49.)

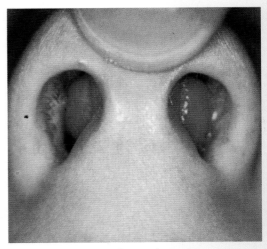

Figure 23-6 Bilateral septal hematoma. Bilateral erythematous masses arising from the nasal septum.
(Used with permission from Handler SD, Myer CM. *Atlas of eat nose and throat disorders in children*. Ontario, Canada: BC Decker; 1998:52.)

DIAGNOSIS	ICD-9	DISTINGUISHING CHARACTERISTICS	DISTRIBUTION	DURATION/ CHRONICITY
Viral Rhinorrhea	478.1	Thin and clear or thick white or yellow rhinorrhea	Any age More frequent in daycare attendees	Lasts 5–10 days Occurs most often in winter
Allergic Rhinitis	477.9	Thin, profuse, watery rhinorrhea	Unusual in children less than 3 years Peak incidence in adolescence	Occurs more seasonally or upon exposure to allergens or irritants, such as smoke, animals, and dust
Impetigo	684	Golden "honey-crusted" erythematous area	Any age but may be associated with children who pick their noses Usually near the nares but may be seen anywhere on the body	Easy to treat but contagious May recur if child is colonized with *Staphylococcus aureus*
Nasal Foreign Body	932	Unilateral purulent nasal discharge	Most common in children of preschool age	N/A
Nasal Polyp	471.9	Glistening gray, yellow, or erythematous mass in nares	Usually solitary Unusual in children less than 10 years	Long lasting unless removed
Septal Hematoma	920	Purple or dark fluctuant mass on mucosa of nasal septum	No age or gender predilection	Should be treated within 48 hours of occurrence to avoid necrosis

ASSOCIATED FINDINGS	COMPLICATIONS	PREDISPOSING FACTORS	TREATMENT GUIDELINES
Sore throat Cough Fever Enlarged cervical lymph nodes	Rhinosinusitis	Exposure to others with upper respiratory tract infections	Supportive treatment Nasal saline washes
Associated with ocular symptoms of tearing and itchiness Often associated with atopic dermatitis	Headaches from sinus pressure Postnasal drip with or without halitosis	Allergens Familial predisposition with other allergic symptoms	Systemic antihistamines and/or nasal corticosteroids Environmental allergen elimination
May have skin lesions in other areas	Rarely, invasive infection with S. aureus Generally does not result in scarring	Nasal colonization with S. aureus Nose picking	Topical antibiotic cream if lesions are small and localized Oral antibiotics if lesions are widespread
Malodorous nasal discharge, sometimes bloody	Nasal septum erosion with retained foreign body	Behavior of child Follows foreign body placement into a nare	Removal of foreign body
May be associated with epistaxis	Persistent nasal congestion and decreased ability to breathe through affected side	Recurrent infections and persistent inflammation Associated with cystic fibrosis	Decrease inflammation by use of nasal steroids Removal of polyps
Facial tenderness or contusions over other facial bones	Nasal septum erosion	Trauma	Prompt evacuation of hematoma

OTHER
DIAGNOSES
TO CONSIDER

- Cerebrospinal fluid leak

- Rhinitis medicamentosa

- Nasal glioma or encephalocele

- Craniofacial anomalies

- Nasopharyngitis from gastroesophageal reflux

- Choanal atresia

- Anterior nasal stenosis

- Cocaine use

WHEN TO
CONSIDER
FURTHER
EVALUATION
OR TREATMENT

- Recurrent or chronic sinusitis should prompt consideration and investigation of diagnoses including cystic fibrosis, specific immunodeficiencies, and ciliary dysmotility syndromes.

- Allergic rhinitis unresponsive to treatment may be secondary to enlarged adenoids or lack of allergen control in the child's environment.

- Impetiginous skin lesions near the nares that are painful or associated with fever must be considered as possibly representing invasive staphylococcal or streptococcal infections. Treatment for invasive disease warrants consideration of methicillin-resistant *Staphylococcus aureus* (MRSA) when choosing antibiotic coverage.

- Nasal polyps in a child with growth failure, malabsorption, and/or frequent lower respiratory tract infections or inflammation should prompt a work-up for cystic fibrosis.

- Nasal foreign body removal can be attempted in the pediatrician's office, but failure to accomplish removal necessitates prompt referral to the otolaryngologist.

- Erosion through or perforation of the nasal septum following the resolution of a nasal septal hematoma necessitates referral to the otolaryngologist.

SUGGESTED READINGS

Handler SD, Myer CM. *Atlas of ear, nose and throat disorders in children*. Ontario, Canada: BC Decker, Inc.; 1998:49, 52, 59.

Osborn L, DeWitt T, First L, et al. *Pediatrics*. Philadelphia, PA: Elsevier Mosby, Inc.; 2005:454–460.

Schoem SR, Josephson GD, Mendelson LM, et al. Why won't this child's nose stop running? *Contemp Pediatr*. 2002;19:48–63.

Yellon RF, McBride TB, Davis HVV. Otolaryngology. In: *Atlas of pediatric physical diagnosis*. 4th ed. Philadelphia, PA: Mosby; 2002:832–838.

Mouth

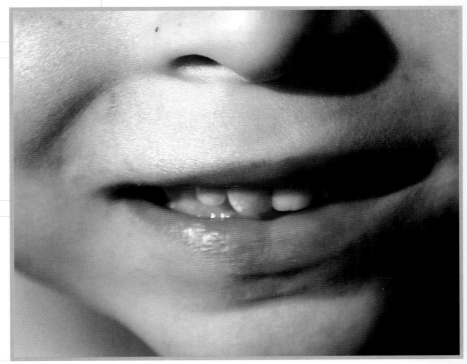

(Courtesy of Daniel R. Taylor, DO.)

ROBERT L. BONNER, JR.

Mouth Sores and Patches

24

APPROACH TO THE PROBLEM

In the pediatric patient, lesions of the oral cavity may range from those that are asymptomatic to those that are extremely painful and uncomfortable. Oral lesions may present at any age and are often self-limited. An oral lesion often occurs in isolation, but a systemic infection or disorder should always be considered when arriving at a diagnosis. A thorough history and complete examination are necessary for an accurate diagnosis and appropriate treatment. Managing pain is particularly important to prevent dehydration because children often refuse to eat or drink when painful oral lesions are present.

KEY POINTS IN THE HISTORY

- Aphthous ulcers are the most common cause of mouth ulceration in childhood with an increasing prevalence in late childhood and adolescence.

- The presence of aphthous ulcers and systemic symptoms, such as fever, may be an indication of an inflammatory, autoimmune, or connective tissue disease.

- Fever, headaches, and erythematous oral vesicles in the posterior pharynx during the summer months are suggestive of herpangina resulting from coxsackievirus infection.

- Viral etiologies of oral ulcerations usually present as vesicles before becoming ulcerated.

- Herpes simplex virus (HSV) gingivostomatitis most commonly presents in children younger than 4 years of age.

- White nodules on the palate of a neonate are consistent with Epstein pearls. These self-limited benign cysts, containing sebaceous and keratin material, are extremely common.

- Thrush will have an insidious onset, and parents may report decreased oral intake as the presenting symptom.

- Palatal burns typically will have an acute onset with localization to the palate.

- Lip-licking dermatitis may occur in isolation, but is often seen in patients with atopic dermatitis.

KEY POINTS IN THE PHYSICAL EXAMINATION

- HSV gingivostomatitis is characterized by vesicles in the anterior and posterior oropharynx, while herpangina presents with vesicles predominately in the posterior oropharynx.

- The ulcers of herpangina have erythematous borders with a white to gray base, whereas the ulcers of HSV gingivostomatitis are erythematous and associated with gingival erythema and edema.

- Aphthous ulcers present on nonkeratinized mucosa of the mouth, which includes the buccal and labial mucosae and the floor of the mouth.

- Ulcerative lesions may be so painful that drooling may be apparent on examination.

- Epstein pearls are seen in the first few weeks of life as white, nodular lesions of the palatal mucosa. Similarly, Bohn nodules are 2 to 3 mm nodular lesions on the gum mucosa.

- Koplik spots are often missed because these lesions arise only during the prodrome of measles.

- Thrush is typically seen throughout the oropharynx on the buccal and labial mucosae. Scraping of the white plaque-like lesion of thrush will reveal an erythematous superficial ulceration of the mucosae.

PHOTOGRAPHS OF SELECTED DIAGNOSES

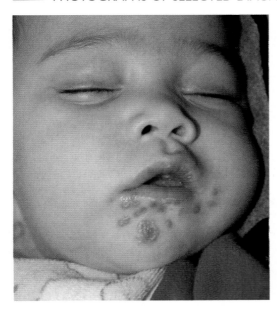

Figure 24-1 Herpes simplex viral stomatitis. An infant with extraoral HSV lesions.
(Courtesy of George A. Datto, III, MD.)

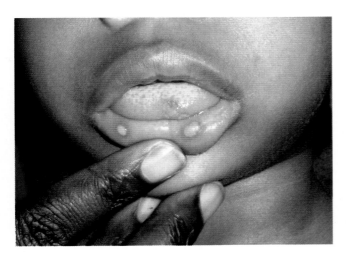

Figure 24-2 Herpes simplex viral stomatitis. Lesions are visible on the tongue and labial mucosa.
(Courtesy of Paul S. Matz, MD.)

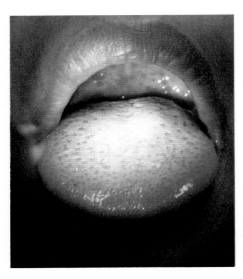

Figure 24-3 Herpangina. Posterior pharyngeal lesions, as seen with coxsackievirus.
(Courtesy of Paul S. Matz, MD.)

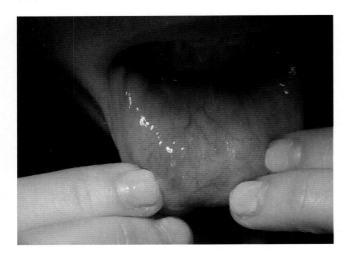

Figure 24-4 Aphthous ulcers. Lesions visible on the inner lip.
(Courtesy of Michael Lemper, DDS.)

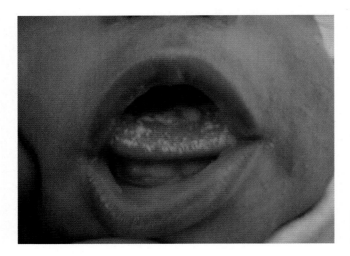

Figure 24-5 Oral thrush. An infant with numerous whitish tongue plaques.
(Courtesy of Paul S. Matz, MD.)

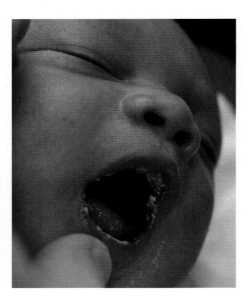

Figure 24-6 Oral thrush. Note the whitish plaques on the labial mucosae.
(Courtesy of George A. Datto, III, MD.)

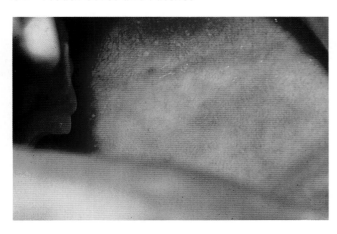

Figure 24-7 Koplik spots. Fine white spots with red rings seen on the buccal mucosa.
(Used with permission from The Wellcome Trust, National Medical Slide Bank, London, UK.)

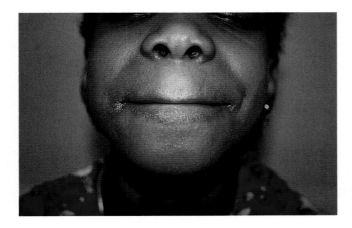

Figure 24-8 Lip-licking dermatitis. Rash visible in a child with a history of chronic lip licking.
(Courtesy of George A. Datto, III, MD.)

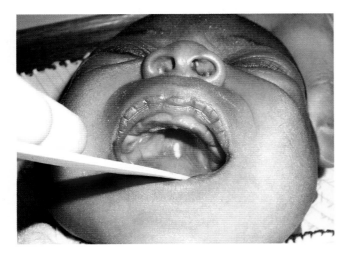

Figure 24-9 Epstein pearls. Whitish cysts visible on the midline palate of a neonate.
(Courtesy of Paul S. Matz, MD.)

DIFFERENTIAL DIAGNOSIS

DIAGNOSIS	ICD-9	DISTINGUISHING CHARACTERISTICS	DISTRIBUTION
HSV Gingivostomatitis	054.2	Clusters of erythematous, painful vesicles Edematous gingiva Yellow exudative ulcers with an erythematous halo	Anterior oral pharynx: • Lips • Gingiva • Tongue • Buccal mucosa • Palate
Herpangina	074.0	Discrete erythematous vesicles Painful gray ulcers on an erythematous base	Posterior pharynx: • Soft palate • Tonsillar pillars • Uvula
Aphthous Ulcers	528.2	Ulcers with pseudomembrane and erythematous halo	Buccal and labial mucosae, floor of mouth and ventral surface of tongue
Palatal Erosion (Burn, Sucking Blister)	947.0	Erythematous ulcerated lesions	Palate
Thrush	771.7	White plaques on an erythematous base	Throughout anterior and posterior oral pharynx, including buccal and labial mucosae
Koplik Spots	055.9	Bluish-white papules on an erythematous base	Buccal mucosa opposite the first molar and soft palate
Lip-Licking Dermatitis	528.5	Perioral dryness Scaly and lichenified Hyperpigmentation	Perioral
Epstein Pearls	528.4	Small, white pearly cysts	Midline of palate Gums may have similar lesions that are referred to as "Bohn nodules."

ASSOCIATED FINDINGS	COMPLICATIONS	PRECIPITATING FACTORS	TREATMENT GUIDELINES
High fever Irritability Odynophagia	Dehydration Recurrent presentation	Exposure to HSV, most commonly type I Age less than 4 years	Supportive care with topical or systemic analgesics Early oral acyclovir for immunocompromised patients or those with severe disease
Fever Headache Malaise	Dehydration	Exposure to coxsackievirus group A	Supportive care with topical or oral analgesics
Fever May manifest systemic symptoms	Recurrent presentation	Associated with local trauma, infection, GI disorders, food allergy, vitamin deficiencies, stress	Supportive care Chlorhexidene rinses, and oral and topical steroids have been beneficial.
Pain Decreased intake	Dysphagia Facial scarring	Age less than 2 years	Antibiotics for mild burns and erosions Oral burn splints for severe burns
Often concurrent with candidal diaper dermatitis	Poor feeding	Infants less than 12 months Use of broad-spectrum antibiotics Steroid therapy Immunocompromise	Oral nystatin applied topically to lesions
Fever Cough Coryza Conjunctivitis Morbilliform rash	None from lesions	Exposure to rubeola	Supportive care
May have eczematous changes to skin elsewhere	None	Mouth breathing Atopic disease	Moisturizing creams, topical steroids
None	None	None	No therapy

OTHER DIAGNOSES TO CONSIDER

- Mucoceles or ranulas
- Hemangiomas
- Leukoplakia
- White sponge nevus

WHEN TO CONSIDER FURTHER EVALUATION OR TREATMENT

- Oral thrush should be treated with an oral antifungal agent, such as nystatin. If examination also reveals candidal diaper dermatitis, it should be treated with topical nystatin.

- Lesions of viral stomatitis may be treated with oral analgesics, as well as topical analgesics, such as the combination of diphenhydramine liquid and aluminum and magnesium hydroxide, with or without viscous lidocaine, especially before meals.

- Oral or intravenous acyclovir should be reserved for severe cases of HSV gingivostomatitis or for patients with an immunodeficiency.

- Patients with oral lesions that frequently recur despite appropriate therapy should be evaluated for conditions associated with recurrent oral lesions, such as immunodeficiencies or rheumatologic disease.

- Recurrent aphthous ulcers may be treated with saline rinses, chlorhexidine rinses, or oral or topical corticosteroids.

SUGGESTED READINGS

Milano M. Oral electrical and thermal burns in children: review and report of case. *ASDC J Dent Child.* 1999;66:85, 116–119.
Patel NJ, Sciubba J. Oral lesions in young children. *Pediatr Clin North Am.* 2003;50:469–486.
Perry RT, Halsey NA. The clinical significance of measles: a review. *J Infect Dis.* 2004;189(Suppl 1):S4–S16.
Peter JR, Haney HM. Infections of the oral cavity. *Pediatr Ann.* 1996;25:10:572–576.
Witman PM, Rogers RS. Pediatric oral medicine. *Dermotol Clin.* 2003;21:157–170.

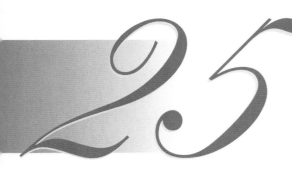

NANCY D. SPECTOR

Focal Gum Lesions

APPROACH TO THE PROBLEM

Oral lesions are very common in newborns, infants, and young children. Parents may be particularly concerned when there is a focal swelling on their child's gum. Fortunately, most of these lesions are benign. The prevalence and incidence of the most commonly noted gum lesions, Bohn nodules and eruption cysts, are unknown. Both typically resolve without intervention, and their presence does not have adverse effects. Some lesions, however, represent infections that are the result of untreated dental caries and poor oral hygiene. Dental abscesses, if left untreated, may extend to involve the adjacent tissue, resulting in the formation of a fistula to the gum surface, facial cellulitis, and even osteomyelitis involving the facial bones.

KEY POINTS IN THE HISTORY

- Eruption cysts are common in infants and children during the mixed-dentition stage, when primary and permanent teeth are present in the mouth.

- Eruption cysts tend to rupture spontaneously.

- A deflection in the path of tooth eruption (e.g., crowding or over-retention of primary teeth) may result in a mucogingival defect.

- Bohn nodules and alveolar cysts, often present at birth, generally do not interfere with feeding.

- Parents may confuse Bohn nodules with oral thrush.

- Poor dental hygiene and dental caries are risk factors for dental abscesses.

- Children with dental abscesses may have a history of fever or mouth pain.

- Some children with a fistula between a dental abscess and the gum may report drainage, a funny taste in their mouth, or both.

KEY POINTS IN
THE PHYSICAL
EXAMINATION

- Bohn nodules are smooth, translucent, pearly white, and approximately 1- to 3-mm cysts.

- Alveolar cysts are visible along the alveolar ridges.

- Eruption cysts are usually found in the region of the incisors on the edge of the alveolar ridge where a tooth is erupting.

- Eruption cysts may feel rubbery and have a bluish hue.

- Natal teeth are erupted teeth that are present at the time of birth.

- A retrocuspid papilla, often bilateral, is a firm, round, pink to red 2- to 3-mm papule attached to the gingiva lingual to the mandibular canines.

- The presence of fever in association with a focal gum lesion should raise suspicion for a dental abscess.

- Dental abscesses may appear as a swelling of the gum, often in the region of a dental caries.

- Dental abscesses may cause swelling of the overlying cheek.

- Dental abscesses may develop a fistula between the tooth apex and the oral cavity.

PHOTOGRAPHS OF SELECTED DIAGNOSES

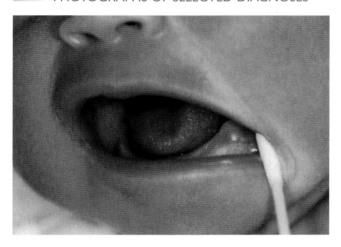

Figure 25-1 Bohn nodule. Pearly nodule on the gum of a neonate.
(Used with permission from Fletcher MA. *Physical diagnosis in neonatology.* Philadelphia, PA: Lippincott–Raven Publishers; 1998:216.)

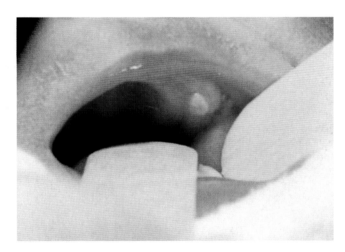

Figure 25-2 Alveolar cyst. Cyst on the alveolar ridge of a newborn.
(Used with permission from Fletcher MA. *Physical diagnosis in neonatology.* Philadelphia, PA: Lippincott–Raven Publishers; 1998:216.)

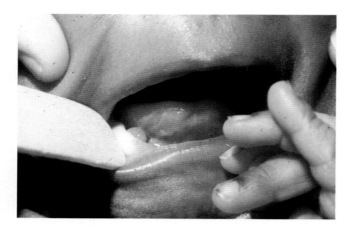

Figure 25-3 Alveolar cyst. Cyst on the alveolar ridge of a newborn.
(Courtesy of the late Peter Sol, MD.)

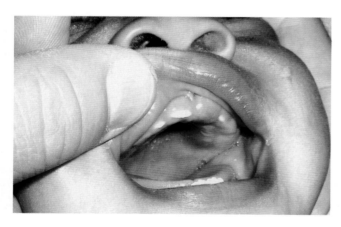

Figure 25-4 Eruption cyst. Swelling and blue discoloration are visible along the alveolar ridge shortly before the upper left central incisor erupts.
(Courtesy of Paul S. Matz, MD.)

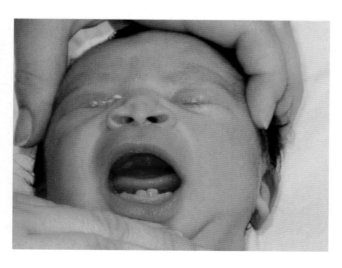

Figure 25-5 Natal teeth. Bilateral lower central incisors in a neonate.
(Courtesy of Denise A. Salerno, MD, FAAP.)

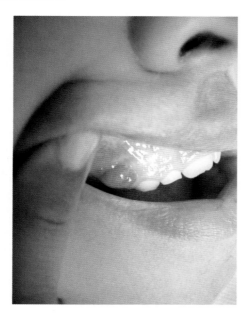

Figure 25-6 Dental abscess with fistula to the gum. Spongy mass on the gum associated with nearby caries. (Courtesy of Paul S. Matz, MD.)

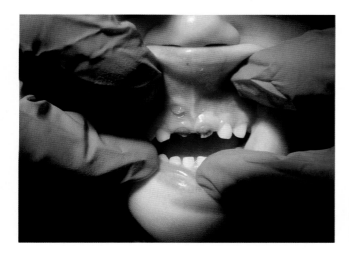

Figure 25-7 Dental abscess and fistula associated with severe dental caries. Note the fistula above the upper right central incisor, associated with severe caries of that tooth. (Courtesy of Michael Lemper, DDS.)

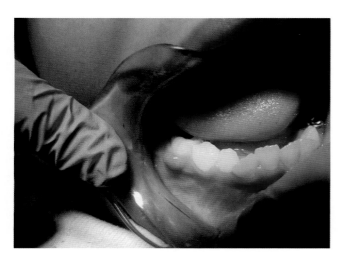

Figure 25-8 Gingival abscess. Erythematous mass on the lower gum, associated with dental caries. (Courtesy of Michael Lemper, DDS.)

DIFFERENTIAL DIAGNOSIS

DIAGNOSIS	ICD-9	DISTINGUISHING CHARACTERISTICS	DISTRIBUTION
Bohn Nodule	528.4 (oral cyst)	Occurs commonly in up to 85% of newborns Smooth, translucent, pearly white, keratin-filled, 1–3-mm cyst	Buccal or alveolar surface of the gums
Eruption Cyst	526.0	Common in infants and children during the mixed-dentition phase Dome-shaped, fluid-filled, rubbery cyst Bluish hue Ruptures spontaneously	On the edge of the alveolar ridge where the tooth is erupting Usually, in the region of the incisors Less often in the region of the permanent molars
Alveolar Cyst	525.5	Gingival cysts that appear in up to 50% of newborns Smooth, translucent, pearly white, keratin-filled, 1–3-mm cyst Single or multiple Discrete or clustered	Alveolar mucosa, most commonly on the maxillary mucosa
Retrocuspid Papilla	523.8	Fibroepithelial papule Firm, round, pink to red 2–3 mm in diameter Usually bilateral	Attached to gingiva lingual to the mandibular canines
Dental Abscess with Fistula to the Gum	522.7	Dental caries progresses to involve the tooth pulp, causing an abscess, which may progress to the development of a fistula to the gum Tooth and gum pain	Fistula between the tooth apex and the oral cavity

DURATION/CHRONICITY	ASSOCIATED FINDINGS	COMPLICATIONS	TREATMENT GUIDELINES
Ruptures spontaneously in the first month of life	None	None	No intervention required
Related to tooth eruption	Mixed dentition Tooth eruption Hematoma	May precede neonatal teeth	No intervention required. Resolves spontaneously as the tooth erupts through the lesion
Ruptures spontaneously in first 3 months of life	None	None	No intervention required
Decreases in size with age	None	None	No intervention required
Takes months to develop Will not resolve without intervention	Dental caries Pain Discharge from the gum	Facial space infection Sepsis Primary tooth infection may disrupt normal development of the secondary tooth Destruction of underlying bone	Refer to dentistry. Administer oral antibiotics

- Congenital epulis (granular cell tumor of the alveolar ridge)

- Teratomas and dermoid cysts

- Peripheral giant cell granuloma

- Alveolar lymphangioma

- Rhabdomyosarcoma

- Osteogenic sarcoma

- Fibrosarcoma

- Mucoepidermoid carcinoma

- Oral lymphoepithelialized cyst

- Most focal gum lesions in newborns, children, and adolescents are benign, do not interfere with feeding, and do not require intervention.

- Consider referral to dentistry for eruption cysts that do not resolve spontaneously.

- The presence of a dental abscess requires referral to dentistry and the administration of oral antibiotics.

- Consider referral to dentistry for any painful, localized gum lesions.

- A focal gum lesion that continues to enlarge or is associated with systemic symptoms or signs warrants further evaluation for an oncologic process.

SUGGESTED READINGS
Caufield PW, Griffen AL. Dental caries: an infectious and transmissible disease. Pediatr Clin North Am. 2000;47(5):1001–1019.
Fleisher GR, Ludwig S, Baskin MN. Atlas of pediatric emergency medicine. Philadelphia, PA: Lippincott Williams & Wilkins; 2004:78.
Fletcher MA. Physical diagnosis in neonatology. Philadelphia, PA: Lippincott–Raven Publishers; 1998:216.
Krol DM, Keels MA. Oral conditions. Pediatr Rev. 2007;28:15–22.
Pinkham JR, Casamassimo PS, McTigue DJ, et al., eds. Pediatric dentistry: infancy through adolescence. 4th ed. St. Louis, MO: Elsevier Science; 2005:9–60.
Wright JT. Normal formation and development defects of the human dentition. Pediatr Clin North Am. 2000;47(5):975–1000.

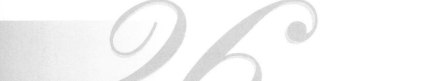

DANIEL R. TAYLOR
AND HAROLD V. SALVATI

Discoloration of the Teeth

APPROACH TO THE PROBLEM

Discoloration of the teeth may result from congenital abnormalities, dental trauma, medications, diets, systemic illnesses, genetic syndromes, or infections. Historically, tooth discoloration is usually classified as intrinsic or extrinsic according to the location of the stain. *Intrinsic* tooth staining occurs with changes in the composition or thickness of the tooth. *Extrinsic* discoloration refers to staining on a tooth's exterior. Appropriate dental hygiene, oral infection control, establishment of a "dental home," and the avoidance of specific medications and cariogenic diets during critical moments in tooth development will reduce the risks of tooth staining.

KEY POINTS IN THE HISTORY

- A caries risk potential should be performed in infancy for all children. Children at high caries risk include children with special needs, children of mothers with multiple caries, children who sleep with a bottle or breastfeed throughout the night, and children of low-income families.

- Deciduous incisors and canines are most susceptible to tetracycline staining between 4 months gestation and 5 months postnatally, while permanent dentition is most susceptible from 4 months to approximately 7 years of age.

- Cosmetically important fluorosis of the permanent maxillary central incisors is most likely to occur when excess fluoride is ingested between 15 and 30 months of age.

- Common sources of fluoride include fluoride-supplemented water, fluoridated tooth-paste, polyvitamins with fluoride, and many topical whitening products.

- Exposure to metal salts, most commonly iron, can cause extrinsic discoloration.

- Tooth discoloration in infancy may be indicative of developmental defects of the teeth.

- Coffee, tea, red wine, cigarette smoking, and chewing tobacco can all cause extrinsic staining.

- Dental trauma is also a common cause of tooth discoloration.

- Opaque white spots are a common presentation of early caries.

- Tetracycline causes a brown/yellow permanent discoloration of the teeth.

- The discoloration due to fluorosis may vary from mild pale discolorations to more intense dark stains, which may also be associated with pitting.

- Iron causes a distinctive black stain that may be cleaned by a dentist.

- Staining and damage limited to maxillary teeth suggest bottle caries. The mandibular dentition is believed to be spared because of the protective barrier formed by the presence of the lower lip and tongue.

- The presence of other symptoms—involving the eyes, hair, or musculoskeletal areas—in a child with dental staining should prompt further evaluation for a genetic or autoimmune process.

PHOTOGRAPHS OF SELECTED DIAGNOSES

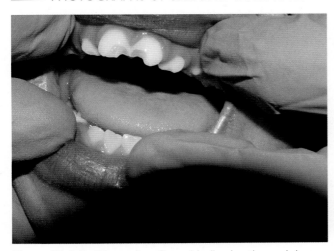

Figure 26-1 Bottle caries. Brownish discoloration and decay of the upper central incisors.
(Courtesy of Michael Lemper, DDS.)

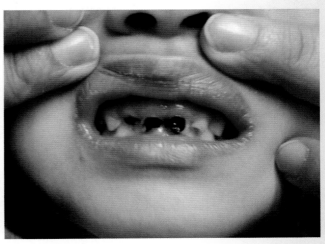

Figure 26-2 Bottle caries. Severe erosion of the upper incisors, associated with black staining.
(Courtesy of Philip Siu, MD.)

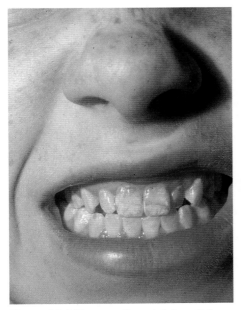

Figure 26-3 Tetracycline staining. Yellow-brown discoloration, most notably on the upper central incisors.
(Courtesy of the late Peter Sol, MD.)

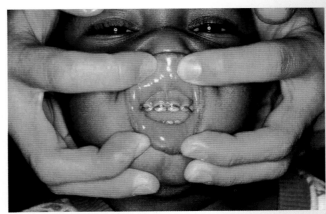

Figure 26-4 Tetracycline staining. Brown, band-like staining visible on all four maxillary incisors.
(Courtesy of Jan Edwin Drutz, MD.)

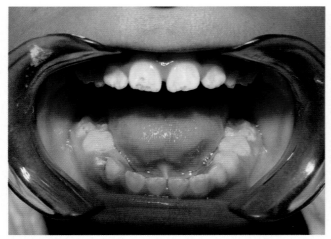

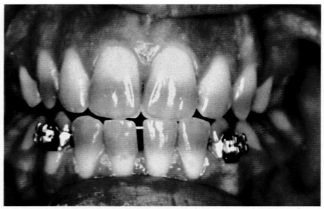

Figure 26-6 Dental erosion. Diffuse gray-brown discoloration.
(Courtesy of the American Academy of Pediatrics.)

Figure 26-5 Fluorosis. Brown spots, associated with pitting of
the central maxillary incisors.
(Courtesy of Michael Lemper, DDS.)

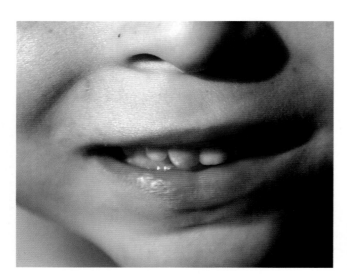

Figure 26-7 Enamel hypoplasia. Gray discoloration of the
right central maxillary incisor following dental trauma that occurred
during mineralization of the tooth.
(Courtesy of Daniel R. Taylor, DO.)

DIAGNOSIS	ICD-9	DISTINGUISHING CHARACTERISTICS	DISTRIBUTION	PREDISPOSING FACTORS	ASSOCIATED FINDINGS	TREATMENT GUIDELINES
Bottle Caries	521.0	Brown, decayed teeth	Maxillary incisors most affected	Protracted use of bottles, including bottle use throughout the night Poor dental hygiene	Halitosis Gingivitis Tooth abscess Mouth pain Failure to thrive School problems	Dental fillings Tooth extraction Reconstructive surgery
Iron Staining	521.7	Black stain that can be scraped off	Lingual tooth surfaces	Exposure to vitamins or other products with iron	Gastrointestinal symptoms Dark stools	Microabrasion Bonding
Tetracycline Staining	520.8	Brown-yellow discoloration that cannot be removed	Earlier exposure affects primary teeth; later exposure affects secondary teeth	Exposure to tetracycline prenatally or in the first 7 years of life	Photosensitivity Gastrointestinal symptoms	Bleaching Veneers
Fluorosis	520.3	White-to-brown staining that is not removable	Predominantly permanent central incisors	Excess fluoride exposure Sources of fluoride might include water, fluoridated toothpaste, and supplemental fluoride.	N/A	Bleaching Veneers
Enamel Hypoplasia	520.4	Diffuse gray tooth	Traumatized tooth	Trauma or infection	Associated trauma	Bonding

OTHER
DIAGNOSES
TO CONSIDER

- Enamel hypoplasia

- Pseudohypoparathyroidism

- Rickets

- Dentinogenesis imperfecta

- Alkaptonuria

- Congenital porphyria

- Trauma

WHEN TO
CONSIDER
FURTHER
EVALUATION
OR TREATMENT

- Children at high risk for dental caries should be referred to a pediatric dentist 6 months after the first tooth eruption or at 12 months of age, whichever comes first.

- The development and eruption of permanent teeth should be monitored carefully in children with a history of trauma to their primary teeth.

- Discoloration affecting all teeth necessitates a search for systemic disorders such as vitamin D deficiency, hypophosphatasia, or fluorosis.

SUGGESTED READINGS
Lewis CS, Milgrom P. Fluoride. *Pediatr Rev.* 2003;24:327–336.
Martof A. Consultation with the specialist: dental care. *Pediatr Rev.* 2001;22:13–15.
Watts A, Addy M. Tooth discolouration and staining: a review of the literature. *Br Dent J.* 2001;190:309–316.
Weiss PA, Czerepak CS, Hale KJ, et al. American Academy of Pediatrics Policy Statement. Oral health risk assessment timing and establishment of the dental home. *Pediatrics.* 2003;111:1113–1116.

KEITH HERZOG
AND PAUL S. MATZ

Oral Clefts and Other Variants

APPROACH TO THE PROBLEM

The formation of the nose and mouth during embryogenesis occurs as a result of selective cell proliferation, cell death, and tissue fusion; the disruption of these processes may result in congenital clefts. Both genetic and nongenetic (e.g., teratogenic) factors impact the development of clefts. While there are familial predilections, most clefts (75%) are sporadic. Combined cleft lip and palate occur more frequently (50%) than either alone. Isolated cleft palate appears to be a distinct entity in terms of inheritance patterns and a greater association with other anomalies. The repair of cleft lip is usually undertaken at approximately 10 weeks of age and the repair of cleft palate occurs between 9 and 12 months. Velopharyngeal incompetence of varying severity often accompanies cleft palate and may result in speech problems; tonsillectomy and adenoidectomy may worsen this functional problem.

KEY POINTS IN THE HISTORY

- While there is a familial predilection for clefts, there is no simple pattern of inheritance.

- Maternal exposure to teratogens may result in cleft lip or palate.

- A cleft lip or palate may interfere with the infant's ability to create the oral vacuum necessary for bottle-feeding or breastfeeding. As a result, the infant may have poor intake and hence fail to thrive.

- Excessive air intake, nasal regurgitation, fatigue, coughing, choking, gagging on fluids, and prolonged feeding times are negative consequences of the oral-nasal coupling seen with cleft palate.

- Patients with isolated cleft palate, cleft lip and palate, submucosal cleft palate, or a bifid uvula may demonstrate impaired articulation, nasal speech, and poor enunciation of certain consonant sounds.

- Conductive hearing loss from recurrent otitis media is common among children with cleft palate.

- Some infants with ankyloglossia may have difficulty with breastfeeding.

- Ankyloglossia in older children may be associated with speech articulation problems; however, ankyloglossia does not cause speech delay. It may also be associated with problems with oral hygiene (cleaning lips and oral buccal gutters).

KEY POINTS IN THE PHYSICAL EXAMINATION

- Cleft lip may vary from a small notch on the vermillion border to a complete separation that extends to the floor of the nose.

- In a newborn presenting with a cleft lip, a careful examination should be performed to rule out associated cleft palate.

- Isolated cleft palate without cleft lip may be associated with other congenital anomalies (20% to 30% of the time). Bilateral cleft lip has a higher association with other congenital anomalies than unilateral cleft lip.

- In some cases, a bifid uvula may be associated with a submucosal cleft palate, often only diagnosed by direct palpation (including a palpable "notch" on the back of the hard palate). One fifth of such patients may have velopharyngeal incompetence.

- A cleft palate may also involve the teeth, maxilla, and labial musculature.

- Cleft palate predisposes affected individuals to frequent acute otitis media (AOM) because of eustachian tube dysfunction.

- Ankyloglossia leads to decreased tongue movement in all directions, most notably with tongue protrusion, and may be associated with a notched or heart-shaped appearance.

PHOTOGRAPHS OF SELECTED DIAGNOSES

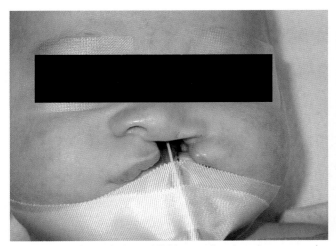

Figure 27-1 Cleft lip in a child immediately prior to repair.
(Courtesy of Wellington Davis, MD.)

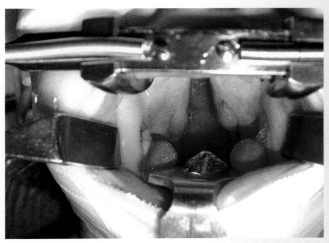

Figure 27-2 Cleft palate visualized intraoperatively.
(Courtesy of Wellington Davis, MD.)

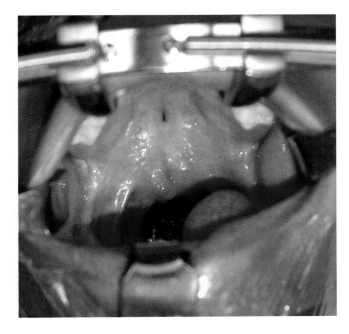

Figure 27-3 Operative photo of a submucosal cleft palate with a small palatal perforation.
(Courtesy of Wellington Davis, MD.)

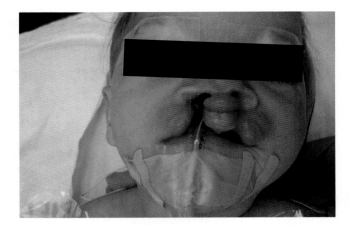

Figure 27-4 Bilateral cleft lip and palate.
(Courtesy of Scott VanDuzer, MD.)

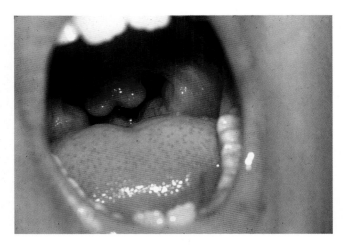

Figure 27-5 An isolated bifid uvula without other oral clefting.
(Courtesy of the late Peter Sol, MD.)

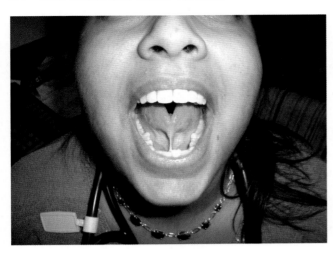

Figure 27-6 Ankyloglossia—note the lingual frenulum extending to the tip of the tongue.
(Courtesy of Paul S. Matz, MD.)

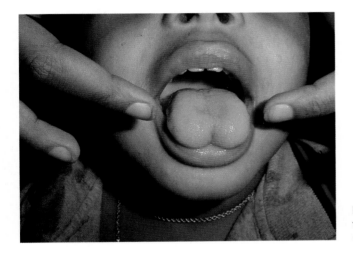

Figure 27-7   Ankyloglossia—notched or heart-shaped tongue visible on protrusion of the tongue.
(Courtesy of Michael Lemper, DDS.)

DIFFERENTIAL DIAGNOSIS

DIAGNOSIS	ICD-9	DISTINGUISHING CHARACTERISTICS	DISTRIBUTION	
Cleft Lip	749.10–14 w/ cleft palate: 749.20–25	Fissure in the upper lip, may be unilateral or bilateral Variation in presentation from a notch on the vermillion border to a large separation extending to the floor of the nose	Upper lip, may involve the maxilla or the gums	
Cleft Palate	749.00	Unilateral or bilateral clefting of the hard and/or soft palate May involve just the uvula and soft palate (incomplete clefts) or the entire palate	Hard palate Soft palate Uvula	
Bifid Uvula	749.02	Notched or cleft uvula	Uvula	
Ankyloglossia (Tongue Tie)	750.0	Very short frenulum; may be fibrous or thin, membranous tissue Limited tongue protrusion Tongue, when protruding, with notched appearance	Tongue	

ASSOCIATED FINDINGS	COMPLICATIONS	PREDISPOSING FACTORS	TREATMENT GUIDELINES
Deformed, absent, or supernumerary teeth Cleft palate	Difficulty feeding	Intrauterine drug exposure (teratogens): phenytoin, valproic acid, thalidomide, alcohol, cigarettes, isotretinoin, digoxin Genetic syndromes	Multidisciplinary evaluation Orthodontic management preoperatively Surgical repair at approximately 3 months Bilateral deformities more likely to require repeat surgery
Velopharyngeal insufficiency Cleft lip Dental dysgenesis Occasional (5%) development of growth hormone deficiency	Hypernasal speech Difficulty feeding	Teratogen exposures Genetic syndromes	Multidisciplinary evaluation Orthodontic management preoperatively Timing of repair is controversial, but it is generally done before 12 months.
Submucosal cleft palate Velopharyngeal incompetence	N/A	N/A	N/A
Usually isolated	Abnormal speech Difficulty feeding Poor oral hygiene	N/A	Surgical repair should be reserved for breastfeeding problems, articulation problems, or dental disease.

OTHER
DIAGNOSES
TO CONSIDER

- Pierre-Robin sequence
- Orofacial digital syndrome
- Fetal alcohol syndrome
- Stickler syndrome
- Velocardiofacial syndrome
- Treacher Collins syndrome
- Goldenhar syndrome

WHEN TO
CONSIDER
FURTHER
EVALUATION
OR TREATMENT

Early evaluation and management of patients with clefts by a multidisciplinary team is paramount:

- A geneticist to evaluate for other anomalies and for genetic counseling
- A speech pathologist to assist with feeding technique early on and phonation
- An otorhinolaryngologist, with consideration of myringotomy tube placement
- An audiologist to assess conductive hearing loss due to frequent AOM
- A plastic and/or oromaxillofacial surgeon for surgical correction

If ankyloglossia appears to be causing functional problems, evaluation by a speech pathologist may help determine whether operative correction may be warranted.

SUGGESTED READINGS

Kliegman RM, Behrman RE, Jenson HB, Stanton BF. Cleft lip and palate. In: Kliegman RM, Behrman RE, Jenson HB, Stanton BF, eds. *Nelson Textbook of Pediatrics*. 18th ed. Philadelphia, PA: Saunders Elsevier; 2007: Chap 307.

Lalakea ML, Messner AH. Ankyloglossia: does it matter? *Pediatr Clin North Am*. 2003;50(2):381–397.

Moore KL, Dalley AF. *Clinical oriented anatomy*. 4th ed. Baltimore, MD: Lippincott Williams & Wilkins; 1999:929.

Morris H, Ozanne A. Phonetic, phonological, and language skills of children with a cleft palate. *Cleft Palate Craniofac J*. 2003;40(5):460–469.

Murray JC. Gene/environment causes of cleft lip and/or palate. *Clin Genet*. 2002;61:248–256.

Redford-Badwal DA, Mabry K, Frassinelli JD. Impact of cleft lip and/or palate on nutritional health and oral-motor development. *Dent Clin North Am*. 2003;47:305–317.

Shprintzen RJ, Schwartz RH, Daniller A, et al. Morphologic significance of bifid uvula. *Pediatrics*. 1985;75(3):553–561.

Tongue Discoloration and Surface Changes

APPROACH TO THE PROBLEM

The surface of the tongue may develop changes in color or texture because of intrinsic or extrinsic factors. Discolorations may be related to chewed, ingested, or topical products, or certain infections. It is important to be familiar with some of the more common benign tongue abnormalities that may present in the pediatric patient so that reassurance and appropriate guidance may be given to families.

KEY POINTS IN THE HISTORY

- Medications, such as antibiotics, antifungal agents, antimalarial drugs, psychotropic agents (including selective serotonin reuptake inhibitors), phenothiazines, benzodiazepines, and phenytoin, may cause tongue discoloration.

- Chewing betel leaf, which is common in some Southeast Asian countries, may stain the tongue red.

- Use of coffee, tea, tobacco, and cola products may cause brown discoloration of the tongue.

- Ingestion of bismuth-containing products may lead to black tongue staining.

- Hairy tongue, or elongated filiform papillae in the midline tongue, is associated with the use of tobacco, tea, coffee, antibiotics, griseofulvin, or certain mouthwashes containing an oxidizing agent, such as sodium perborate, sodium peroxide, or hydrogen peroxide.

- Immunodeficiency, recent radiation, or cytotoxic therapy predisposes patients to oral thrush and oral hairy leukoplakia. Hairy leukoplakia is seen more commonly in adults affected by human immunodeficiency virus (HIV), but is rare in children affected by HIV.

- Glossitis may be precipitated by the use of cytotoxic agents.

- Syphilis and lichen planus may be associated with white plaques on the tongue.

- The use of antibiotics, immunosuppressive agents, systemic steroids, or inhaled corticosteroids may predispose patients to oral thrush.

- Minocycline-associated pigmentary changes may persist for years.

KEY POINTS IN THE PHYSICAL EXAMINATION

- A white plaque that wipes off easily may be due to milk or food. If it cannot be scraped off easily, bleeds, or leaves a denuded surface after scraping, the white plaque is generally the result of a fungal infection.

- Oral hairy leukoplakia generally cannot be scraped off and is often located on the lateral surface of the tongue.

- A red tongue that is smooth indicates glossitis, while a red tongue with enlarged papillae is more consistent with strawberry tongue.

- The enlarged papillae of strawberry tongue may briefly persist after the redness has resolved.

- Patches of hyperpigmentation on the tongue may be a normal variant in darkly pigmented individuals.

- The raised papillae of strawberry tongue may be visualized better with indirect lighting from the side.

- A tongue with small smooth areas of denuded papillae surrounded by annular loops of normal papillae is geographic tongue.

- Median rhomboid glossitis is a reddened and smooth rhomboid-shaped area of papillary atrophy just anterior to the circumvallate papillae.

- Hairy tongue discoloration may be brown, black, green, or yellow; hence, it is no longer known as "black hairy tongue."

PHOTOGRAPHS OF SELECTED DIAGNOSES

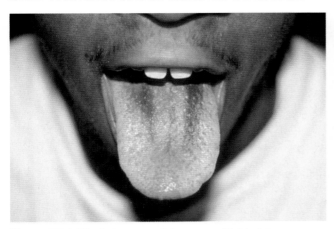

Figure 28-1 Black tongue. A teenager with black tongue staining after bismuth ingestion.
(Courtesy of Kathleen Cronan, MD.)

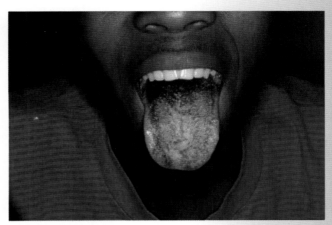

Figure 28-2 Black tongue. A teenager experiencing black tongue discoloration after exposure to bismuth.
(Courtesy of Jan Edwin Drutz, MD.)

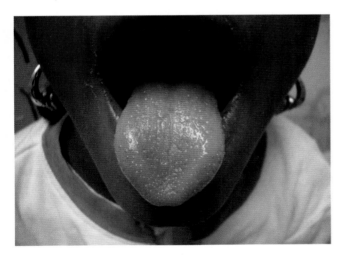

Figure 28-3 Strawberry tongue. Note the prominent fungiform papillae in this child with streptococcal pharyngitis.
(Courtesy of Paul S. Matz, MD.)

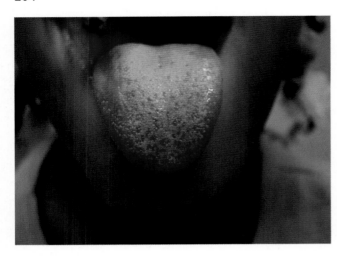

Figure 28-4 Strawberry tongue. The prominent white papillae appear like strawberry seeds in a child with streptococcal pharyngitis.
(Courtesy of Esther K. Chung, MD, MPH.)

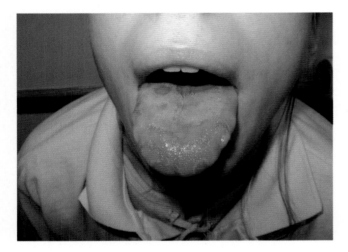

Figure 28-5 Geographic tongue. Irregular areas of denuded papillae are surrounded by normal tongue mucosa.
(Courtesy of Paul S. Matz, MD.)

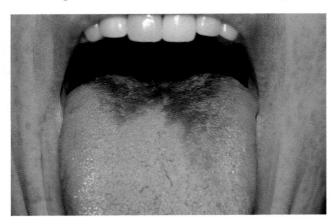

Figure 28-6 Black hairy tongue. Elongated papillae associated with black discoloration.
(Used with permission from Goodheart HP. *Goodheart's photoguide of common skin disorders.* 2nd ed. Philadelphia, PA: Lippincott Williams & Wilkins; 2003:228.)

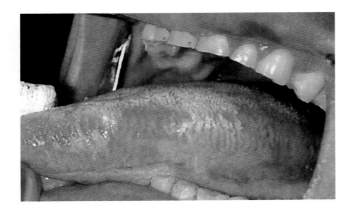

Figure 28-7 Oral hairy leukoplakia. Raised white plaques on the lateral surface of the tongue.
(Used with permission from Weber J, Kelley J. *Health assessment in nursing.* 2nd ed. Philadelphia, PA: Lippincott Williams & Wilkins; 2003:244.)

DIAGNOSIS	ICD-9	DISTINGUISHING CHARACTERISTICS	DISTRIBUTION	
Blackening from Medication	529.3	Typically black discoloration of dorsal surface without changes in size or distribution of papillae	Affects dorsal surface May affect lateral edges especially in Addison disease	
White Plaques from Thrush	112.0 771.7 (newborn candidal infection)	When scraped off the tongue, bleeds or reveals a denuded surface Mostly in infants—peak prevalence is in the fourth week of life	Localized plaques may occur throughout oral cavity	
Strawberry Tongue	529.3	Reddened dorsal surface with enlarged fungiform papillae White or yellow papillae resembling seeds on a strawberry's surface	Usually generalized and found on the anterior two thirds of the dorsal and lateral tongue surfaces	
Geographic Tongue	529.1	White areas of normal papillae surrounding reddened areas of atrophic papillae	Dorsal surface, widespread Appears to migrate across the tongue as it waxes and wanes	
Hairy Tongue	529.3	Elongated filiform papillae in the midline dorsally with a plaque of discoloration over this (the color depends on the offending agent) Discoloration is the result of chromogenic bacteria, fungi, or trapped particles underneath hyperplastic layers of keratin on the filiform papillae.	Medial aspect of dorsal surface just anterior to circumvallate papillae	

DURATION	ASSOCIATED FINDINGS	PRECIPITATING FACTORS	TREATMENT GUIDELINES
Resolves within days of discontinuation of the offending agent Some cases have prolonged staining	Staining of the dentitia	Hydroxychloroquine Crack cocaine Tobacco Linezolid Risperidone (orally disintegrating form) Chlorhexidine Terbinafine Fluconazole Activated charcoal Bismuth	Brushing the tongue, discontinuation of the offending agent
Persistent unless treated	N/A	Erythema multiforme Fifth disease Viral stomatitis Antimalarial agents Lichen planus (rare) Secondary syphilis (rare) Oral hairy leukoplakia Stevens-Johnson syndrome	Antifungal agent
Resolves along with other symptoms of underlying illness	Conjunctival erythema in Kawasaki disease and adenoviral infection Palatal petechiae in group A streptococcal pharyngitis	Streptococcal pharyngitis Adenoviral infection Kawasaki disease Toxic shock syndrome Ehrlichiosis *Yersinia pseudotuberculosis* Candy tongue Glossitis Pernicious anemia Antiepileptic drug hypersensitivity (a reaction to one of the aromatic antiepileptic drugs—phenytoin, carbamazepine, phenobarbital, and primidone)	Group A streptococcal pharyngitis requires antibiotic treatment to prevent rheumatic fever.
Hours to weeks but may wax and wane for months to years	Fissured tongue Atopic diseases Psoriasis Pain, rarely	Case reports associated with lithium treatment	Reassurance
Persists without discontinuation of offending agent	Halitosis Gagging sensation	Penicillin Oxytetracycline Chloramphenicol Olanzapine Chlortetracycline Smoking Alcohol Xerostomia Tea Coffee	Smoking cessation Brushing the tongue with a soft toothbrush

OTHER
DIAGNOSES
TO CONSIDER

- Glossitis

- Dyskeratosis congenita

- Peutz-Jeghers syndrome

- Malignant melanoma

- Addison disease

WHEN TO
CONSIDER
FURTHER
EVALUATION
OR TREATMENT

- Recurrent thrush is an indication for immunological evaluation, including HIV testing.

- Strawberry tongue is one potential finding in Kawasaki disease. A detailed history and physical examination should be performed to prove or disprove Kawasaki disease so that appropriate therapy may be initiated.

- Hairy tongue has been associated with trigeminal neuralgia. It is postulated that the pain associated with the movement or manipulation of the tongue prevents normal desquamation of the filiform papillae.

- If brushing the tongue does not successfully treat hairy tongue, other therapies such as topical 40% urea, retinoids, salicylic acid, CO_2 laser therapy, or electrodessication may be tried.

- Rare cases of painful geographic tongue may be treated with oral rinses of mucosal anesthetic solutions, such as diphenhydramine, or with topical steroid creams, with the latter being less well tolerated.

SUGGESTED READINGS

Addy M, Moran J. Mechanisms of stain formation on teeth, in particular associated with metal ions and antiseptics. Adv Dent Res. 1995;9:450.

Assimakopoulos A, Patrikakos G, Fotika C, et al. Benign migratory glossitis or geographic tongue: an enigmatic oral lesion. Am J Med. 2002;113:751–755.

Cleveland DB, Rinaggio J. Oral and maxillofacial manifestations of systemic and generalized disease. Endod Top. 2003;4:69–90.

Mirowski GW ,Waibel JS. Pigmented lesions of the oral cavity. Dermatol Ther. 2002;15:218–228.

Poulopoulos AK, Antoniades DZ, Epivatianos A, et al. Black hairy tongue in a 2-month-old infant. J Paediatr Child Health. 2008;44:377–379.

Shulman JD. Prevalence of oral mucosal lesions in children and youths in the USA. Int J Paediatr Dent. 2005;15:89–97.

NANCY D. SPECTOR

Swellings within the Mouth

APPROACH TO THE PROBLEM

A variety of swellings exist that may occur in the mouths of newborns, children, and adolescents. These swellings range from benign lesions to very serious infections. The incidence and prevalence of many of the benign lesions are unknown. The more serious swellings of the mouth are secondary to bacterial infections of the deep soft tissues of the mouth and the pharynx. These more serious entities may be distinguished from benign lesions by the presence of systemic signs of illness. Peritonsillar abscess and Ludwig's angina have potentially life-threatening complications.

KEY POINTS IN THE HISTORY

- Bohn nodules and Epstein pearls are present in newborns (see Chapter 25).
- Mucoceles and ranulas arise acutely and rupture spontaneously.
- Mucoceles and ranulas are painless and asymptomatic.
- Systemic signs of infection, such as fever and throat pain, help differentiate benign swellings of the mouth from more serious infections.
- Peritonsillar abscess is generally preceded by acute tonsillopharyngitis.
- Patients with Ludwig angina have a history of high fever and an inability to handle their secretions.

KEY POINTS IN THE PHYSICAL EXAMINATION

- Epstein pearls are smooth, translucent, pearly white, 1- to 3-mm cysts on the palate at the roof of the mouth. When such lesions occur on the gums, they are referred to as Bohn nodules.

- Mucoceles and ranulas are nontender, mobile, glistening, and have a bluish hue.

- Mucoceles are most common on the lower lip.

- Ranulas are found on the floor of the mouth.

- Peritonsillar abscess is characterized by swelling of tissues lateral and superior to the affected tonsil, anterior and medial displacement of the affected tonsil, and displacement of the uvula toward the contralateral side.

- Patients with peritonsillar abscess have a muffled, or "hot potato," voice.

- Ludwig angina always has bilateral involvement of the submandibular spaces.

- Ludwig angina is characterized by tongue elevation and an inability to depress the tongue.

- Trismus, or difficulty in opening the mouth, is a frequent finding in patients with peritonsillar abscess and Ludwig angina.

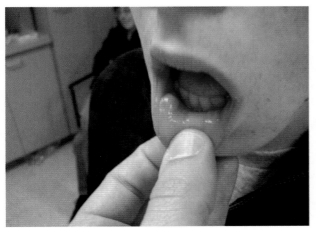

Figure 29-1 Mucocele. Fluid-filled pseudocyst protruding from lower lip.
(Courtesy of Paul S. Matz, MD.)

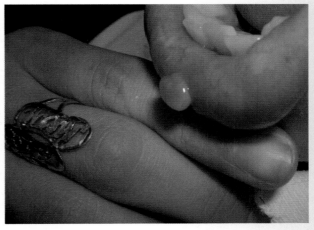

Figure 29-2 Mucocele. Fluid-filled pseudocyst protruding from lower lip.
(Courtesy of Michael Lemper, DDS.)

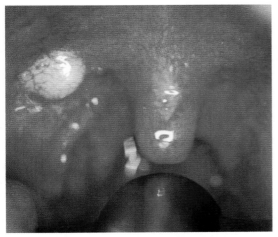

Figure 29-3 Mucocele of soft palate. Whitish pseudocyst on the right side of the soft palate.
(Used with permission from Handler SD, Myer CM. *Atlas of ear, nose and throat disorders in Children.* Ontario: BC Decker; 1998:85.)

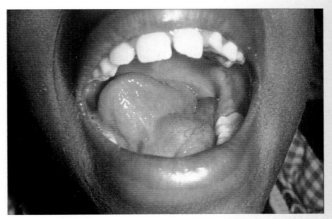

Figure 29-4 Ranula. Fluid-filled mass on the floor of the mouth.
(Courtesy of Kathleen Cronan, MD.)

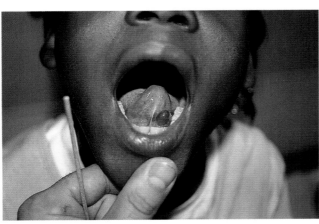

Figure 29-5 Ranula. Fluid-filled cyst on the base of the tongue.
(Courtesy of George A. Datto, III, MD.)

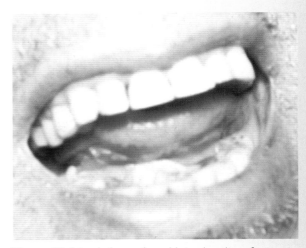

Figure 29-6 Ludwig angina. Note elevation of tongue secondary to swelling of the floor of the mouth.
(Used with permission from Greenberg MI. *Greenberg's atlas of emergency medicine.* Philadelphia, PA: Lippincott Williams & Wilkins; 2005:7.)

DIFFERENTIAL DIAGNOSIS

DIAGNOSIS	ICD-9	DISTINGUISHING CHARACTERISTICS	DISTRIBUTION	DURATION/ CHRONICITY
Mucocele	527.6	Pseudocyst resulting from mucus extravasation into the surrounding tissues Minor salivary gland in origin Acute onset of painless, asymptomatic swelling May fluctuate in size May rupture spontaneously	Most commonly on the lower lip Less commonly on the upper lip, palate, buccal mucosa, tongue, or the floor of the mouth	Recurrence rate of 14% Can be present for weeks to months before rupture
Ranula	527.6	Pseudocyst resulting from mucus extravasation into the surrounding tissues Most arise from sublingual gland Nontender, mobile, glistening, broad-based enlargement Bluish hue May fluctuate in size May rupture spontaneously	Floor of the mouth	Recurrence rate of 14% May be present for weeks to months before rupture
Peritonsillar Abscess (see Chapter 30)	475	Throat pain, fever, dysphagia, "hot potato voice," and drooling Occurrence of trismus in 63% of cases Tonsils are erythematous, enlarged, and covered with exudate.	Swelling of the tissues lateral and superior to the tonsil with medial and anterior displacement of the tonsil	Develops over several days after acute tonsillopharyngitis Recurrence rate of 6–36%
Ludwig Angina	528.3	Acute life-threatening cellulitis Trismus, high fever, halitosis, unable to handle secretions Feels woody on palpation Unable to depress tongue Caused by gingival bacteria (anaerobic streptococci, bacteroides species, fusobacteria, and spirochetes)	Bilateral involvement of the submandibular spaces	Develops over several days

ASSOCIATED FINDINGS	COMPLICATIONS	PREDISPOSING FACTORS	TREATMENT GUIDELINES
None	None	Trauma to the salivary gland and excretory duct Obstruction to salivary gland duct flow Trauma to salivary glandular parenchymal cells	No intervention is required
None	Large ranulas—may interfere with speech, swallowing, or respiration	Trauma to the salivary gland excretory duct Obstruction to salivary gland duct flow Trauma to salivary glandular parenchymal cells	Generally, no intervention is required. Consider consultation with otolaryngology for ranulas that interfere with speech, swallowing, or respiration.
Tender cervical adenopathy	Airway compromise Aspiration, if spontaneous rupture of abscess Spread of infection resulting in retropharyngeal abscess, parapharyngeal abscess, mediastinitis Septic thrombi leading to osteomyelitis, meningitis, or brain abscess	Acute tonsillopharyngitis	Antibiotics Pain management Consider hospitalization. Consider consultation with otolaryngology for possible drainage.
Overlying skin erythema, pitting edema, and tenderness	Spread of infection resulting in mediastinitis Laryngeal or subglottic edema Respiratory distress Difficult intubation	Poor oral hygiene Dental extractions Sialadenitis	Immediate hospitalization, evaluation for airway compromise, antibiotics, consultation with otolaryngology

OTHER
DIAGNOSES
TO CONSIDER

- Hemangioma

- Lymphangioma

- Fibroma

- Parulis (gum abscess)

WHEN TO
CONSIDER
FURTHER
EVALUATION
OR TREATMENT

- Most mucoceles and ranulas will rupture spontaneously and will not require further intervention.

- Large ranulas that interfere with speech, swallowing, or respiration should be referred for evaluation by otolaryngology.

- Peritonsillar abscesses require antibiotic administration and pain management.

- A peritonsillar abscess is a condition that usually requires hospitalization and consultation with otolaryngology for possible abscess drainage.

- Ludwig angina is a life-threatening condition and requires immediate hospitalization, evaluation for airway compromise, intravenous antibiotics, and evaluation by otolaryngology.

SUGGESTED READINGS

Bluestone CD, Casselbrant ML, Stool SE, et al., eds. *Pediatric otolaryngology*. 4th ed. Philadelphia: WB Saunders; 2003:1261, 1272, 1688–1699.
Delaney, J, Keels MA. Pediatric oral pathology. *Pediatr Clin North Am*. 2000;47(5):1125–1147.
Greenberg MI. *Greenberg's atlas of emergency medicine*. Philadelphia: Lippincott Williams & Wilkins; 2005:7.
Handler SD, Myer CM. *Atlas of ear, nose and throat disorders in children*. Ontario: BC Decker; 1998:85.
Krol DM, Keels MA. Oral conditions. *Pediatr Rev*. 2007;28:15–22.
Patel NJ, Sciubba J. Oral lesions in young children. *Pediatr Clin North Am*. 2003;50:469–486.
Pinkham JR, Casamassimo PS, McTigue DJ et al., eds. *Pediatric dentistry: infancy through adolescence*. 4th ed. St. Louis: Elsevier Science; 2005:9–60.
Wetmore RF, Muntz HR, McGill TJ, eds. *Pediatric otolaryngology: principles and practice pathways*. New York: Thieme Medical Publishers; 2000:555–614.

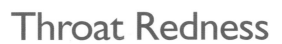

ROBERT L. BONNER, JR.

Throat Redness

APPROACH TO THE PROBLEM

Erythema of the posterior oropharynx suggests an inflammatory process, most commonly caused by infection. In most cases, the inflammation may be attributed to viral pharyngitis. Bacterial pharyngitis from group A beta-hemolytic streptococcus is very common in school-aged children. These disorders may present with or without exudates. Obtaining a throat culture is important when considering the diagnosis of strep throat or scarlet fever. Noninfectious causes of pharyngeal erythema are rare, but they should be considered in patients with a prolonged course or with treatment failure.

KEY POINTS IN THE HISTORY

- Throat redness associated with upper respiratory tract symptoms such as rhinorrhea, cough, and conjunctivitis is characteristic of a viral infection and rarely represents a bacterial infection.

- Throat redness in association with conjunctivitis, otitis media, or both suggests infection with adenovirus.

- Infectious mononucleosis—Epstein-Barr virus (EBV) infection—should be considered in adolescents with fever, throat pain, swollen lymph nodes, and significant fatigue.

- Streptococcal pharyngitis, which peaks in the late winter and early spring, presents with a sudden onset of pain, fever, and redness in the throat.

- Children younger than 3 years of age with throat redness and exudates are less likely to have a streptococcal infection.

- Throat redness with progressive unilateral throat pain and dysphagia may suggest a peritonsillar abscess.

- Children with pharyngitis may complain of neck pain and stiffness.

| 215

KEY POINTS IN THE PHYSICAL EXAMINATION

- Severe viral pharyngitis and streptococcal pharyngitis may be clinically indistinguishable, because both may present with fever, pharyngeal erythema, and cervical lymphadenopathy.

- Infectious mononucleosis may present with pharyngeal and tonsillar erythema, fever, and posterior cervical lymphadenopathy.

- Children with a peritonsillar abscess may have pharyngeal erythema accompanied by unilateral tonsillar hypertrophy, uvular deviation toward the unaffected side, fever, and trismus. In addition, they typically have a "hot potato" voice.

- Ulcerations are typically seen with viral pharyngitis and stomatitis. Ulcerations on the tonsillar pillars suggest the diagnosis of herpangina, typically caused by coxsackievirus.

- Drooling occurs from the inability to swallow one's secretions, and it typically occurs as a result of pain. Drooling may be seen with severe pharyngitis, pharyngeal ulceration, and retropharyngeal abscess.

- Sitting in a tripod position, inspiratory stridor, difficulty breathing, and dehydration are findings that may accompany pharyngeal erythema and require prompt attention and evaluation to rule out epiglottitis.

- Retropharyngeal cellulitis/abscess should be considered in an ill-appearing, young child with pharyngeal erythema and drooling.

PHOTOGRAPHS OF SELECTED DIAGNOSES

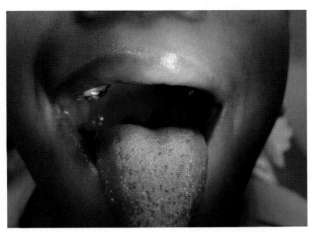

Figure 30-1 Group A streptococcal pharyngitis. Note the marked erythema posteriorly in this patient with scarlet fever. (Courtesy of Esther K. Chung, MD, MPH.)

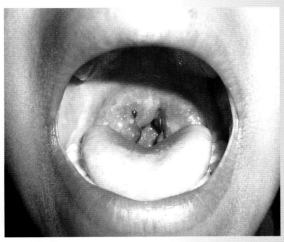

Figure 30-2 Viral pharyngitis. Mild erythema and erythematous papules on both tonsils. (Courtesy of Paul S. Matz, MD.)

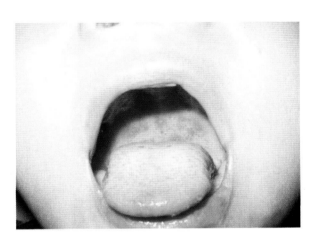

Figure 30-3 Herpangina. Erythematous papules and vesicles on the posterior pharynx. (Courtesy of Philip Siu, MD.)

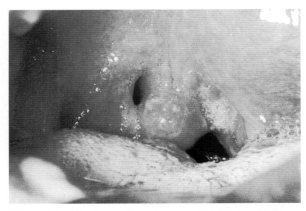

Figure 30-4 Peritonsillar abscess of the left tonsil.
(Used with permission from Handler SD, Myer CM. *Atlas of ear, nose and throat disorders in children.* Ontario: BC Decker; 1998:90.)

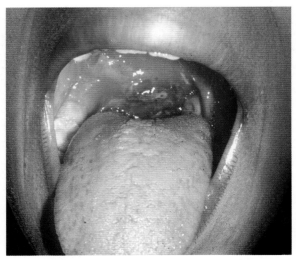

Figure 30-5 Peritonsillar abscess of the right tonsil.
Note the swelling and distortion of the area around the right tonsil.
(Courtesy of the late Peter Sol, MD.)

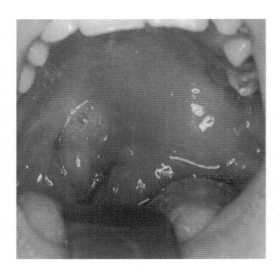

Figure 30-6 Peritonsillar abscess. Note the erythema and swelling on the left and the right deviation of the uvula.
(Courtesy of Seth Zwillenberg, MD.)

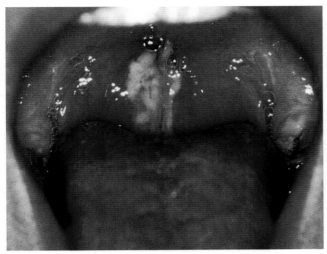

Figure 30-7 Acute tonsillitis secondary to infectious mononucleosis. Note the marked tonsillar enlargement with erythema and the large white-gray patches.
(Used with permission from Handler SD, Myer CM. *Atlas of ear, nose and throat disorders in children.* Ontario: BC Decker; 1998:91.)

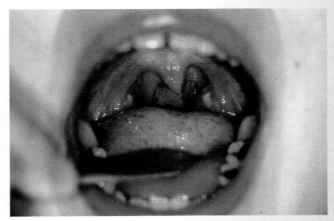

Figure 30-8 Acute tonsillar inflammation due to infectious mononucleosis. Note the tonsillar enlargement with erythema and white exudates.
(Courtesy of the late Peter Sol, MD.)

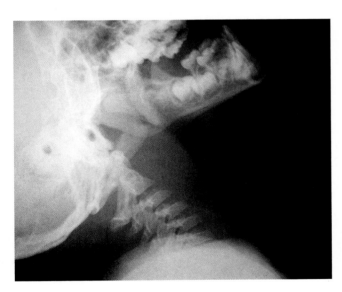

Figure 30-9 Retropharyngeal abscess. Neck extension radiograph showing a retropharyngeal space wider than the cervical vertebral bodies.
(Courtesy of Paul S. Matz, MD.)

DIAGNOSIS	ICD-9	DISTINGUISHING CHARACTERISTICS	DISTRIBUTION
Streptococcal Pharyngitis	034.0	Posterior pharyngeal erythema Palatal petechiae Tonsillar enlargement Erythema	Posterior oropharynx
Viral Pharyngitis	462.0	Mild to severe pharyngeal erythema Vesicles or ulcers	Posterior oropharynx
Herpangina	074.0	Discrete erythematous ulcers Painful gray ulcers on an erythematous base	Posterior oropharynx
Infectious Mononucleosis	075	Pharyngeal and tonsillar erythema	Posterior oropharynx
Peritonsillar Abscess	475.0	Unilateral tonsillar enlargement Uvular deviation	Tonsils

ASSOCIATED FINDINGS	COMPLICATIONS	PRECIPITATING FACTORS	TREATMENT GUIDELINES
Fever Throat pain Cervical lymphadenopathy Abdominal pain	Rheumatic fever Glomerulonephritis Cervical adenitis Peritonsillar and retropharyngeal abscesses	Exposure to *Streptococcus pyogenes*	Oral penicillin or amoxicillin for 10 days
Cough Coryza Conjunctivitis Hand and foot papulovesicles in hand-foot-and-mouth disease	None	Exposure to precipitating virus	Supportive care Topical or oral analgesics
Fever Headache Malaise	None	Exposure to coxsackievirus A	Supportive care Topical or oral analgesics
Fever Fatigue Cervical lymphadenopathy	Splenomegaly Hepatomegaly Jaundice Splenic rupture Guillain-Barré syndrome Myocarditis Arthritis Meningoencephalitis	Exposure to EBV	Supportive care Oral steroids if respiratory compromise from tonsillar obstruction
Fever Trismus "Hot potato" voice	Cellulitis	Streptococcal pharyngitis	Oral antibiotic therapy Incision and drainage of abscess

OTHER DIAGNOSES TO CONSIDER

- Pharyngitis resulting from *Neisseria gonorrhoeae*

- Diphtheria

- Pharyngitis resulting from *Mycoplasma pneumoniae*

WHEN TO CONSIDER FURTHER EVALUATION OR TREATMENT

- Patients with persistent streptococcal pharyngitis after 48 hours of appropriate antimicrobial therapy should be seen to rule out suppurative complications. Broad-spectrum antibiotics should be considered.

- Viral pharyngitis and herpangina require repeat evaluation if the symptoms persist more than 10 days.

- Urgent evaluation of infectious mononucleosis and treatment with corticosteroids are warranted if signs of airway obstruction develop.

- Symptoms, such as jaundice, irritability, mental status change, chest pain, or limp, may indicate the development of complications of mononucleosis.

- A peritonsillar abscess or cellulitis requires emergent otolaryngologic evaluation. Patients may require incision and drainage and parenteral antibiotics.

SUGGESTED READINGS

Attia MW, Bennett JE. Pediatric pharyngitis. *Pediatr Case Rev.* 2003;3(4):203–210.

Bisno AL. Acute pharyngitis. *N Engl J Med.* 2001;344(3):205–211.

Feldman WE. Pharyngitis in children. *Postgrad Med.* 1993;93(3):141–145.

Handler SD, Myer CM. *Atlas of ear, nose and throat disorders in children.* Ontario, Canada: BC Decker; 1998:90–91.

McCracken GH. Diagnosis and management of children with streptococcal pharyngitis. *Pediatr Infect Dis J.* 1986;5(6):754–759.

Steyer TE. Peritonsillar abscess: diagnosis and treatment. *Am Fam Physician.* 2002;65(1):93–96.

Vincent MT, Celestin N, Hussain AN. Pharyngitis. *Am Fam Physician.* 2004;69(6):1465–1470.

Section

EIGHT

Neck

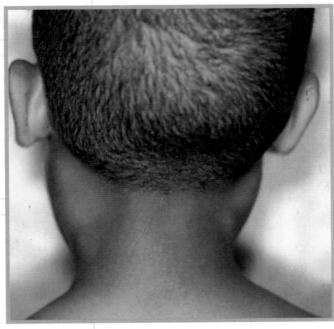

(Courtesy of Ellen Deutsch, MD.)

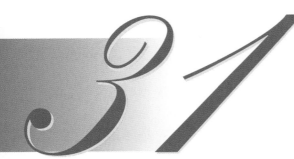

SERENA YANG

Neck Masses and Swelling

APPROACH TO THE PROBLEM

The major causes of childhood neck masses, the majority of which are benign, may be categorized as congenital, inflammatory, neoplastic, and trauma-related. Many neck masses represent cervical adenopathy or adenitis. To determine the etiology of a neck mass, it is helpful to determine whether the swelling is acute versus chronic, unilateral versus bilateral, or associated with focal versus generalized lymphadenopathy. Although malignancies are uncommon, one should be able to recognize the signs and symptoms of these lesions so that an early diagnosis may be made.

KEY POINTS IN THE HISTORY

- A history of a painless mass noted at birth or shortly after birth suggests a congenital etiology.

- Acute onset of erythema, tenderness, and rapid progression in size suggests an inflammatory etiology, particularly when these symptoms are in association with an upper respiratory tract infection.

- More than 90% of patients with cat scratch disease have a history of contact with a cat, and up to 75% of patients have a history of being scratched by a cat. Three to ten days after inoculation, 60% to 93% of patients develop a vesicle or pustule at the inoculation site that may persist for days to months. Cervical lymphadenopathy typically appears proximal to the inoculation site 2 to 4 weeks later.

- Malignant masses are typically firm and painless, and they may be associated with systemic symptoms such as weight loss.

- When a malignancy is suspected, the patient's age is an important factor when considering the differential diagnosis. Those younger than 6 years presenting with neck swelling are at greatest risk for neuroblastoma; those aged 7 to 12 years, for Hodgkin and non-Hodgkin lymphomas; and those who are adolescents, for Hodgkin lymphoma.

KEY POINTS IN THE PHYSICAL EXAMINATION

- The majority of branchial cleft sinuses and cysts present laterally, along the anterior border of the sternocleidomastoid muscle.

- Thyroglossal duct cysts usually are midline at or next to the hyoid bone. Rarely, they may be sublingual or suprasternal.

- Dermoid cysts, which contain sebaceous material, are also found in the midline. Compared to thyroglossal duct cysts, they are more superficial. In addition, they typically do not have connections to the hyoid bone or tongue.

- Congenital torticollis is associated with a hard fibrotic mass in the sternocleidomastoid muscle that may be detected at 2 to 8 weeks of life.

- Cystic hygromas are soft, mobile, nontender, cystic masses usually found in the posterior triangle of the neck, and they transilluminate when a light source is applied.

- Hemangiomas are soft, mobile, painless masses that are initially bluish to fiery-red, and then they turn gray during the involution phase.

- In children, palpable cervical lymph nodes less than 1 cm may be normal. In infants, palpable nodes are rare, and the possibility of an underlying disease should be considered.

- The chronic cervical lymphadenitis caused by *Mycoplasma tuberculosis* (often associated with fluctuance, a draining sinus, and/or supraclavicular adenopathy) usually represents an extension of primary pulmonary disease.

- The most common site of inoculation for cat scratch disease is the upper extremity, resulting in epitrochlear or axillary adenopathy, or both.

- Any of the following should raise suspicion for malignancy: overlying skin ulceration; supraclavicular adenopathy; and a nontender, fixed, rubbery cervical mass greater than 3 cm.

PHOTOGRAPHS OF SELECTED DIAGNOSES

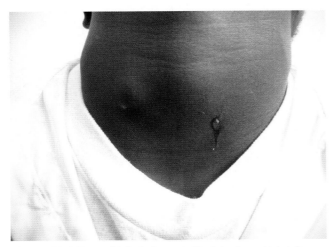

Figure 31-1 Branchial cleft cyst. Draining branchial cleft sinus.
(Courtesy of Paul S. Matz, MD.)

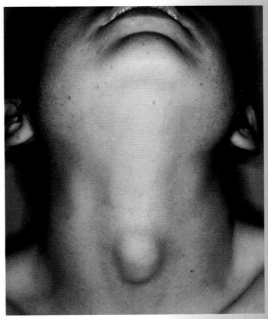

Figure 31-2 Thyroglossal duct cyst. A midline cervical mass presenting in a 6-year-old child.
(Used with permission from Snell RS. *Clinical anatomy*, 7th ed. Baltimore, MD: Lippincott Williams & Wilkins; 2005:CD418.)

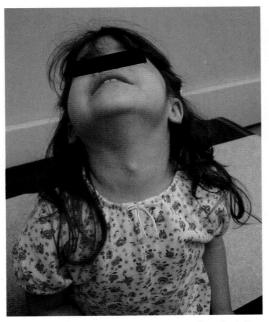

Figure 31-3 Dermoid cyst. A mass found midline overlying the hyoid bone in a 4-year-old child.
(Courtesy of Mary L. Brandt, MD.)

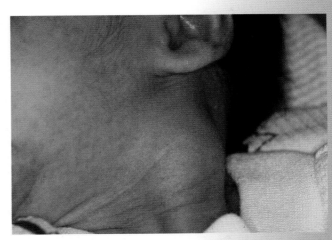

Figure 31-4 Congenital torticollis. A fibrotic mass located in the sternocleidomastoid muscle of a 1-month-old infant whose mother was concerned about the infant's head tilt to one side.
(Courtesy of Ellen Deutsch, MD.)

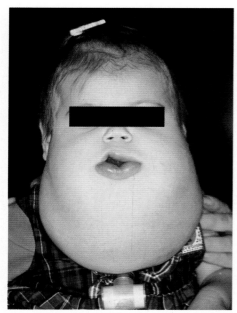

Figure 31-5 Cystic hygroma. A large, soft cervical mass in a 9-month-old infant. Tracheostomy was placed at birth.
(Courtesy of Ellen Deutsch, MD.)

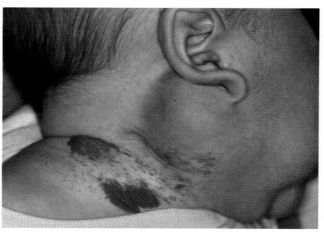

Figure 31-6 Hemangioma. A soft, nontender mass with bluish as well as bright-red aspects of color presents in this 1-month-old infant.
(Courtesy of Ellen Deutsch, MD.)

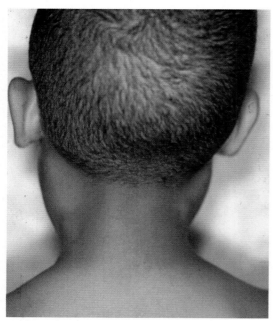

Figure 31-7 Cervical adenopathy. A posterior view of bilateral adenopathy in a 7-year-old male with a 1- to 2-week history of malaise, sore throat, and low-grade fevers.
(Courtesy of Ellen Deutsch, MD.)

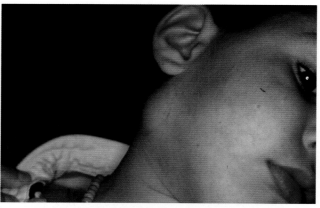

Figure 31-8 Cervical adenitis. This case of acute unilateral adenitis in this 3-year-old child is most likely caused by *Staphylococcus aureus* or group A streptococcus.
(Courtesy of Jan Edwin Drutz, MD.)

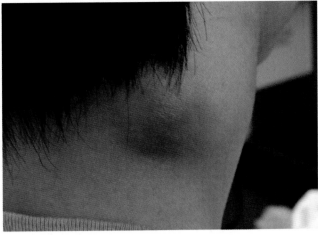

Figure 31-9 Tuberculous adenitis. Note the erythematous swelling in this 13-year-old recent immigrant from southeast Asia who presented with bilateral posterior cervical neck masses. (Courtesy of Esther K. Chung, MD, MPH.)

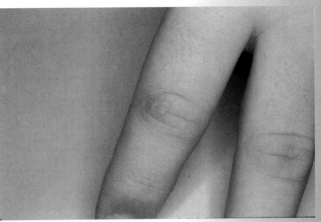

Figure 31-10 Cat scratch inoculation site on the extremity of a 9-year-old child. (Courtesy of Mark A. Ward, MD.)

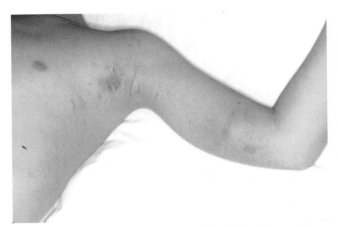

Figure 31-11 Cat scratch adenopathy. Epitrochlear and axillary adenopathy that developed proximal to the inoculation site on the finger shown in the previous photo. (Courtesy of Mark A. Ward, MD.)

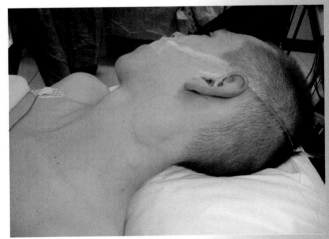

Figure 31-12 Hodgkin lymphoma. Large, fixed cervical masses in a 14-year-old adolescent with weight loss. (Courtesy of Mary L. Brandt, MD.)

DIAGNOSIS	ICD-9	DISTINGUISHING CHARACTERISTICS	ASSOCIATED FINDINGS
Congenital			
Branchial Cleft Cyst	744.42	Most originate from second branchial cleft. May be an associated fistula in the mid-to-lower anterior border of the sternocleidomastoid muscle Cyst forms when a fistula becomes occluded.	Recurrent cyst Infection
Thyroglossal Duct Cyst	759.2	Most common congenital neck mass Commonly presents after age 2, when infected, and drains externally Located anywhere along line of descent of the thyroid (midline or next to the hyoid bone)	Ectopic thyroid tissue Papillary adenocarcinoma
Dermoid Cyst	229.9	Contains sebaceous material Soft, mobile, nontender, superficial mass Can be found midline over the hyoid bone and confused with a thyroglossal duct cyst	Infection Malignancy is rare.
Congenital Torticollis	754.1	Noted at 2–8 weeks of age when head tilts toward affected side Fibrotic mass associated with shortening of the sternocleidomastoid muscle May be associated with a difficult delivery	Congenital hip dislocation Tibial torsion
Cystic Hygroma	228.1	Twice the likelihood of presenting on left side of neck because the thoracic duct enters the left subclavian vein on this side Soft, mobile, nontender, cystic mass associated with gradual or rapid enlargement and compression of surrounding structures Most commonly in posterior triangle of neck Transilluminates when light source applied Spontaneous resolution is rare.	When infected, may become warm, erythematous, and tender
Hemangioma	228.01	Most common head and neck lesion detected during early infancy Soft, mobile, nontender, bluish to fiery-red color turning to gray or beige during involution phase Proliferates during first year of life, then regresses over the next 3–4 years (80% resolve by age 5)	Hemangiomatosis Internal hemangiomas
Inflammatory			
Cervical Adenopathy	785.6	In children, palpable cervical lymph nodes <1 cm are typically benign. In infants, palpable nodes are rare and should raise suspicion for an underlying disease.	When recurrent, consider chronic granulomatous disease. When associated with supraclavicular adenopathy, consider malignancy.
Cervical Adenitis	683	Tenderness Erythema Swelling Warmth May be associated with fever	Acute bilateral adenitis is most often due to viruses that infect the upper respiratory tract. Acute unilateral adenitis is most often caused by *S. aureus* and group A streptococcus. Chronic adenitis is associated with EBV, CMV, mycobacteria, and *Bartonella henselae*.
Mycobacterial Cervical Adenitis	031.8	A chronic, suppurative adenitis that may develop a draining sinus Tuberculous mycobacterial infection presents in school-aged children and adolescents via person-to-person spread Nontuberculous mycobacterial infection presents in those aged <5 years; no definitive person-to-person spread	Tuberculous mycobacteria: supraclavicular nodes, pulmonary infection Nontuberculous mycobacteria: no systemic symptoms (unless immunocompromised)
Cat Scratch Disease	078.3	Caused by *B. henselae* Chronic, tender adenitis that forms 2–4 weeks after inoculation Papule often found at inoculation site	Mild constitutional symptoms Suppuration Parinaud oculoglandular syndrome (resulting from conjunctival inoculation by rubbing eye after handling cat)
Neoplastic			
Lymphoma	202.81	Hodgkin and non-Hodgkin lymphoma are the most common types of tumor found in the neck for children aged 7–12 years. Hodgkin lymphoma is the most common tumor in the neck for adolescents. Unilateral clusters of firm, fixed, rubbery, nontender masses	Non-Hodgkin: extranodal involvement (i.e., bone marrow, CNS) common Hodgkin: systemic signs and symptoms (e.g., anorexia, fever) common

COMPLICATIONS	PREDISPOSING FACTORS	TREATMENT GUIDELINES
Recurrence rate following resection: 7%	N/A	Antibiotics if infected Surgical resection of fistula and cyst
Recurrence rate after resection: <10% Previous infection or incomplete excision are risk factors for recurrence.	N/A	Incision and drainage and antibiotics if infected Surgical resection of cyst, cylinder of tissue above cyst, and central portion of hyoid bone
N/A	N/A	Surgical resection
Facial hemihypoplasia	N/A	Passive range of motion exercises Physical therapy Surgery if facial hemihypoplasia
Airway compromise Dysphagia Failure to thrive	Rapid enlargement resulting from infection, trauma, or hemorrhage into lesion	Surgical resection, sclerotherapy, or observation
Airway obstruction Hemorrhage Thrombocytopenia Congestive heart failure Infection Ulceration Necrosis Kasabach-Merritt syndrome (consumptive coagulopathy) Visual impairment	Female:male prevalence ratio (3:1)	Observation If associated with complications, treatment options include corticosteroids (first line), interferon, chemotherapy, radiation, excision, and cryotherapy.
N/A	Upper respiratory tract infections Epstein-Barr virus (EBV) Cytomegalovirus (CMV) Human immunodeficiency virus (HIV)	Dependent on etiology
N/A	At 3–7 weeks of age, males are at greater risk of cervical adenitis due to late-onset group B streptococcal infection.	Select antibiotics based on patient's age, clinical status, and the epidemiology of local microbiology and antibiotic resistance patterns.
Scarring Otomastoiditis Sinusitis	Contact with persons from endemic areas Foreign-born from endemic areas Contact with persons infected with tuberculosis, HIV, or a history of IV drug abuse and/or incarceration Indigent or homeless	Tuberculous mycobacteria: anti-TB medication (compliance should be ensured to reduce the risk of development of multidrug resistant TB). Nontuberculous mycobacteria: surgical excision, antibiotic therapy
Dysphagia Encephalopathy Retinopathy Hemolytic anemia Thrombocytopenic purpura	A history of cat exposure is common but not always present.	Spontaneously resolves in 2–4 months Antipyretics and analgesics Antibiotics for severe or systemic disease Aspiration if tense, painful, suppurative node
Airway obstruction Superior vena cava syndrome Horner syndrome	Male:female prevalence ratio (3:1)	Chemotherapy Radiation

OTHER
DIAGNOSES
TO CONSIDER

- Toxoplasmosis

- Kawasaki disease

- Graves disease

- Hashimoto thyroiditis

- Pyriform sinuses and cysts

- Leukemia

- Rhabdomyosarcoma

- Hematoma

WHEN TO
CONSIDER
FURTHER
EVALUATION
OR TREATMENT

- Infected thyroglossal duct cysts initially are treated with incision and drainage and antibiotics, prior to surgical correction.

- If congenital torticollis is associated with facial hemihypoplasia, surgical intervention should be considered.

- Treatment should be considered for hemangiomas that block the airway, visual axis, or auditory canals; and for those that are ulcerated, bleeding, or associated with congestive heart failure.

SUGGESTED READINGS

Brown RL, Azizkhan RG. Pediatric head and neck lesions. *Pediatr Clin North Am.* 1998;45(4):889–905.

Friedmann AM. Evaluation and management of lymphadenopathy in children. *Pediatr Rev.* 2008;29(2):53–60.

Gampper TJ, Morgan RF. Vascular anomalies: hemangiomas. *Plast Reconstr Surg.* 2002;110(2):572–585.

Gross E, Sichel JY. Congenital neck lesions. *Surg Clin North Am.* 2006;86(2):383–392.

Peters TR, Edwards KM. Cervical lymphadenopathy and adenitis. *Pediatr Rev.* 2000;21(12):399–405.

Stechenberg BW. Cat scratch disease. In: Kliegman RM, Behrman RE, Jensen HB, Stanton BF, eds. *Nelson textbook of pediatrics.* 18th ed. Philadelphia, PA: WB Saunders; 2007:1219–1222.

Velez MC. Consultation with the specialist: lymphomas. *Pediatr Rev.* 2003;24(11):380–386.

Section

NINE

Chest

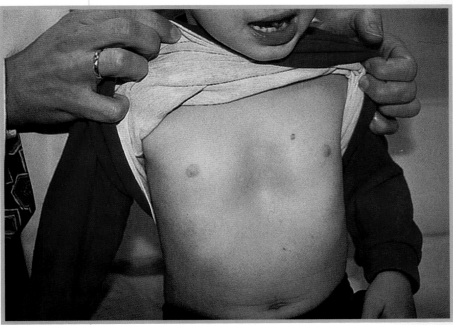

(Courtesy of George A. Datto, III, MD.)

Abnormal Chest Shape

APPROACH TO THE PROBLEM

Several elements contribute to chest shape, including muscles, bones (ribs, sternum, clavicles, and spine), and underlying organs. Deficiency, hypertrophy, or malformation of any of these structures may produce abnormalities in the appearance of the chest wall. Abnormalities in lung form or function may cause changes in the chest shape; conversely, alterations in the size or shape of the thorax may significantly affect pulmonary function. Rarely, chronic cardiac enlargement may produce a prominence in the precordial chest wall. Pectus excavatum is the most common pediatric chest wall deformity; most of the others are quite rare.

KEY POINTS IN THE HISTORY

- Pectus excavatum and pectus carinatum are more common in males.
- Family history is often positive in patients with pectus excavatum.
- Asymmetry in the immediate neonatal period may be the result of intrauterine compression.
- Children who have symptoms of severe exercise intolerance with abnormal chest shape may have underlying pulmonary or cardiac disease.

KEY POINTS IN THE PHYSICAL EXAMINATION

- Tall stature, arachnodactyly, and joint laxity suggest Marfan syndrome in patients with pectus excavatum or pectus carinatum.
- Syndactyly and brachydactyly are associated with Poland syndrome.
- Short stature and webbed neck with shield chest (broad, with widely spaced nipples) may be seen in Turner or Noonan syndrome. Patients with Noonan syndrome also may have pectus excavatum or pectus carinatum.
- Narrow shoulders with various anomalies of the clavicles and upper extremities occur in Holt-Oram syndrome (which is also associated with cardiac and sternal defects) and cleidocranial dysplasia (in which delays in fontanel closure and tooth eruption also may be seen).
- A narrow or bell-shaped thorax is associated with many osteochondrodysplasias, such as achondroplasia, cleidocranial dysplasia, and Jeune thoracic dystrophy. It may also be seen in patients with neuromuscular disorders.
- Skin overlying a sternal cleft may be thin, scarlike, and hyperpigmented.

DIFFERENTIAL DIAGNOSIS

DIAGNOSIS	ICD-9	DISTINGUISHING CHARACTERISTICS	ASSOCIATED FINDINGS
Pectus Excavatum	754.81	Sternal depression Sternum may rotate to right, making right-sided structures smaller Deformity worsens during puberty	Increased incidence of scoliosis, congenital heart disease May be associated with Marfan syndrome, homocystinuria, Noonan syndrome, and other genetic disorders
Pectus Carinatum	754.82	Sternal protrusion Generally noted later in childhood than pectus excavatum	As for pectus excavatum
Barrel Chest	738.3	Anteroposterior diameter of chest increased relative to transverse diameter. (Normal ratio is 1:1 in infancy, with transverse diameter increasing with age.)	Digital clubbing
Shield Chest	754.89	Wide chest with broadly spaced nipples	Turner syndrome Noonan syndrome
Poland Sequence	756.81	Unilateral deficiency of pectoralis muscles and breast structures Usually right-sided	May also have rib defects Ipsilateral syndactyly of hand
Sternal Cleft	756.3	Complete or partial separation of sternum May manifest as U-shaped or V-shaped depression, or with bulge from underlying structures May change with respiration Pulsations of heart may be visible. If there is overlying skin, it is often thin and hyperpigmented.	Usually an isolated anomaly Ectopia cordis Pentalogy of Cantrell Facial hemangiomas Cleft lip or palate
Cleidocranial Dysplasia	755.59	Absent or hypoplastic clavicles resulting in abnormal shoulder movement Narrow thorax	Variety of other skeletal anomalies Delayed closure of sutures and anterior fontanel Abnormal teeth Delayed tooth eruption Deafness

COMPLICATIONS	PREDISPOSING FACTORS	TREATMENT GUIDELINES
Rarely interferes with cardiac or respiratory function, though some children have exercise limitations May be a significant cosmetic problem Can give false appearance of cardiomegaly on chest x-ray	Excessive growth of costal cartilage Male:female prevalence ratio 3:1	Treatment is often not necessary. Surgical correction may have psychological benefits. Physiological benefits of surgery are controversial.
Rarely interferes with cardiac or respiratory function, though some children have exercise limitations May be a significant cosmetic problem	Excessive growth of costal cartilage More common in males	Treatment is often not necessary. Surgical correction may have psychological benefits. Physiological benefits of surgery are controversial.
According to underlying cause	Severe asthma or other obstructive lung disease (e.g., meconium aspiration syndrome) Genetic disorders such as spondyloepiphyseal dysplasia, Smith-McCort dysplasia, Costello syndrome	Address underlying cause if possible.
According to underlying cause	N/A	N/A
Respiratory problems when significant rib defects are present Breast tissue also is typically absent on affected side	Male:female prevalence ratio 3:1 Abnormal blood flow through subclavian artery	Breast reconstruction may be considered, particularly for females.
None (unless associated defects)	None	Surgical repair in infancy
Respiratory problems in infancy	Autosomal dominant inheritance	Extensive dental work often necessary Evaluate for hearing loss

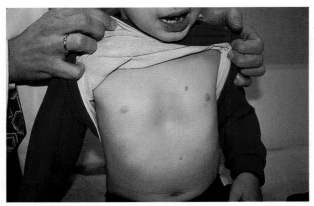

Figure 32-1 Pectus excavatum. Anterior view of child with pectus excavatum.
(Courtesy of George A. Datto, III, MD.)

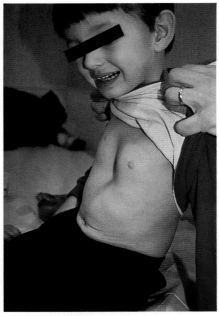

Figure 32-2 Pectus excavatum. Lateral view of child with pectus excavatum.
(Courtesy of George A. Datto, III, MD.)

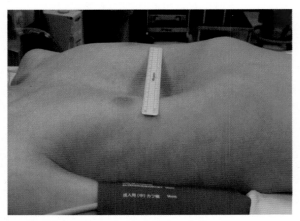

Figure 32-3 Pectus excavatum. Severe pectus in an adolescent with significant exercise intolerance.
(Courtesy of Christopher D. Derby, MD.)

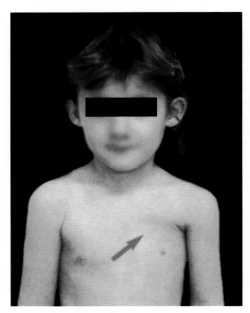

Figure 32-4 Poland syndrome. Absence of pectoralis major muscle.
(Used with permission from Staheli LT. *Practice of pediatric orthopedics.* Philadelphia, PA: Lippincott Williams & Wilkins; 2001:192.)

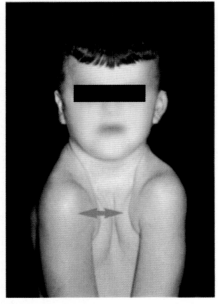

Figure 32-5 Cleidocranial dysplasia.
Narrow chest with drooping shoulders.
(Used with permission from Staheli LT. *Practice of pediatric orthopedics.* Philadelphia, PA: Lippincott Williams & Wilkins; 2001:192.)

OTHER
DIAGNOSES
TO CONSIDER

- Vertebral deformities

- Acute or healed injuries

- Isolated rib anomalies

- Isolated clavicular anomalies

- Other genetic syndromes or congenital malformations

WHEN TO
CONSIDER
FURTHER
EVALUATION
OR TREATMENT

- Surgical intervention may be considered for patients with significant psychosocial concerns relating to pectus excavatum or pectus carinatum.

- Perceived limitations of exercise tolerance in patients with pectus excavatum or pectus carinatum can be evaluated with pulmonary function testing or exercise tolerance testing.

- Definitive evidence of improvement in exercise tolerance and other measures of cardiorespiratory function after surgery to correct pectus excavatum or pectus carinatum is lacking.

- Patients with sternal cleft should be evaluated for other midline abnormalities.

- Sternal clefts are usually repaired in infancy.

- Breast reconstruction may be performed for patients, especially females, with Poland syndrome.

- Patients with cleidocranial dysplasia should have a hearing evaluation, and often require extensive dental work.

SUGGESTED READINGS

Grissom LE, Harcke HT. Thoracic deformities and the growing lung. *Semin Roentgenol.* 1998;33:199–208.

Jones K. *Smith's recognizable patterns of human malformation.* 6th ed. Philadelphia, PA: Elsevier Saunders; 2006.

McGuigan RM, Azarow KS. Congenital chest wall defects. *Surg Clin North Am.* 2006; 86:353–370.

Myers NA. An approach to the management of chest wall deformities. *Prog Pediatr Surg.* 1991;27:170–190.

Ravitch M. *Congenital deformities of the chest wall and their operative correction.* Philadelphia, PA: WB Saunders; 1977.

Staheli LT *Fundamentals of pediatric orthopedics.* 3rd ed. Philadelphia, PA: Lippincott Williams & Wilkins; 2003:112.

Welch KJ. Chest wall deformities. In: Holder TM, Ashcraft KW, eds. *Pediatric surgery.* Philadelphia, PA: WB Saunders; 1980:162–182.

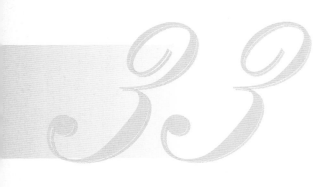

D'JUANNA WHITE-SATCHER

Breast Swelling and Enlargement

APPROACH TO THE PROBLEM

Disorders involving breast swelling most often present during the pubertal years, although they may occur in infancy and early childhood. It is important to consider the age of the patient and his/her stage of pubertal development while assessing the cause of breast enlargement. It is not uncommon for an individual's breasts to develop at different rates. Many patients may be uncomfortable bringing up their breast concerns; therefore, related abnormalities may be only coincidentally identified during routine physical examinations. A comprehensive breast examination should be performed as part of every well child visit.

Some of the most common breast concerns, such as breast asymmetry and gynecomastia, may not be true disorders but rather normal physiological variants. Breast enlargement and swelling may also be congenital, infectious, or hormonal in etiology. In male patients, the most common cause of breast tissue development is benign physiological gynecomastia.

KEY POINTS IN THE HISTORY

- Breast tissue development occurring in females less than 8 years is generally considered to be abnormal; although there may be race/ethnic variation. Some use a younger acceptable age for African American children.

- Benign gynecomastia often begins as unilateral enlargement and involves the right side twice as often as the left.

- Breasts in gynecomastia tend to be tender/painful at or soon after onset.

- Development of gynecomastia either before or after puberty would not be consistent with benign physiological gynecomastia.

- In a teenager with gynecomastia, the history should include any medications or recreational drugs that the patient might be using as they might be the cause of the gynecomastia. Some drugs associated with gynecomastia include anabolic steroids, marijuana, heroin, isoniazid (INH), metronidazole, dilantin, ketoconazole, H_2 blockers, and omeprazole.

- Rapid painful growth of breast tissue in a female in early adolescence is seen with juvenile breast hypertrophy.

- A history of significant chest wall trauma in the prepubertal female may predispose to underdevelopment of the breast on the side of the trauma and thus result in breast asymmetry.

- A history of breastfeeding, nipple piercing, or breast trauma often precedes the development of an infectious breast process.

KEY POINTS IN THE PHYSICAL EXAMINATION

- It is important to note that there is considerable variability in size, shape, and consistency of breasts among individuals.

- Normal breasts in an individual may develop at different rates, which might result in a different Tanner stage for each breast.

- Although breast asymmetry may be a normal physiological variant, breast palpation should be done to rule out a mass in the larger breast.

- Erythema, warmth, and tenderness of the breast would support the diagnosis of an infectious process such as mastitis or breast abscess.

- In the evaluation of premature thelarche, the patient must be examined for other signs of pubertal development, such as the presence of pubic hair or a growth spurt.

- In an overweight patient, fatty tissue may be confused with breast development. Palpation is necessary to determine if breast tissue is present.

- Physiological gynecomastia in males, if it occurs, usually presents when a male is Tanner Stages II–III for pubic hair and genitalia.

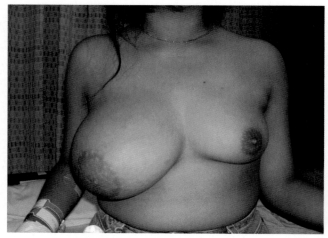

Figure 33-1 Breast asymmetry. Adolescent female with Tanner III breast development and significantly asymmetric breasts. (Courtesy of Mary L. Brandt, MD.)

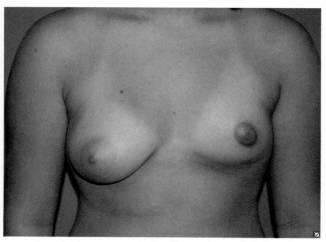

Figure 33-2 Breast asymmetry. Note the left breast is smaller although with a normal appearance. (Courtesy of Jeff Friedman, MD.)

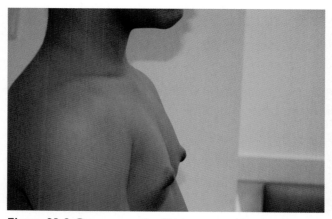

Figure 33-3 Gynecomastia. Thirteen-year-old male with gynecomastia Tanner Stage II breasts. (Courtesy of D'Juanna White-Satcher, MD, MPH.)

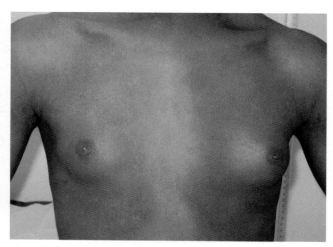

Figure 33-4 Gynecomastia. Adolescent male with Tanner III–IV genital staging and bilateral breast development with palpable breast buds, front view. (Courtesy of Christine Finck, MD.)

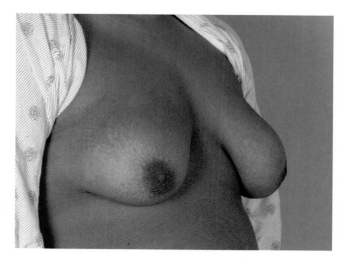

Figure 33-5 Gynecomastia. Fourteen-year-old male with cosmetically significant benign gynecomastia—both breasts Tanner Stage III. (Courtesy of Lior Heller, MD.)

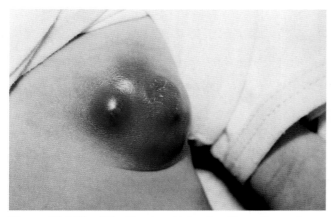

Figure 33-6 Mastitis. Ten-day-old female with swelling and erythema of the left breast.
(Used with permission from Fleisher GR, Ludwig S, Baskin MN, et al. *Pictorial review of pediatrics.* Baltimore, MD: Lippincott Williams & Wilkins; 1998:185.)

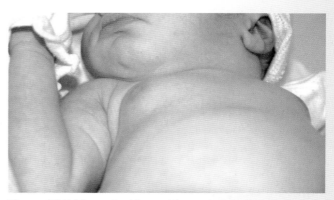

Figure 33-7 Neonateal breast hypertrophy. Two-week-old female with right breast hypertrophy.
(Courtesy of D'Juanna White-Satcher, MD, MPH.)

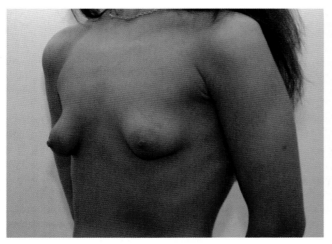

Figure 33-8 Tuberous breast. Note hypoplasia and sagging of breast tissue at chest wall on right breast.
(Courtesy of David A. Horvath, MD.)

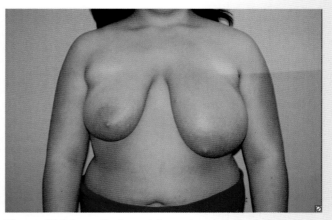

Figure 33-9 Juvenile breast hypertrophy. Note pendulous left breast in this 13-year-old female. Patient also with asymmetric breasts.
(Courtesy of Jeff Friedman, MD.)

DIFFERENTIAL DIAGNOSIS

DIAGNOSIS	ICD-9	DISTINGUISING CHARACTERISTICS	DURATION	ASSOCIATED FINDINGS	PREDISPOSING FACTORS	TREATMENT GUIDELINES
Breast Asymmetry	611.8/ 757.6	Size differential between breasts No palpable mass in larger breast	May resolve after puberty 25% persists into adulthood	Left breast more often larger	May have history of prepubertal trauma or surgery involving the smaller breast	Breast pads Cosmetic surgery, if severe, after breast development is complete
Gynecomastia	611.1	Rubbery or firm breast tissue Size may vary from a small nodule beneath areola to a size resembling female Tanner stage II–III breast	Physiological: 1–2 years Nonphysiological: may resolve if causal agent could be removed	More prevalent in obese patients	Physiological: puberty, family history Nonphysiological: variety of therapeutic and recreational drugs, liver disease, Klinefelter syndrome, hormone-secreting tumor	Surgery if not resolved after puberty or after discontinuation of involved medicine or resolution of medical condition
Mastitis/ Neonatal Mastitis	611.0/ 771.5	Erythema, warmth, induration, pain Unilateral Fever may be present.	Resolves with appropriate therapy	N/A	Breast or nipple trauma Breastfeeding	Antibiotics Warm compresses
Premature Thelarche	259.1	Breast development in a non-African-American female <8 years (<6 years in African American) No other signs of pubertal development present	Evolves into normal pubertal development	No other signs of pubertal development should be present.	Family history Exogenous estrogen exposure	N/A
Pseudo-gynecomastia (Lipomastia)	611.1	No breast tissue present Fatty tissue or excessive muscular development in breast region	Lifelong unless weight loss occurs	Obesity	Obesity	Weight loss, although may not completely resolve
Neonatal Breast Hypertrophy	778.7	Unilateral or bilateral Present at birth or shortly thereafter	Weeks to 2–3 months of age	May be associated with white milky discharge	Present in 70% newborns	Self resolves
Tuberous Breast	757.9	Breast base is limited in size but nipple-areola is overdeveloped.	Lifelong	None	Although congenital, becomes notable with puberty	Surgical after full breast development for cosmesis
Juvenile Breast Hypertrophy	611.1	Rapid growth Painful May be associated with thinning of skin and overlying venous distension	N/A	N/A	Puberty Family history	Hormonal manipulation and/or surgery may be considered after complete breast development.
Polymastia/ Polythelia (Supernumerary Nipple; Accessory Breast)	757.6	Unilateral or bilateral	Since birth May not become notable until puberty or lactation	Occasionally associated with genitourinary or cardiovascular anomalies	Family history	Surgical excision if desired for cosmetic reasons

OTHER
DIAGNOSES
TO CONSIDER

- Fibroadenoma

- Breast cyst

- McCune Albright syndrome

- Klinefelter syndrome

WHEN TO
CONSIDER
FURTHER
EVALUATION
OR TREATMENT

- If surgical intervention is being considered, it should be delayed until breast development is complete.

- Patients with gynecomastia, breast tissue greater than 4 cm, before the onset of puberty should be evaluated for underlying pathology.

- In a patient with isolated premature thelarche, consider obtaining a bone age especially if a growth spurt has been noted.

- In a patient with premature thelarche who has other secondary signs of sexual maturation, further evaluation for precious puberty is recommended.

SUGGESTED READINGS

Diamantopoulos S, Bao Y. Gynecomastia and premature thelarche: a guide for practitioners. *Pediatr Rev.* 2007;28(9):e57–e66.

Emans SJ, Laufer MR, Goldstein DP, eds. *Pediatric and adolescent gynecology.* 4th ed. Philadelphia, PA: Lippincott Williams & Wilkins; 1998:587–610.

Goldstein DP, Emans SJ, Laufer MR. The breast: examination and lesion. In: Greydanus D, Matytsina L, Gains M, eds. Breast disorders in children and adolescents. *Prim Care Clin Office Pract.* 2006;33(2):455–502.

Macdonald HR. Breast disorders. In Neinstein LS, ed. *Adolescent health care: a practical guide.* 5th ed. Philadelphia, PA: Lippincott Williams & Wilkins; 2008:754–763.

BARBARA W. BAYLDON
AND TOMITRA LATIMER

34 Chest Lumps

APPROACH TO THE PROBLEM

Chest wall lumps may be divided into those of skeletal origin, by far the most common, and those of nonskeletal origin. Skeletal causes of lumps include accidental and nonaccidental trauma, rickets, and less commonly malignancy, infection, or congenital anomalies. Nonskeletal lumps represent abnormalities of other chest wall elements resulting in accessory nipples, precocious puberty, male gynecomastia, hemangiomas, or infection. Skeletal lumps, other than a prominent xyphoid process, should be evaluated by medical imaging, and child physical abuse should be considered in the differential diagnosis of traumatic or unexplained injuries.

KEY POINTS IN THE HISTORY

- In a neonate, a chest lump likely represents a clavicular callus, from a missed clavicular fracture, or a congenital skeletal anomaly.

- Although dark-skinned infants and toddlers are most at risk, rickets should be considered in any infant who has been breast-fed without receiving vitamin D supplementation and in older children with a vitamin D intake of less than 400 IU per day.

- Children with acquired skeletal chest lumps should be evaluated for nonaccidental trauma or child physical abuse.

- Rib fractures in an infant or child, usually posterior, strongly suggest child physical abuse. Significant force is needed to fracture children's ribs as the thoracic cage is particularly compliant and elastic in children.

- In preadolescents, trauma represents the most likely cause of a skeletal swelling or lump, usually resulting from a motor vehicle accident or a fall from a height.

- Parents may bring their preadolescents for evaluation of chest lumps that represent precocious thelarche, precocious puberty, or pseudo-precocious puberty in obese children.

- Adolescent males with gynecomastia may present with a chief complaint of chest lumps.

- Congenital and asymptomatic lumps are usually benign. Bone malignancies rarely present in the first decade.

- Pectus carinatum is a rare condition often not diagnosed at birth. It can be associated with an underlying ventriculo-septal defect (VSD).

- Growth of a chest lump over time raises concern for trauma, infection, or malignancy.

- A hemangioma will typically grow over time and then involute.

- Pain, redness, or other associated symptoms raise concern for trauma, infection, or malignancy.

KEY POINTS IN THE PHYSICAL EXAMINATION

- Tenderness or erythema at the location is concerning for trauma, infection, or malignancy.

- Other areas of skeletal tenderness, bruising, or unexplained marks on the skin are highly suggestive of child physical abuse.

- Rickets is characterized by a "rachitic rosary" (swelling at the costochondral junction of numerous ribs bilaterally) and can be accompanied by widening at the wrists and ankles, genu varus or valgus, frontal bossing, and delayed fontanelle closure and tooth eruption.

- Newborn clavicular fractures are associated with brachial plexus injuries 10% of the time; therefore, a careful examination of the ipsilateral upper extremity should be performed.

- A nonskeletal chest lump located along the mammary (or milk) line is usually an accessory or supernumerary nipple. Supernumerary nipples are typically smaller than normal nipples, may be bilateral, and may range from hyperpigmented macules to well-formed nipples.

- Pseudo-precocious puberty, which represents fat deposition (the areola is small and the nipple is flat), needs to be differentiated from precocious puberty.

DIFFERENTIAL DIAGNOSIS

DIAGNOSIS	ICD-9	DISTINGUISHING CHARACTERISTICS	DISTRIBUTION	DURATION/ CHRONICITY
Precocious Thelarche	259.1	Breast bud	Nipple area	Months
Supernumerary or Accessory Nipple	757.6	Small often underdeveloped nipple	Mammary or milk line	Congenital and persists
Clavicular Fracture	810.0	Crepitus or swelling over clavicle	Clavicle	Short
Rickets	268.0	"Rachitic rosary," beads or knobs at costochondral junction	Costochondral junction Wrists Ankles Long bones	Months
Rib Fractures	807.0	Pain, tenderness, shallow breathing	Anywhere over ribs but more likely lower ribs In child physical abuse, posterior ribs	Short

ASSOCIATED FINDINGS	COMPLICATIONS	PRECIPITATING FACTORS	TREATMENT GUIDELINES
Other signs of puberty	If associated with precocious puberty, short stature	If central precocious puberty, activation of the hypothalamic, pituitary gonadal axis	Usually none Serial examinations are recommended to see if this becomes associated with precocious puberty
None	None except cosmetic	Congenital	None, except for elective surgical removal
Brachial plexus injury	Misalignment, long-term brachial plexus deficits	Trauma	None
Bowing of legs Widening, splayed wrists	Hypotonia and delayed motor milestones, hypocalcemic seizures	Inadequate intake of vitamin D, or lack of necessary enzyme or renal wasting depending on etiology	Initiation of adequate intake of vitamin D with maintenance of calcium intake. In cases of genetic abnormality, calcitriol.
With child physical abuse, look for associated fractures, bruises, and retinal hemorrhages in young children	Ineffective breathing, pulmonary contusion, or abdominal organ injury	Trauma With predisposing conditions, such as cancer or osteogenesis imperfecta, history and evidence of trauma may be minimal	Ensure adequate breathing, pain control

PHOTOGRAPHS OF SELECTED DIAGNOSES

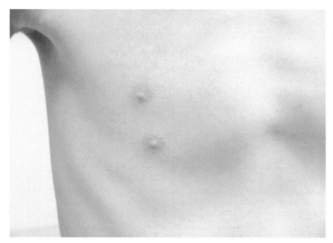

Figure 34-1 Supernumerary nipple. Fully developed nipple in embryonic milk line.
(Courtesy of Philip Siu, MD.)

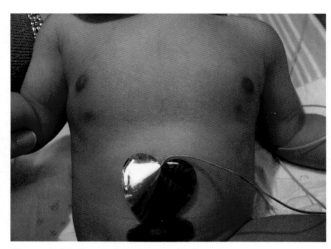

Figure 34-2 Supernumerary nipples. Bilateral supernumerary nipples in a newborn.
(Courtesy of Esther K. Chung, MD, MPH.)

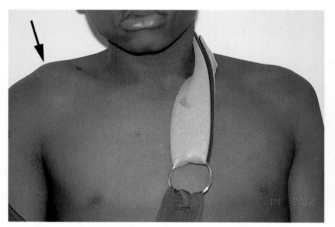

Figure 34-3 Clavicular fracture. Distal clavicular fracture with swelling over child's acromioclavicular joint.
(Used with permission from Fleisher GR, Ludwig S, Baskin MN, eds. *Atlas of pediatric emergency medicine*. Philadelphia, PA: Lippincott Williams & Wilkins; 2004:362.)

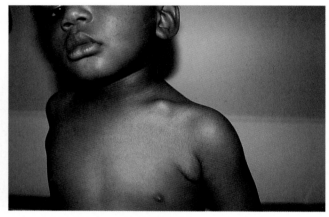

Figure 34-4 Pseudoarthrosis (nonunion of fracture with healing) of clavicle. Painless swelling of mid-clavicle.
(Courtesy of George A. Datto, III, MD.)

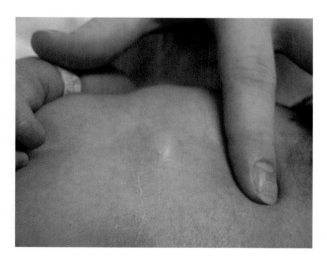

Figure 34-5 Prominent xyphoid process. Firm, painless palpable xyphoid process in an infant.
(Courtesy of Esther K. Chung, MD, MPH.)

OTHER DIAGNOSES TO CONSIDER

- Bifid rib

- Osteochondroma

- Osteomyelitis, which rarely occurs in the chest

- An underlying heart condition, causing a precordial bulge

- Pathologic fracture, which may be seen with osteogenesis imperfecta

- Malignancies including the following:

  - Osteosarcoma

  - Ewing sarcoma

  - Rhabdomyosarcoma

  - Metastatic bone disease

WHEN TO CONSIDER FURTHER EVALUATION OR TREATMENT

- Most noncongenital lumps warrant further evaluation.

- A chest lump associated with pain, erythema, and soft tissue swelling or any constitutional symptoms warrants further evaluation.

- Precocious puberty deserves further evaluation and/or referral to an endocrinologist.

- Gynecomastia in prepubertal males, other than in infancy, warrants further evaluation.

- When a fracture, malignancy, or rickets is suspected, radiographic imaging may be diagnostic.

- Whenever child physical abuse is suspected as a cause of a chest lump, a skeletal survey is indicated. In young children, an ophthalmologic examination is also warranted to rule out retinal hemorrhages.

SUGGESTED READINGS

Jewell JA, McElwain LL, Blake AS. Picture of the month. Nutritional Rickets. *Arch Pediatr Adolesc Med.* 2006;160(9):983–985.

Kocher MS, Kasser JR. Orthopedic aspects of child abuse. *J Am Acad Orthop Surg.* 2000;8(1)10–20.

Nield LS, Kamat D. Refracture of the clavicle in an infant: case report and review of clavicle fractures. *Clin Pediatr.* 2005; 44 (1):77–83.

Nimkin K, Kleinman PK. Imaging of child abuse. *Pediatr Clin North Am.* 1997;44:615–635.

Schweich P, Fleisher G. Rib fractures in children. *Pediatr Emerg Care.* 1985;1(4):187–189.

Yaw KM. Pediatric bone tumors. *Semin Surg Oncol.* 1999;16(2):173–183.

TEN

Abdomen

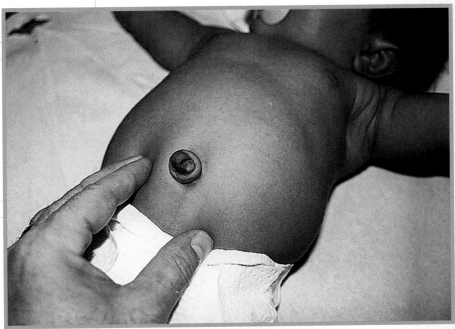

(Courtesy of George A. Datto, III, MD.)

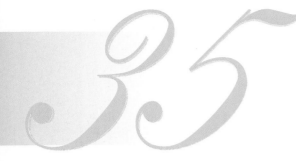

ANTHONY E. BURGOS

Abdominal Midline Bulge

APPROACH TO THE PROBLEM

A variety of midline bulges can be seen in children and, because an underlying abdominal mass may cause a bulge, severity may range from being entirely benign to being acutely life-threatening. Fortunately, midline presentation and age of the child limit the list of potential causes. In the newborn, more than 80% of abdominal masses are nonsurgical and more than two thirds of lesions arise from the genitourinary tract. The most common causes result from incomplete fetal development, fetal remnants, and/or persistence of structures that fail to obliterate before or at the time of birth. Umbilical hernias are common in the neonatal period and represent a central fascial gap beneath the umbilicus, arising secondary to the delayed contraction of the encircling fibromuscular umbilical ring. Defects less than 1.5 cm in size usually close spontaneously. Omphalomesenteric remnants and urachal remnants require surgical excision.

KEY POINTS IN THE HISTORY

- Diastasis recti is common in newborns and pregnant women.

- Umbilical hernias are more common in African-American children, preterm infants, infants with Down syndrome, and in children with increased intra-abdominal pressure and congenital hypothyroidism.

- Umbilical hernias are usually present shortly after cord separation and protrude when the infant sits up, cries, or bears down. An umbilical hernia should be easily reducible.

- Patent urachus should be suspected if persistent or intermittent umbilical cord drainage is persistent.

- Urachal cysts and sinuses are usually asymptomatic and undetectable until they become infected.

- Pain and retraction of the umbilicus during urination suggest an urachal anomaly.

- An umbilical fistula, and frequently an umbilical polyp, will be apparent in the newborn period, while a sinus enteric cyst may not be apparent until it becomes infected later in childhood.

- Umbilical granulomas occur in the first few weeks of life and respond to silver nitrate cauterization, while umbilical polyps do not.

- Obstructive genital anomalies may present at birth with mucocolpos, but the obstructive anomaly often is asymptomatic.

- Gastroschisis and omphalocele are rare conditions that are generally diagnosed prenatally.

- Although gastrointestinal anomalies are rare, feeding difficulties or emesis may indicate intestinal obstruction from intestinal duplication.

KEY POINTS IN THE PHYSICAL EXAMINATION

- Diastasis recti presents as a midline ridge protruding from the xiphoid process to the umbilicus. Both sides of the rectus muscle are palpable during relaxation.

- The size of an umbilical hernia is determined by the size of the defect in the abdominal wall, not by the size of the protruding skin. Large hernias, greater than 2.5 cm (1 in.), are less likely to close on their own and may require surgical closure.

- A paraumbilical hernia is usually situated just above the umbilicus, and an epigastric hernia presents as a tender lump in the midline of the epigastrium.

- In contrast to inguinal hernias, umbilical hernias are rarely incarcerated. A tender erythematous, irreducible umbilical hernia suggests an incarcerated hernia, which is a surgical emergency.

- A patent urachus may present with serosanguinous or purulent discharge, periumbilical swelling, and tenderness.

- If connected to the terminal ileum, a patent vitelline/omphalomesenteric fistula may present with leakage of intestinal contents or stool, or even with intestinal prolapse.

- Urachal cysts and enteric sinus cysts present as tender, erythematous masses at the midline below the umbilicus.

- Pelvic enlargement may occur with bladder distention or obstruction, vaginal outlet obstruction, or an ovarian cyst.

- Neuroblastoma usually presents with a fixed, irregularly shaped mass that crosses the midline.

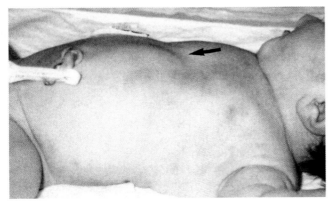

Figure 35-1 Diastasis recti.
(Used with permission from Fletcher MA. *Physical diagnosis in neonatology.* Philadelphia, PA: Lippincott–Raven Publishers; 1998:357.)

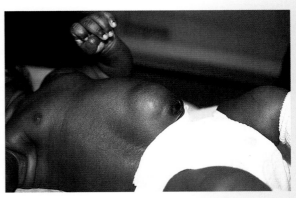

Figure 35-2 Umbilical hernia and diastasis recti.
(Courtesy of George A. Datto, III, MD.)

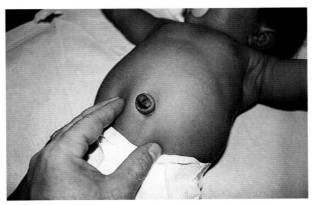

Figure 35-3 Umbilical granuloma. Pink granulation tissue at the base of the umbilicus.
(Courtesy of George A. Datto, III, MD.)

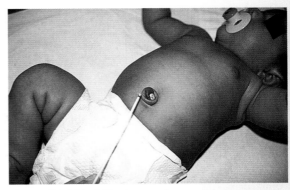

Figure 35-4 Umbilical granuloma. Umbilical granuloma after treatment with silver nitrate.
(Courtesy of George A. Datto, III, MD.)

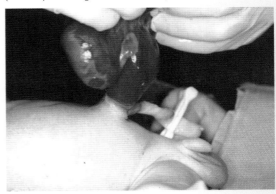

Figure 35-6 Gastroschisis.
(Courtesy of Douglas Katz, MD.)

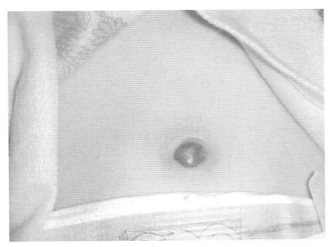

Figure 35-5 Urachal cyst. Infected urachal cyst in a 3-month-old infant.
(Courtesy of Ben Alouf, MD.)

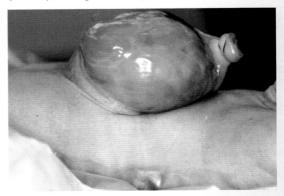

Figure 35-7 Omphalocele.
(Courtesy of Douglas Katz, MD.)

DIAGNOSIS	ICD-9	DISTINGUISHING CHARACTERISTICS	DISTRIBUTION
Diastasis Recti	728.84	Increased intra-abdominal pressure usually from Valsalva maneuver exhibits a midline ridge Common in newborns and pregnant women	From xiphoid process to umbilicus
Umbilical Hernia	553.1	Soft protruberance of skin-covered bowel at umbilicus The edge of the surrounding fascia can be felt.	Occurs at the umbilicus
Epigastric Hernia	55.29	Skin-covered protrusion in the mid-abdomen above the umbilicus	From rib cage to umbilicus
Paraumbilical Hernia	553.1	Skin-covered protrusion of the midline in any area adjacent to the umbilicus	From rib cage to anterior iliac crests
Umbilical Granuloma	771.4	Granulation tissue often arising from the base of the umbilicus Usually pink in color with seropurulent discharge	Umbilicus
Patent Urachus	753.7	Persistent wet or draining cord with thin, clear discharge	Umbilicus, with primary lesion in deep anterior abdominal wall, in the midline, between the bladder and the umbilicus
Urachal Cyst	753.7	Usually diagnosed when symptomatic with pain and erythema with a mass in the infraumbilical region. If there is an open sinus, drainage may be present.	Deep anterior abdominal wall, in the midline, between the bladder and the umbilicus
Omphalomesenteric Cyst	751.0	May present as umbilical cyst or abdominal mass	Umbilicus or anterior abdominal wall
Omphalomesenteric Fistula	751.0	Persistent drainage of bilious or fecal matter from the umbilicus	Deep anterior abdominal wall, communication between intestine and umbilicus
Gastroschisis	756.7	Extrusion of the gastrointestinal tract through a defect in the abdominal wall. Often a small defect on the right side of the intact umbilical cord. The intestine has no covering sac.	Any part of the gastrointestinal tract—from the stomach to the sigmoid colon—can be eviscerated.
Omphalocele	756.79	Extruded abdominal contents covered by a sac consisting of amnion and peritoneum. The umbilical cord is usually near the center. This often replaces the normal umbilicus.	The defect in the abdominal fascia can range in size from 4 to 14 cms. Intestinal bowel and liver may be extruded into the sac.
Hydrocolpos	623.8	Lower abdominal mass or soft, fluctuant bulge from vaginal introitus, especially with crying or straining	Vaginal vault
Ovarian Cyst	620.2	Smooth, immobile mass in the lower abdomen	Lower abdomen and pelvis
Posterior Urethral Valves	753.6	Typically diagnosed antenatally Abdominal distention or lower abdominal mass Potter syndrome	Bladder, ureters, and kidneys
Intestinal Duplication	751.5	Abdominal distention	Any portion of the gastrointestinal tract from esophagus to rectum
Urinary Ascites	789.59	Abdominal distention, shifting dullness to percussion Potter syndrome	Peritoneum
Neuroblastoma	194.0	Fixed abdominal mass, may cross midline	Retroperitoneum

ASSOCIATED FINDINGS	COMPLICATIONS	PRECIPITATING FACTORS	TREATMENT GUIDELINES
None	None	None	None
Diastasis recti	Incarceration rare, but should be suspected if not easily reducible	Low birth weight, female gender, African-American race/ethnicity	None, if small If still present at 4 years of age and greater than 1 cm, refer to pediatric surgeon
None	Incarceration rare, but should be suspected if not easily reducible	None	Refer to pediatric surgeon for nonurgent surgery, although severe cases with incarceration require emergent surgical correction.
None	Incarceration rare, but should be suspected if not easily reducible	None	Refer to pediatric surgeon for nonurgent surgery, although severe cases with incarceration require emergent surgical correction.
None	Occasionally does not completely resolve after treatment and may need excision	None	Silver nitrate cauterization for granulation that persistently drains
None	Urinary tract infection	None	Cystogram is recommended to rule out obstructive lesion. Refer to pediatric surgeon for evaluation, exploration, and repair.
Infected cysts present with fever, pain, or erythema at the site and purulent exudate	May rupture intraperitoneally and result in acute abdomen Rare case reports of development of urachal carcinoma from urachal remnants	Persistence of allantoic duct	Refer to pediatric surgeon for evaluation, exploration, and repair.
Pain and swelling when infected	May become infected Less commonly results in intestinal obstruction	Male gender	Refer to pediatric surgeon for evaluation and repair.
None	Intestinal obstruction	Male gender	Refer to pediatric surgeon for evaluation, exploration, and repair.
Occasionally genital tissue—testes, ovaries, or fallopian tubes—may be extruded as well. Solid organs are usually not extruded. Intestinal atresia may be present, approximately 10% of the time.	Short bowel syndrome Third-trimester fetal demise Mortality rate, 10%–15% due to complications from short bowel syndrome	Vascular accident or atrophy involving the right umbilical vein	Refer to pediatric surgeon for evaluation and repair.
Associated with chromosomal disorders such as: Trisomy 13, 14, 15, 18, and 21, and Beckwith-Wiedemann syndrome. Associated anomalies including cardiac, renal, and skeletal (limb) defects, and pulmonary hypoplasia (see with large omphaloceles)	Difficulty in achieving full closure Large omphaloceles disrupt lung development, and pulmonary hypoplasia may be present.	Arises from abnormal formation of the umbilical ring	Refer to pediatric surgeon for evaluation and repair.
Genital, urinary tract, gastrointestinal, cardiac, and limb abnormalities	Urinary tract obstruction, intestinal obstruction, respiratory distress, poor perfusion of lower extremities all may occur due to compression of surrounding structures.	High circulating maternal estrogens	Ultrasound to confirm diagnosis followed by simple incision and catheter drainage. Refer to OB/Gyn to confirm structural integrity of vaginal components.
Abdominal distention, tachypnea	Rupture, torsion, hemorrhage, or necrosis of the cyst, loss of ipsilateral ovary and/or fallopian tube	None	Refer to pediatric surgeon for evaluation and removal.
Respiratory distress, pulmonary hypoplasia, ascites, voiding dysfunction, urinary tract infection	Urosepsis, dehydration, electrolyte abnormalities, failure to thrive, renal parenchymal damage and renal failure if undiagnosed and untreated	Males only	Refer to pediatric urologist for evaluation and repair.
Nausea, vomiting, respiratory distress, vertebral anomalies, intestinal atresias, genitourinary malformations	Intestinal obstruction, gastrointestinal bleeding, or perforation, airway compression	None	Refer to pediatric surgeon for evaluation and repair.
Respiratory distress, urinary tract obstruction, bladder or ureter perforation, other complicated urinary abnormalities	Urosepsis, dehydration, electrolyte abnormalities, failure to thrive, renal parenchymal damage and renal failure if obstruction or perforation goes undiagnosed and untreated	Males	Refer to pediatric surgeon for evaluation and treatment.
Flushing, sweating, irritability, subcutaneous blue skin lesions, dark circles under eyes, fever, respiratory difficulty	Depending on treatment modality and patient response, may cause additional cancers, infertility, impaired growth, thyroid problems, neuropsychiatric, and behavioral problems	None	Refer to pediatric oncologist for evaluation, surgical resection, radiation, and/or chemotherapy.

OTHER
DIAGNOSES
TO CONSIDER

- Epigastric hernia

- Paraumbilical hernia

- Patent urachus

- Urachal cyst

- Omphalomesenteric cyst

- Patent vitelline/omphalomesenteric fistula

- Gastroschisis

- Omphalocele

- Hydrocolpos

- Ovarian cyst

- Posterior urethral valves

- Intestinal duplication

- Urinary ascites

- Neuroblastoma

WHEN TO
CONSIDER
FURTHER
EVALUATION
OR TREATMENT

- Any abdominal mass not readily identified on examination should be evaluated further with imaging, including an ultrasound or a CT scan.

- If an abdominal hernia is not reducible or there are signs of an acute abdomen, consider immediate referral to a pediatric surgeon.

- Umbilical hernias that persist at age 4 years should be referred to a pediatric surgeon.

- Urachal cysts and patent urachus should be further evaluated by an ultrasound or a CT scan and referred to a pediatric surgeon for further management.

SUGGESTED READINGS

Chandler JC, Gauderer MW. The neonate with an abdominal mass. *Pediatr Clin North Am.* 2004;51(4):979–997.
Longino LA, Martin LW. Abdominal masses in the newborn infant. *Pediatrics.* 1958;21(4):596–604.
Peppas DS. Pediatric urologic emergencies. In: Gearhart JP, ed. *Pediatric urology.* New York: Humana Press; 2003:23–25.
Pomeranz A. Anomalies, abnormalities, and care of the umbilicus. *Pediatr Clin North Am.* 2004;51(3):819–827.
Wilson RD, Johnson MP. Congenital abdominal wall defects: an update. *Fetal Diagn Ther.* 2004;19:385–398.

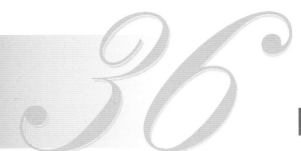

VANI V. GOPALAREDDY
AND DEVENDRA I. MEHTA

Enlarged/Distended Abdomen

APPROACH TO THE PROBLEM

Distension of the abdomen may occur because of feces, flatus, fluid, fat, full urinary bladder, tumors, cysts, organomegaly, and pregnancy. Ileus from many causes or reduced intestinal motility from drugs or metabolic derangements may also lead to acute abdominal distension. The intestinal obstruction of any etiology can lead ultimately to diffuse distension. Lumbar lordosis, whether physiological in a prepubescent child or pathological in neuromuscular disorders, will cause the child to have the appearance of abdominal distension. Rapid recognition of abdominal distension in an ill-appearing child is essential to reduce morbidity and mortality. Imaging studies have their role in determining the etiology of a child's enlarged abdomen.

KEY POINTS IN THE HISTORY

- Failure to thrive or acute weight loss may be a marker for significant pathology causing an enlarged abdomen.

- A child usually will complain of minimal pain with an ileus but will complain of significant pain with an intestinal obstruction.

- Severe infections—including gastrointestinal infections, pneumonia, and peritonitis—and abdominal surgeries may be associated with paralytic ileus and abdominal distension.

- Prior abdominal surgery puts a child at risk for adhesions and small-bowel obstruction.

- Bilious vomiting should be presumed to be secondary to intestinal obstruction until proven otherwise.

- A thorough history assessing for frequency, consistency, and difficulty with stool passage is important for diagnosing constipation.

- Often, bezoars are found in neurologically or psychologically impaired children with pica.

- Children with diseases associated with hemolysis are at risk for splenomegaly.

- Hematemesis, melena, and jaundice can be seen with portal hypertension.

- Parents often note abdominal tumors when their child is in the bathtub, when the abdomen is more relaxed.

- Increased flatus suggests that the abdominal distension may be from increased intestinal air.

- Pregnancy should be considered and ruled out in an adolescent female with secondary amenorrhea and lower abdominal distension.

KEY POINTS IN THE PHYSICAL EXAMINATION

- The overall health and habitus of a child will suggest whether the condition is acute or chronic.

- To detect abdominal organomegaly on palpation, it is important to examine the lower abdomen close to the groin and then proceed upward toward the chest.

- Pallor and nail clubbing are physical findings that suggest chronic malabsorption.

- Ascites, flatus, and ileus present with symmetrical abdominal distension.

- Malignancy, constipation, pregnancy, and organomegaly may present with localized abdominal distension.

- Skin findings of chronic liver disease include spider nevi, palmar erythema, and jaundice.

- Visible peristaltic waves may be seen with intestinal obstruction.

- Bowel sounds are often absent in ileus, but they are hyperactive in intestinal obstruction.

- A child with peritonitis often resists any movement and has involuntary guarding on abdominal examination.

- A large fecal mass palpable in the left lower quadrant with hard stool on rectal exam is suggestive of functional constipation, while constipation with an empty rectal vault is suggestive of Hirschsprung disease.

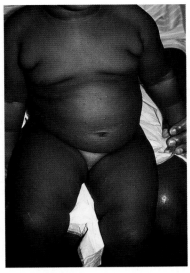

Figure 36-1 Obesity. Enlarged abdomen from increased adiposity.
(Courtesy of George A. Datto, III, MD.)

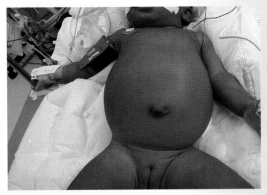

Figure 36-2 Ascites. Large distended abdomen in an infant.
(Courtesy of Vani V. Gopalareddy, MD.)

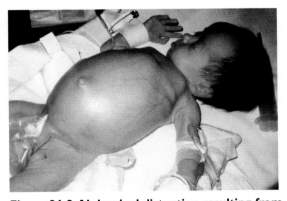

Figure 36-3 Abdominal distention resulting from hepatomegaly in a child with untreated galactosemia. Note that the distention is more prominent in the upper abdomen.
(Used with permission from Fletcher MA. *Physical diagnosis in neonatology.* Philadelphia, PA: Lippincott–Raven Publishers; 1998:353.)

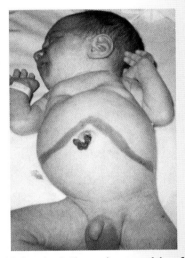

Figure 36-4 Abdominal distention resulting from massive hepatosplenomegaly in an infant with congenital cytomegalovirus infection. Note that the distention is more prominent in the upper abdomen.
(Used with permission from Fletcher MA. *Physical diagnosis in neonatology.* Philadelphia, PA: Lippincott–Raven Publishers; 1998:354.)

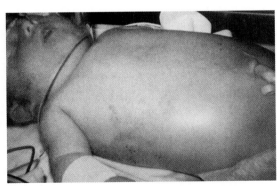

Figure 36-5 Abdominal distention in an infant with anasarca. Note that the distention is more prominent in the flanks.
(Used with permission from Fletcher MA. *Physical diagnosis in neonatology.* Philadelphia, PA: Lippincott–Raven Publishers; 1998:355.)

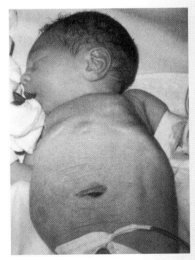

Figure 36-6 Abdominal distention at the flanks in an infant with Prune Belly syndrome.
(Used with permission from Fletcher MA. *Physical diagnosis in neonatology.* Philadelphia, PA: Lippincott–Raven Publishers; 1998:355.)

DIFFERENTIAL DIAGNOSIS

DIAGNOSIS	ICD-9	DISTINGUISHING CHARACTERISTICS	DISTRIBUTION	DURATION/ CHRONICITY
Obesity	278.0	Increased subcutaneous fat	Generalized	Chronic
Constipation	564.0	Indentable abdominal mass Hard stool in rectum	Left lower quadrant and suprapubic pain and enlargement May be generalized if more severe	Chronic—often begins in toddler age
Flatus	787.3	Resonant percussion note	Generalized	Chronic
Ascites	789.5	Dull percussion note Fluid wave Fullness of flanks	Generalized	Acute or nonacute
Hepatomegaly	789.1	Enlarged liver span determined by palpation or percussion	Right upper quadrant, but if severe may appear to be generalized enlargement of the abdomen	Acute or nonacute
Splenomegaly	789.2	Palpable edge in left upper quadrant	Left upper quadrant	Acute or nonacute
Intestinal Obstruction	560.9	Acute abdominal distension	Generalized	Acute
Wilms Tumor	189.0	Asymptomatic flank mass Median age of presentation: 3 years	Flank	Acute
Neuroblastoma	194.0	Large abdominal mass Lymphadenopathy Median age: 2 years	Flank or abdominal	Acute
Prune Belly Syndrome	756.71	Wrinkled abdominal wall skin with abdominal distension	Generalized	Chronic

ASSOCIATED FINDINGS	COMPLICATIONS	PREDISPOSING FACTORS	TREATMENT GUIDELINES
Acanthosis nigricans Polycystic ovary syndrome	Hypertension Diabetes Obstructive sleep apnea	Excessive caloric intake Inactivity	Weight management program
External or internal hemorrhoid Anal fissures	Encopresis Psychological distress	Diet low in fiber Psychological factors	Bowel cleanout—oral, nasogastric or rectal Long-term maintenance program
Periumbilical pain	Psychological distress	Consumption of lactose in lactose-intolerant patient Certain foods	Lactose-free diet or use of lactase supplements if thought to be due to lactose intolerance
Ankle swelling	Patient at risk for developing spontaneous bacterial peritonitis	Liver disease Cardiac disease Infections Lymphoma Ovarian pathology	Treat underlying condition Spironolactone Salt restriction Albumin and lasix
Jaundice Pruritus Skin findings Ascites	Portal hypertension Liver failure Encephalopathy Renal failure	Infection Storage disease Malignancy Autoimmune Vascular disease	Treat underlying conditions, if possible Fat-soluble vitamin supplements Screen for varices
Superficial abdominal venous distension when associated with portal hypertension Pallor	Cytopenias Splenic rupture	Infection Hematologic disorder Neoplasm Storage diseases Congestion Autoimmune disorder	Treat underlying condition Spleen guard Portosystemic shunts Splenectomy
Bilious vomiting Obstipation	Peritonitis	Prior abdominal surgery	Urgent surgical intervention
Hypertension Hematuria Abdominal pain Vomiting	Dependent on stage of tumor	Beckwith-Wiedemann syndrome WAGR syndrome—Wilms tumor, aniridia, genitourinary abnormalities, and mental retardation	Refer to oncologist to treat underlying condition.
Bone pain Proptosis and ecchymosis Opsoclonus myoclonus Horner syndrome	Dependent on stage of tumor	N/A	Refer to oncologist to treat underlying condition.
Urethral obstruction Pulmonary hypoplasia Undescended testes Renal dysplasia Congenital cardiac disease	One third of children are stillborn or die in the first 3 months of life Renal failure	Male	Treat underlying condition Manage constipation, if present

OTHER
DIAGNOSES
TO CONSIDER

- Intussusception

- Volvulus

- Pancreatic pseudocyst

- Mesenteric cysts

- Necrotizing enterocolitis

WHEN TO
CONSIDER
FURTHER
EVALUATION
OR TREATMENT

- Abdominal distension in a neonate always warrants immediate, detailed evaluation for surgical causes and consultation with pediatric surgery.

- Presence of ascites always warrants detailed evaluation for underlying cause and consultation with pediatric gastroenterology.

- Imaging, especially ultrasound, may identify a cause for ascites. A diagnostic paracentesis may be needed to further define the ascites as chylous, exudates, or transudate.

- Presence of a mass that cannot be indented on examination warrants detailed evaluation for organomegaly, abscesses, matted loops of bowel, tumors, or cysts.

SUGGESTED READINGS

Fletcher MA. *Physical diagnosis in neonatology*. Philadelphia, PA: Lippincott–Raven Publishers; 1998:353–355.

Squires RH Jr. Abdominal masses. In: Walker WA, Durie PR, Hamilton JR, et al., eds. *Pediatric gastrointestinal disease*. 3rd ed. Ontario, Canada: B.C. Decker; 2000:150–163.

Youssef NN, Di Lorenzo C. Childhood constipation: evaluation and treatment. *J Clin Gastroenterol*. 2001;33:199–205.

Back

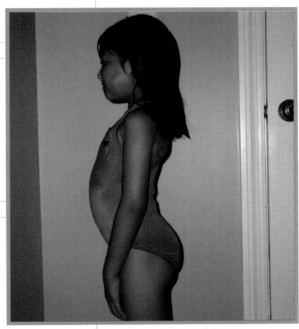

(Courtesy of Esther K. Chung, MD, MPH.)

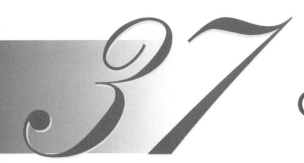

SHAREEN F. KELLY

Curvature of the Back

APPROACH TO THE PROBLEM

Curvature of the spine is described by the plane of curvature and the position of the curve relative to the spine. Kyphosis is an exaggerated curve of the thoracic spine in the sagittal plane with the apex of the curve directed posteriorly. Lordosis refers to a marked curvature that occurs in the sagittal plane of the lumbar spine, the apex of which is directed anteriorly. The term scoliosis describes lateral spinal curvature in the coronal plane and necessarily involves a rotational component as well. The rotational component is visualized most often as a rib hump viewed posteriorly. Curvature of the spine can present with varying severity and may progress with age and time. Beyond skeletal maturity, scoliosis generally does not progress; however, kyphosis and lordosis may progress into adulthood.

KEY POINTS IN THE HISTORY

- Family history of scoliosis is present in approximately 30% of new cases of scoliosis.

- Sports participation and day-to-day functioning usually are not affected by the curvature of scoliosis unless it is very severe.

- Complaints of back pain are not characteristic of idiopathic scoliosis and should prompt the physician to rule out other treatable diseases.

- Nonambulatory patients are more likely to have progressive scoliosis than ambulatory patients.

- The curvature of idiopathic scoliosis is more likely to progress during times of rapid growth.

- Rapidly progressing curves are more likely to require treatment.

- Fixed kyphosis may cause pain with neck motion.

- Radicular pain, changes in bowel or bladder function, sensory abnormalities, and problems with balance and/or coordination all point to an underlying neurologic problem.

- Constitutional symptoms—including prolonged fever, weight loss, night sweats, and malaise—may provide clues regarding malignancies or inflammatory diseases.

KEY POINTS IN THE PHYSICAL EXAMINATION

- Bony deformities detected upon palpation along the spine suggest vertebral anomalies or spinal dysraphism.

- Skin overlying the lumbar spine marked with hemangiomas, hair tufts, clefts, and/or other macular discolorations may be the only clinical clue to occult spinal dysraphism.

- The most common presentation of idiopathic scoliosis is that of a thoracic curve with a right thoracic rib hump when viewed from behind on the Adams forward bending test.

- Lower extremity muscular weakness, tightness of hamstrings, and decreased deep tendon reflexes are indicative of a neurological abnormality.

- Patients with more advanced sexual maturity ratings are less likely to have progression of their scoliosis.

- Range of motion assessment is critical in children with kyphosis or lordosis.

PHOTOGRAPHS OF SELECTED DIAGNOSES

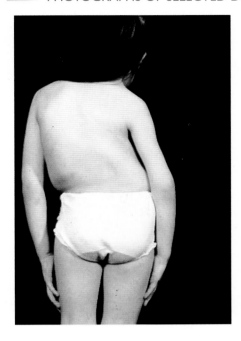

Figure 37-1 Scoliosis.
(Used with permission from SIU/Biomedical Communications/Custom Medical Stock Photography.)

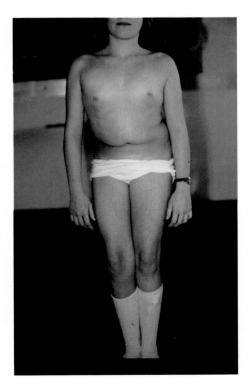

Figure 37-2 Scoliosis, anterior view. Note the pelvic tilt and abnormal skin folds.
(Courtesy of the late Peter Sol, MD.)

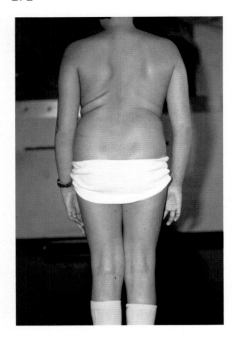

Figure 37-3 Scoliosis, posterior view. Note the abnormal skin folds and scapula position.
(Courtesy of the late Peter Sol, MD.)

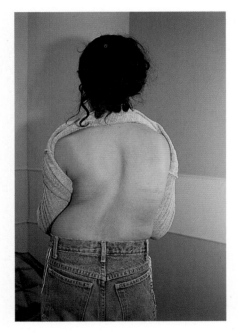

Figure 37-4 Scoliosis, standing. Dramatic spinal curvature in an adolescent.
(Courtesy of George A. Datto, III, MD.)

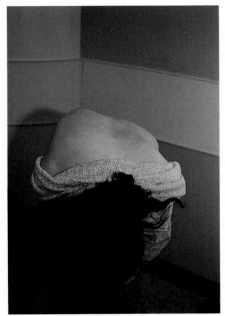

Figure 37-5 Scoliosis, bending forward. Note the marked asymmetry of the back.
(Courtesy of George A. Datto, III, MD.)

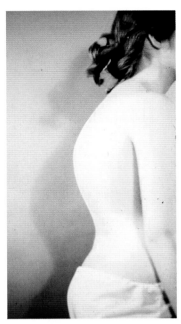

Figure 37-6 Kyphosis.
(Courtesy of Martin Herman, MD.)

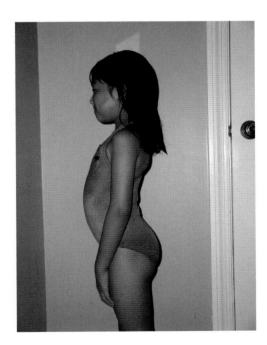

Figure 37-7 Lordosis. Note the thoracolumbar curvature on side view of this child in her normal stance.
(Courtesy of Esther K. Chung, MD, MPH.)

DIFFERENTIAL DIAGNOSIS

DIAGNOSIS	ICD-9	DISTINGUISHING CHARACTERISTICS	DISTRIBUTION	DURATION/ CHRONOCITY
Scoliosis	737.30	Lateral curvature of the spine Right (most often) thoracic rib hump on Adams forward-bending test	Female:male ratio is 4:1 Idiopathic scoliosis presents most often in adolescence.	Curve progresses through puberty Usually no decrease in function
Kyphosis	737.10	Convex curvature of the upper thoracic spine Best viewed from the side with the child standing	Postural kyphosis more common in prepubertal children Structural kyphosis may affect any age.	Postural kyphosis corrects with physical therapy. Structural kyphosis may progress into old age.
Lordosis	737.20	Concave curvature of the lumbar spine Best viewed from the side while child is standing or when child is lying supine on a firm, flat surface	All age groups Physiologic lordosis most often occurs in pre-pubertal children.	Depends on underlying cause—physiologic lordosis will resolve with growth

ASSOCIATED FINDINGS	COMPLICATIONS	PREDISPOSING FACTORS	TREATMENT GUIDELINES
Asymmetry of clavicles and/or scapulae Asymmetry of back skin folds Leg length discrepancy Asymmetric iliac crests when standing upright	Severe cases (mostly nonambulatory) may result in restrictive lung disease and/or cor pulmonale.	Most often idiopathic Congenital scoliosis may result from vertebral anomalies.	Observation for mild curves Bracing for moderate and progressive curves Surgical spinal fusion for extreme curves
Postural kyphosis often seen with compensatory lordosis Fixed kyphosis is often painful	When associated with osteoporosis, painful and may cause symptoms of compression	Postural kyphosis: poor posture Scheuermann disease has no known etiology.	Depending on etiology—bracing or surgical correction or no treatment
Buttocks appear more prominent. Curve may correct with forward bending. May be associated with hip flexor muscle contractures	Pain Decreased flexibility and movement	Poor posture, obesity, hip flexor contracture Congenital lordosis: vertebral or neuromuscular problems Acquired lordosis: diskitis or spondylolisthesis	Physical therapy

OTHER
DIAGNOSES
TO CONSIDER

- Marfan syndrome

- Ehlers-Danlos syndrome

- Leg length discrepancy

- Spasm of the spinous or paraspinous muscles with compensatory splinting

- Bone dysplasias

- Metabolic diseases, including rickets, osteoporosis, homocystinuria, and osteogenesis imperfecta, may be associated with scoliosis.

- Spinal tumors

- Neuromuscular disorders

- Spondylolisthesis

WHEN TO
CONSIDER
FURTHER
EVALUATION
OR TREATMENT

- Left-sided thoracic scoliosis in an otherwise normal teenager should prompt further evaluation to rule out an underlying lesion.

- A tall, thin child with scoliosis and marfanoid features should have genetic, cardiac, and ophthalmologic evaluations.

- Congenital scoliosis mandates orthopedic evaluation.

- Scoliosis associated with constitutional symptoms warrants evaluation to uncover possible rheumatologic disorders or malignancies.

SUGGESTED READINGS

Chin KR, Price JS, Zimbler S. A guide to early detection of scoliosis. *Contemp Pediatr.* 2001;18:77–103.

Marsh JS. Screening for scoliosis. *Pediatr Rev.* 1993;14:297–298.

Staheli, L. *Fundamentals of pediatric orthopedics.* Philadelphia/New York: Lippincott-Raven Publishers; 1998: 73–83.

Ward T, Davis HW, Hanley EN. Orthopedics. In: *Atlas of pediatric physical diagnosis.* 2nd ed. New York, NY: Gower Medical Publishing; 1992:21.25–27.30.

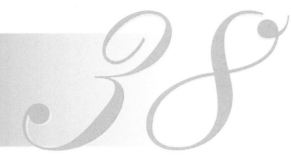

Midline Back Pits, Skin Tags, Hair Tufts, and Other Lesions

APPROACH TO THE PROBLEM

Up to 5% of children have congenital back dimples, pits, skin tags, or hair tufts. Additionally, lipomas and hemangiomas may occur along the midline area of the back. The history and physical examination should focus on the location of the lesion and associated neurological symptoms and signs. A small percentage of these lesions are associated with underlying spinal pathology, which includes spinal dysraphism, or failure of the neural folds to fuse in utero (such as myelomeningocele or spina bifida), or other abnormalities, such as tethered spinal cord or spinal lipomas. A tethered cord occurs when the spinal cord is abnormally fixed to a mass, the meninges, a vertebra, or the skin. As a child with tethered cord grows, excess tension is placed on the spinal cord and its blood vessels, leading to damage of the nerve fibers. It is important to remember that delayed diagnosis can lead to permanent neurological damage in these conditions. Early diagnosis and treatment are associated with a better prognosis. In the absence of underlying spinal pathology, superficial back lesions other than infected pilonidal cysts rarely require treatment.

Spina bifida and sacrococcygeal teratoma are distinct from the other midline lesions. They usually present as sacral masses prenatally or at birth, and require immediate intervention.

KEY POINTS IN THE HISTORY

- Nearly all midline back skin tags, pits, and tufts are congenital.

- Presence of neurological symptoms, such as bowel or bladder incontinence in older children or lower extremity weakness, toe walking, pain, or paresthesias, strongly suggests a spinal dysraphism or other spinal pathology.

- Long-standing tethered cord may result in asymmetric lower extremity growth.

- A family history of neural tube defects may increase the likelihood that a midline defect is associated with occult spinal dysraphism.

- Symptoms of localized inflammation, such as pain and redness, in an older child may signify an infected pilonidal cyst.

- Spina bifida and sacrococcygeal teratoma are congenital lesions that are apparent prenatally on ultrasound or on examination in the delivery room.

- A large sacrococcygeal teratoma may be associated with a history of hydrops fetalis during pregnancy.

- Folic acid supplementation in pregnant women greatly reduces the incidence of spinal cord defects.

KEY POINTS IN THE PHYSICAL EXAMINATION

- High thoracolumbar lesions are more likely than low lumbosacral lesions to be associated with underlying spinal cord lesions.

- Pilonidal sinuses or cysts are located below the superior margin of the gluteal cleft and are rarely associated with spinal cord defects.

- Sacral dimples are located above the superior margin of the gluteal cleft and can be associated with spinal cord defects.

- Isolated dimples are rarely associated with spinal dysraphism.

- Midline lesions have an increased risk of spinal cord involvement. Notably, nonmidline lesions, such as skin tags, may also be associated with underlying spinal cord lesions.

- Many newborns have hair on their backs at birth. Further evaluation is warranted only for distinct hair tufts or patches.

- A subcutaneous mass over the lumbar spine is highly suggestive of dysraphism.

- It is important to distinguish shallow dimples, which require no further workup, from deep or "bottomless" pits without a visible base. The latter require further evaluation to rule out occult spinal pathology.

- The presence of any neurological abnormality, such as weakness of the lower extremities, abnormal reflexes, or abnormal gait, suggests spinal cord involvement.

- While an abnormal neurological examination strongly suggests a spinal cord abnormality, a normal examination cannot rule it out.

- Defects may sometimes be palpated along the spine when there is spinal dysraphism.

- Deviation of the gluteal cleft suggests an underlying mass, such as a lipoma or myelomeningocele.

- Spina bifida and sacrococcygeal teratoma are sacral masses that may be covered by skin or have exposed membranes and spinal cord.

- Deep pilonidal sinuses may become blocked with hair, skin, or other debris and may become cystic and infected.

- Signs of acute inflammation, including redness, warmth, and tenderness, suggest an infected pilonidal cyst.

PHOTOGRAPHS OF SELECTED DIAGNOSES

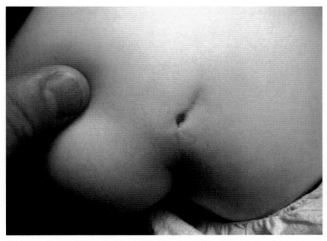

Figure 38-1 Sacral dimple. Shallow dimple visible within the gluteal fold.
(Courtesy of Paul S. Matz, MD.)

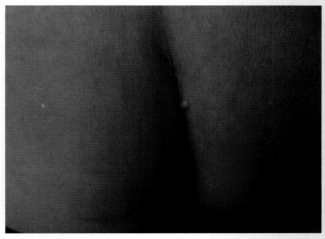

Figure 38-2 Sacral skin tag with no underlying spinal pathology. Note the isolated nodule within the gluteal fold.
(Courtesy of Esther K. Chung, MD, MPH.)

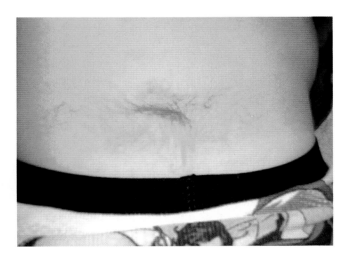

Figure 38-3 Hair tuft.
(Courtesy of Joseph Piatt, MD.)

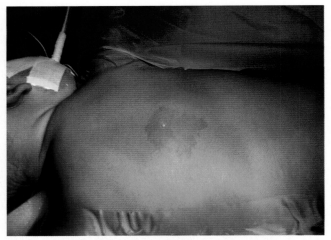

Figure 38-4 Infected dermal sinus connected to intramedullary dermoid cyst. Thoracic sinus associated with purulent discharge.
(Courtesy of Joseph Piatt, MD.)

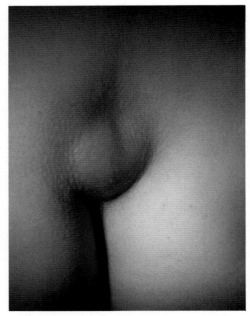

Figure 38-5 Infected pilonidal cyst. A large erythematous fluctuant mass visible at the superior portion of the gluteal fold.
(Courtesy of Scott VanDuzer, MD.)

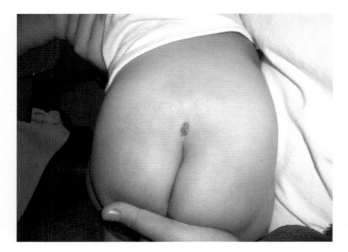

Figure 38-6 Sacral hemangioma. Vascular malformation visible overlying sacral spine.
(Courtesy of Paul S. Matz, MD.)

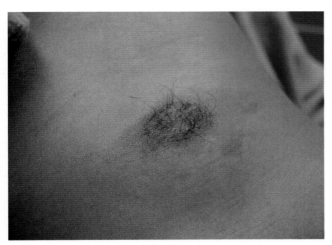

Figure 38-7 Lumbar hemangioma. This midline lesion was associated with a dermal sinus and an underlying tethered cord. (Courtesy of Esther K. Chung, MD, MPH.)

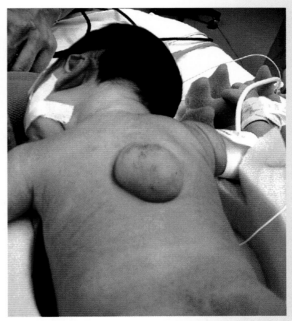

Figure 38-8 Thoracic meningocele. Large skin-covered thoracic mass in an infant. (Courtesy of Joseph Piatt, MD.)

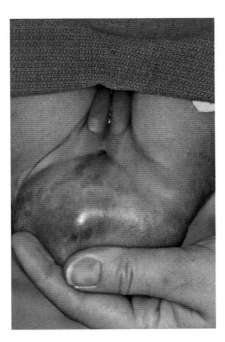

Figure 38-9 Sacrococcygeal teratoma. Large mass protruding from the lower spine of a neonate. (Courtesy of Joseph Piatt, MD.)

DIFFERENTIAL DIAGNOSIS

DIAGNOSIS	ICD-9	DISTINGUISHING CHARACTERISTICS	DISTRIBUTION
Sacral Dimple or Pit	685	Small indentation of the skin, often circular May be shallow or deep ("bottomless")	Mid or lower back, midline or lateral; located above the superior margin of the gluteal cleft
Skin Tag	757.39	Small outgrowth of skin	Mid or lower back
Hair Tufts/Patches	757.4	Cluster of hair, often dark	Mid or lower back
Pilonidal Sinus/Cyst	685	Small indentation or sinus tract in the skin containing hair May appear inflamed if infected	Intergluteal, usually lateral; located below the superior margin of the gluteal cleft
Hemangioma	228.0	Benign neoplasm of proliferating vascular endothelium Rapid growth in infancy followed by involution	May occur anywhere on the back and on other parts of the body
Spina Bifida	741	Sacral mass that may have exposed mucous membranes or spinal cord or may be covered by skin	Midline, lower back
Sacrococcygeal Teratoma	215.6	Large sacral mass that may have exposed membranes or be covered by skin	Overlying the sacrum and coccyx

ASSOCIATED FINDINGS	PREDISPOSING FACTORS	TREATMENT GUIDELINES
Potential for occult spinal pathology with deep, midline dimples	Unknown	Ultrasound/MRI for high, midline, deep lesions or lesions associated with other malformations
Potential for occult spinal pathology	Unknown	Ultrasound/MRI for high or midline lesions Removal for cosmetic concerns
Potential for occult spinal pathology	Unknown	Ultrasound/MRI for distinct tufts
Rarely occult spinal pathology with deep, midline tracts Infection	Sex hormones, obesity, local trauma, and poor hygiene increase the risk of obstruction, which may lead to cyst formation and infection	Incision and drainage for superinfected lesions Intravenous or oral antibiotics depending on the severity of the infection
May be associated with spina bifida, meningomyelocele, tethered cord	Unknown	Ultrasound/MRI for high or midline lesions
Weakness or paralysis of legs May be associated with hydrocephalus or Arnold-Chiari malformation	Inadequate folic acid supplementation during pregnancy	Immediate transfer to a tertiary care Neonatal Intensive Care Unit (NICU) Coverage with a sterile, moist dressing until operative repair is performed Multispecialty evaluation Long-term follow-up with a multispecialty outpatient team
High output heart failure and hydrops fetalis	Unknown	Immediate transfer to a tertiary care NICU Coverage with a sterile, moist dressing until operative repair is performed

- Multiple midline back lesions are more likely to indicate spinal dysraphism.

- In an older child with a midline back lesion and new onset of neurological signs, such as urinary incontinence or weakness, imaging must be done to rule out dysraphism.

- When a sacrococcygeal teratoma is suspected prenatally, perinatology consultation should be undertaken to evaluate for evidence of hydrops fetalis.

- Infants diagnosed with myelomeningocele should undergo head imaging to assess for hydrocephalus.

- Long-term management of infants with myelomeningocele should involve general pediatrics, neurosurgery, orthopedic surgery, urology, and physical and occupational therapy.

SUGGESTED READINGS

Ackerman LL, Menezes AH. Spinal congenital dermal sinuses: a 30-year experience. *Pediatrics.* 2003;112:641–647.

Drolet BA. Cutaneous signs of neural tube dysraphism. *Pediatr Clin North Am.* 2000;47(4):813–823.

Gibson PJ, Britton J, Hall DMB, et al. Lumbosacral skin markers and identification of occult spinal dysraphism in neonates. *Acta Pediatr.* 1995;84:208–209.

Hughes JA, De Bruyn R, Patel K, et al. Evaluation of spinal ultrasound in spinal dysraphism. *Clin Radiol.* 2003;58:227–233.

Pacheco-Jacome E, Ballesteros MC, Jayakar P, et al. Occult spinal dysraphism: evidence-based diagnosis and treatment. *Neuroimag Clin N Am.* 2003:327–334.

TWELVE

Extremities

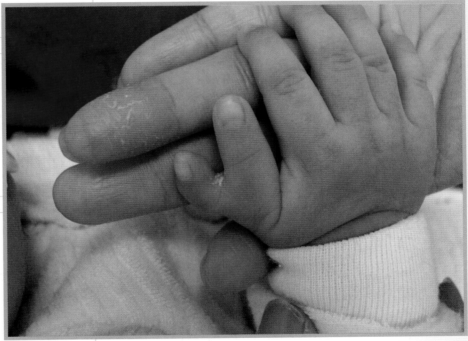

(Courtesy of Esther K. Chung, MD, MPH.)

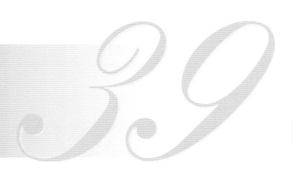

DENISE W. METRY AND
BRANDI M. KENNER

Nail Abnormalities

**APPROACH TO
THE PROBLEM**

Abnormalities of the nail may represent a problem within the nail apparatus itself, an extension of a primary dermatologic disorder, or a systemic disease. The nail grows continuously throughout life and is extremely sensitive to changes in the body and the environment. Anything that disrupts the normal growth and development of the nail or damages its structural components will cause changes in the appearance and function of the nail. Nail abnormalities are sometimes a clue to more serious systemic illness, which may not otherwise be apparent. Most nail abnormalities, however, are benign and primarily of cosmetic concern. It is thus important for the evaluating physician to properly diagnose nail disorders, reassure anxious patients and parents when appropriate, and offer treatment suggestions when available.

**KEY POINTS IN
THE HISTORY**

- Trauma from nail biting, excessive manicuring, or picking is a common contributor to abnormal nails.

- Drug exposure, especially to chemotherapy, tetracycline, chloroquine, or antiretrovirals, is a frequent cause of nail discoloration.

- Longitudinal melanonychia is a common, normal finding among dark-skinned individuals.

- Malignant melanoma should be considered whenever new, solitary nail hyperpigmentation develops in a light-skinned person or when growing or changing hyperpigmentation occurs in a person of any skin type.

**KEY POINTS IN
THE PHYSICAL
EXAMINATION**

- Leukonychia striata is characterized by white spots on the nails that are the result of trauma to the nail as seen with certain grooming techniques.

- Systemic diseases usually produce uniform changes that affect all nails simultaneously.

- Primary dermatologic disorders and fungal infections may affect one or more nails but rarely affect all nails at any given time.

- Schamroth' sign, seen with nail clubbing, refers to the obliteration of the normal, diamond-shaped window formed between the dorsal surfaces of opposed left and right nail bases.

- Hutchinson's sign refers to the periungal extension of longitudinal melanonychia, a potential indicator of malignant melanoma.

- Nail findings of psoriasis, such as pitting and trachyonychia, longitudinal ridging, and roughness, are rare in the absence of cutaneous findings.

- Nail changes associated with alopecia areata, such as pitting and trachyonychia, may appear months to years before the onset of hair loss.

PHOTOGRAPHS OF SELECTED DIAGNOSES

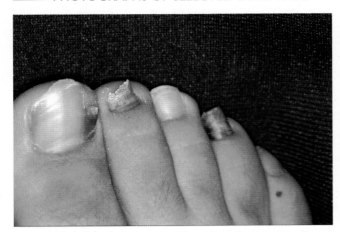

Figure 39-1 Onychomycosis. Note the yellow discoloration and thickening of the nail bed.
(Courtesy of Denise W. Metry, MD.)

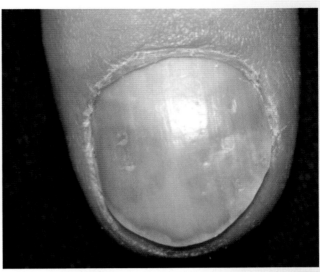

Figure 39-2 Psoriatic nail pitting. The punctate lesions arise from the nail matrix and appear as the nail plate grows.
(Used with permission from Goodheart HP. *Goodheart's photoguide to common skin disorders.* 2nd ed. Philadelphia, PA: Lippincott Williams & Wilkins; 2003:101.)

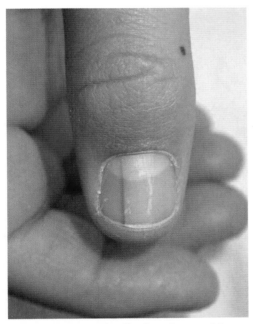

Figure 39-3 Longitudinal melanonychia. Note the longitudinal band of hyperpigmentation with no extension onto surrounding skin.
(Courtesy of Moise L. Levy, MD.)

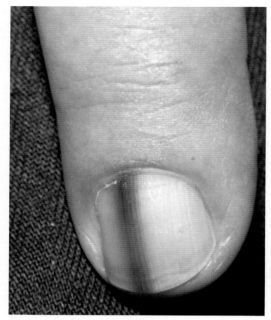

Figure 39-4 Junctional nevus.
(Used with permission from Goodheart HP. *Goodheart's photoguide to common skin disorders.* 2nd ed. Philadelphia, PA: Lippincott Williams & Wilkins; 2003:356.)

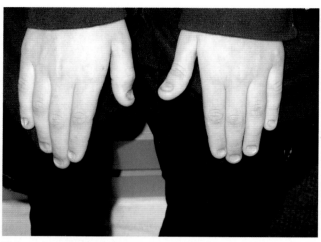

Figure 39-5 Koilonychia/nail spooning. Note the concave shape of the nail bed.
(Courtesy of Moise L. Levy, MD.)

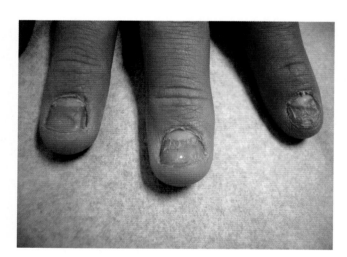

Figure 39-6 Nail dystrophy. A teenager with scaling of the nail suggestive of nail dystrophy.
(Courtesy of Paul S. Matz, MD.)

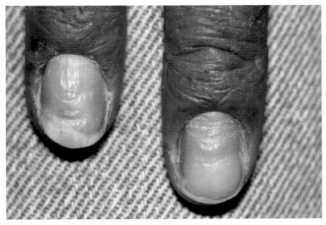

Figure 39-7 Nail dystrophy seen with atopic dermatitis. The eczema of the proximal skin affects the matrix, resulting in nail dystrophy.
(Used with permission from Goodheart HP. *Goodheart's photoguide to common skin disorders.* 2nd ed. Philadelphia, PA: Lippincott Williams & Wilkins; 2003:237.)

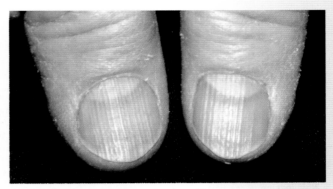

Figure 39-8 Longitudinal ridging. This normal variant is characterized by ridging in all of the nails.
(Used with permission from Goodheart HP. *Goodheart's photoguide to common skin disorders.* 2nd ed. Philadelphia, PA: Lippincott Williams & Wilkins; 2003:233.)

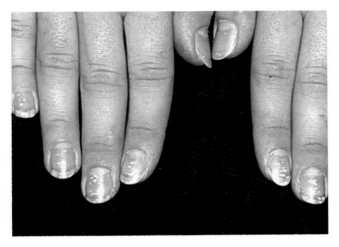

Figure 39-9 Leukonychia striata.
(Used with permission from Goodheart HP. *Goodheart's photoguide to common skin disorders.* 2nd ed. Philadelphia, PA: Lippincott Williams & Wilkins; 2003:240.)

DIFFERENTIAL DIAGNOSIS

DIAGNOSIS	ICD-9	DISTINGUISHING CHARACTERISTICS	DISTRIBUTION
Onychomycosis	110.1	Most common type is distal, lateral subungal: yellow-white discoloration at distal edge near lateral nail fold, extending proximally Thickening of nail plate, may develop dark discoloration with time Less common before puberty	Toenails most frequently affected; usually affects great toenail first Fingernail infection usually associated with toenail infection
Nail Pitting	703.8	Punctate depressions, usually ≤1 mm	Varies from isolated pit involving one nail to uniform pitting of all nails
Longitudinal Melanonychia/ Pigmented Bands	709.09	Brown to black, longitudinal pigmentation	May be solitary or multiple (most commonly a result of normal ethnic pigmentation in darker-skinned persons)
Koilonychia/Nail Spooning	703.8	Flattened, concave nail shape Normal finding in neonates/infants, especially of the great toenails	Usually all 20 nails
Trachyonychia/Nail Dystrophy	681.02 fingers 681.11 toes	Rough nails with sandpapery, opaque appearance; longitudinal ridging with adherent small scales; thinning; fragility; and distal notching Multiple small pits can make nails appear shiny. Peak incidence in ages 3 to 12 years Affects males more than females	May affect 1–20 nails
Clubbing	781.5	Sponginess of proximal nail plate with thickening/swelling of distal digit; onset usually slow and painless Schamroth's sign—obliteration of diamond-shaped space between dorsal sides of opposed, corresponding R and L distal phalanges	Usually all 20 digits, but may be more obvious on thumbs, index finger, and middle fingers

ASSOCIATED FINDINGS	PREDISPOSING FACTORS	TREATMENT GUIDELINES
Distal subungal hyperkeratosis and onycholysis (separation of the nail plate from the nail bed) Tinea pedis and tinea cruris	Warm, moist conditions Commercial manicures and pedicures Prolonged wearing of occlusive footwear	Best cure rates achieved with oral antifungals for 6 weeks (fingernails) or 3 months (toenails)
Randomly distributed shallow pits are common features of psoriasis and eczema. Transverse rows of regularly spaced pits are typically associated with alopecia areata.	May also result from trauma	Treatment of underlying condition
Malignant melanoma (very rare) should be suspected whenever a solitary streak suddenly becomes darker and/or wider, edges become blurred, and/or a family history of melanoma exists	May be caused by infection (fungal or bacterial) or melanin (nevi, normal ethnic pigmentation) Multiple pigmented bands may also be a feature of Addison disease or Cushing disease, Peutz-Jeghers syndrome, or pernicious anemia	Depending on etiology, treatment with antiinfectives or treatment of systemic illness
Nails thin, soft	Feature of iron deficiency with/without anemia, hemochromatosis, hypothyroidism, lichen planus May also be familial	Evaluation and treatment of systemic etiology (e.g., anemia or hypothyroidism) None, if familial
N/A	May be clinical manifestation of • Alopecia areata (most commonly) • Eczema • Lichen planus • Psoriasis	None
Possible acrocyanosis, hypoxia, murmur	Sign of many systemic disorders In children, most commonly recognized in association with cyanotic congenital heart disease, cystic fibrosis, or inflammatory bowel disease	Treatment of underlying systemic condition is recommended, but clubbing is sometimes irreversible.

OTHER DIAGNOSES TO CONSIDER

- Lichen planus

- Yellow-nail syndrome

- Beau's lines

- Mees's lines

- Muehrcke's lines

- Habit tick deformity

WHEN TO CONSIDER FURTHER EVALUATION OR TREATMENT

- Uniform and simultaneous changes of all nails may indicate serious systemic illness.

- Nail clubbing, in particular, is a sign of several serious systemic disorders, and warrants further evaluation.

- Nail changes associated with inflammatory disorders such as psoriasis may require systemic or other therapies. Evaluation by a pediatric dermatologist is recommended.

- Malignant melanoma should be considered whenever new, solitary nail pigmentation develops in a fair-skinned person, or when pigmentary changes occur in a person of any skin type. These changes warrant evaluation by a pediatric dermatologist.

SUGGESTED READINGS

Buka R, Friedman KA, Phelps RG, et al. Childhood longitudinal melanonychia: case reports and review of the literature. *Mt Sinai J Med.* 2001;68(4–5): 331–335.

Fawcett RS, Linford S, Stulberg DL. Nail abnormalities: clues to systemic disease. *Am Fam Physician.* 2004;69(6):1417–1424.

Goodheart HP. *Goodheart's photoguide to common skin disorders.* 2nd ed. Philadelphia, PA: Lippincott Williams & Wilkins; 2003:101, 233, 237, 240, 356.

Noronha PA. Nails and nail disorders in children and adults. *Am Fam Physician.* 1997;55(6):2129–2140.

Nousari HC, Kimyai-Asadi A, Anhalt GJ. Chronic idiopathic acrocyanosis. *J Am Acad Dermatol.* 2001;45(6)(Suppl):S207–S208.

Scheinfeld NS. Trachyonychia: a case report and review of manifestations, associations, and treatments. *Cutis.* 2003;71(4):299–302.

JEOFFREY K. WOLENS
AND MICHAEL C. DISTEFANO

Arm Displacement

APPROACH TO THE PROBLEM

Arm dislocations in children most commonly occur from trauma, but they also may be associated with an underlying abnormality. Congenital musculoskeletal abnormalities that cause joint laxity or conditions that affect nervous system development may be associated with dislocation of the upper extremity. The mechanism of injury must be kept in mind when dealing with traumatic dislocations.

KEY POINTS IN THE HISTORY

- A prior history of dislocation is important to consider because congenital and chronic dislocations are treated differently from acute dislocation.

- Congenital dislocations frequently are seen without a history of trauma and may be associated with an underlying connective tissue disorder.

- Traction injuries of the upper extremity frequently lead to acute radial head subluxation, also known as "nursemaid's elbow."

- Traumatic shoulder dislocations, most of which are due to sports injuries, are typically the result of twisting forces of the arm that are transmitted to the shoulder. Shoulder dislocations are uncommon in young children, who will present more commonly with proximal humeral fractures.

- Elbow dislocations occur most commonly in adolescent boys (75%) and in the left elbow (60%).

- Elbow dislocations are most commonly posterior and secondary to falling on an outstretched arm.

- Radial head subluxation, commonly occurring in children under 5 years of age, is seen more in girls (65%) and in the left arm (70%).

- Radial head dislocations are seen in children of all ages. These usually are caused by trauma and are often associated with fractures of the ulna.

- Wrist dislocations are uncommon because of the protective cushioning effect of immature bone and usually are associated with carpal or distal radius fractures.

- Habitual dislocations occur in children who have ligamentous laxity and can voluntarily dislocate their joints—typically, the shoulder.

- Brachial plexus injuries may lead to shoulder dislocation as early as 3 months of age.

- Sprengel deformity, a congenital elevation of the scapula, may have multidirectional joint instability, and frequently is associated with other abnormalities of the vertebrae and ribs.

KEY POINTS IN THE PHYSICAL EXAMINATION

- With an anterior dislocation of the shoulder, there is a loss of shoulder contour and the arm is held slightly abducted and externally rotated. The humeral head will be palpable anterior to the glenoid fossa.

- With a posterior dislocation of the shoulder, there is a loss of shoulder contour and the arm is held slightly adducted and internally rotated.

- The assessment of distal nerve function and vascular supply needs to be determined early in the physical examination.

- Lateral proximal radial tenderness with swelling and severe limitation to range of motion of the elbow suggests a fracture.

- Elbow dislocations occur when the radius and ulna dislocate together as a unit.

- Sprengel deformity may lead to the loss of abduction of the shoulder.

PHOTOGRAPHS OF SELECTED DIAGNOSES

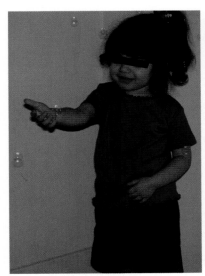

Figure 40-1 Nursemaid's elbow. Child holding left arm slightly flexed and pronated toward body. Note child reaching for bubbles freely with right arm, but not with affected arm. (Courtesy of Jeoffrey K. Wolens, MD.)

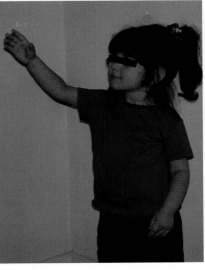

Figure 40-2 Nursemaid's elbow. Child holding left arm slightly flexed and pronated toward body. Note child reaching for bubbles freely with right arm over head, but not with affected arm. (Courtesy of Jeoffrey K. Wolens, MD.)

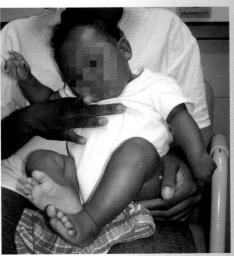

Figure 40-3 Brachial plexus injury. An infant with left arm held in adduction with internal rotation of the arm and pronation of the forearm. (Courtesy of Joseph Piatt, MD.)

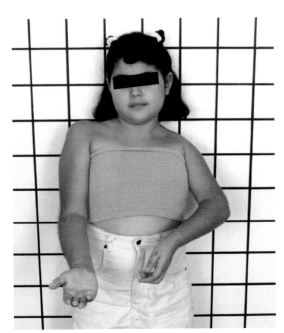

Figure 40-4 Brachial plexus injury. Patient attempting to extend and supinate arms. Compare to the normal movement of right arm. (Courtesy of Shiners Hospitals for Children, Houston, Texas.)

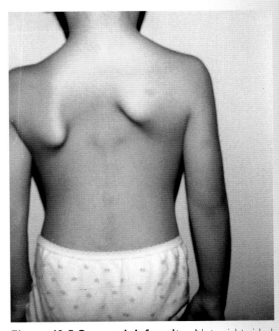

Figure 40-5 Sprengel deformity. Note right-sided deformity with elevation of scapula and asymmetry of shoulders and neck when compared to normal left side. (Courtesy of Shriners Hospitals for Children, Houston, Texas.)

DIFFERENTIAL DIAGNOSIS

DIAGNOSIS	ICD – 9	DISTINGUISHING CHARACTERISTICS	COMPLICATIONS	PRECIPITATING FACTORS	TREATMENT GUIDELINES
Radial Head Subluxation (also Nursemaid's Elbow)	832.00	Elbow held slightly flexed Occurs in children up to 5 years of age, but most commonly in children 1–3 years of age	None	Traction of extended arm	Hyperpronate and extend the affected arm. If unsuccessful, then flex and supinate the arm. The physician should feel a "pop" once it is reduced and the patient should be able to resume using the arm within 15 minutes. The arm does not need immobilization.
Brachial Plexus Injury	953.4 New born 767.6	Painless Displaced humeral head may be palpated posteriorly Swelling of the entire elbow Fracture of the distal humerus	N/A	Birth injury leads to imbalance of musculature that pulls the shoulder posteriorly.	Surgical repair of injured nerve
Shoulder Dislocation	831.0 Anterior 831.02 Posterior	Anterior dislocation—arm held abducted and externally rotated Posterior dislocation—arm adducted and internally rotated Rare in young children	Axillary nerve damage Hill Sachs lesion is a cortical depression of the humeral head secondary to impact on the glenoid. This can lead to shoulder instability.	Twisting of arm or direct trauma to humerus and shoulder. Dislocations from neurological disorders (such as brachial plexus injury) tend to be posterior.	Procedural sedation is highly recommended. Anterior dislocation: With the elbow held at 90 degrees, the arm is externally rotated and then abducted. Posterior dislocation: Arm is adducted with traction. The humeral head is massaged anteriorly. Shoulder immobilizer for 3 weeks
Elbow Dislocation	832.00	Both ulna and radius dislocate as a unit. Usually adolescent males	Median, ulnar, or radial nerve damage Vascular injury	Hyperextension of the elbow	Procedural sedation is highly recommended. Posterior dislocations—Counter-traction and stabilization of distal humerus while traction to distal arm and flexion of the elbow
Radial Head Dislocation	831.01	Pain (typically proximal ulna) Swelling Severe limitation to range of motion of elbow	Ulnar fracture (Monteggia fracture) Ulnar nerve injury	Hyperextension of elbow Fall on an outstretched arm Direct trauma to posterior forearm	An orthopedic surgeon should be consulted for reduction.
Wrist Dislocation	833.00	None	Ligamentous injury	Severe trauma to distal radius or carpals	An orthopedic surgeon should be consulted for reduction.
Sprengel Deformity	755.52	Elevation of scapula	None	None	Physical therapy to strengthen muscles Surgical treatment is best between 3 and 8 years of age.

<table>
<tr><td>

OTHER
DIAGNOSES
TO CONSIDER

</td><td>

- Cerebral palsy

- Ehlers-Danlos syndrome

- Larsen syndrome

- Familial joint instability syndrome

- Marfan syndrome

- Radioulnar synostosis

</td></tr>
<tr><td>

WHEN TO
CONSIDER
FURTHER
EVALUATION
OR TREATMENT

</td><td>

- A child with a history consistent with radial head subluxation but with focal swelling or tenderness should have radiographs to evaluate for a fracture.

- Radiographs of the clavicle and arm should be obtained for any patient with a suspected radial head subluxation that is not reducible. If they are negative, the child should be placed in a sling and followed up in 3 to 4 days. The majority of these subluxations will self-reduce. If reduction is unsuccessful on the second visit, the patient should be referred to an orthopedic surgeon.

- Any child with a joint dislocation should have prereduction and postreduction films to evaluate for fracture. Shoulder dislocations should include an axillary "Y" view to best define the direction of the displacement.

- Unsuccessful shoulder reduction should be referred immediately to an orthopedic surgeon. All other patients who have a successful reduction should be referred to an orthopedic surgeon because of the high incidence of shoulder instability.

- Isolated radial head dislocation is rare; radiographs of the entire forearm should be obtained to look for an associated ulnar fracture.

</td></tr>
</table>

SUGGESTED READINGS

Cramer CE, Sheri SA, eds. *Pediatrics: orthopedic surgery essentials*. Philadelphia, PA: Lippincott Williams & Wilkins; 2004:104–135.
McDonald J, Whitelaw C, Goldsmith LJ. Radial head subluxation: comparing two methods of reduction. *Acad Emerg Med.* 1999;6(7):715–718.
Moukoko D, Ezaki M, Wilkes D, et al. Posterior shoulder dislocations in infants with neonatal brachial plexus palsy. *J Bone Joint Surg Am.* 2004;86-A(4): 787–793.
Pizzutillo PD, ed. *Pediatric orthopedics in primary practice*. New York: McGraw-Hill; 1997:9–12, 29–32, 37–44, 51–54, 61–64, 325–328.
Staheli L. *Practice of pediatric orthopedics*. Philadelphia, PA: Lippincott Williams & Wilkins; 2001:183–201, 216–219, 244–262.
Young K, Sarwark JF. Proximal humerus, scapula, and clavicle. In: Beaty JH, Kassar JR, eds. *Rockwood and Wilkins fractures in children*. 5th ed. Philadelphia, PA: Lippincott Williams & Wilkins; 2001:741–806.

Arm Swelling

APPROACH TO THE PROBLEM

Arm swelling is a common pediatric complaint. The majority of patients with arm swelling have a preceding traumatic event, leading to a fracture, sprain, or hematoma. It is always important for clinicians to not only do a thorough neurovascular examination of the affected arm but also to examine the torso and other extremities looking for other signs of trauma. In patients with a physical examination consistent with trauma but without a clear history, nonaccidental trauma should be considered. Patients who have a subacute presentation are more likely to have a hemangioma, bone mass, or infection. If there are multiple joints involved, a systemic disease, such as systemic lupus erythematosus or juvenile idiopathic arthritis, is more likely.

KEY POINTS IN THE HISTORY

- Most commonly distal radius and ulnar, Colles and Torus (buckle) fractures occur from falling on an outstretched hand.

- Supracondylar fractures usually have a higher velocity mechanism, such as falling from an object or bicycle, and have high complication rates.

- Supracondylar fractures peak in incidence between 4 and 7 years of age.

- Nonaccidental trauma, or child physical abuse, should be considered for patients less than a year of age or with an inconsistent history.

- Clinicians should *suspect bone* or soft tissue infection secondary to *Staphylococcus aureus* or group A streptococcus (*S. pyogenes*) in patients with subacute arm swelling, erythema, tenderness out of proportion to the examination, and fever.

- A ganglion cyst generally presents as a progressive, nonpainful wrist mass, but some may be painful particularly if they occur near a joint.

- Osteochondromas, the most common bone tumors in children, are benign and typically, slow-growing, nonpainful masses.

- Hemangiomas, red or blue vascular malformations, present shortly after birth and continue to increase in size the first 12 months of life and then regress over the next 1 to 7 years.

KEY POINTS IN THE PHYSICAL EXAMINATION

- Colles and Torus fractures will have distal forearm swelling with tenderness to palpation, though Torus fractures tend to be less severe.

- As supracondylar fractures have a high rate of neuropraxia and nerve damage, the median, radial, and ulnar nerves should be assessed by having the patient make the "OK" sign and testing for strength to assess the median nerve, make an "L" shape with thumb and index finger to assess the radial nerve, and splay the fingers while checking for strength to assess the ulnar nerve.

- Patients with supracondylar fractures who have pain on passive extension of the fingers is suggestive of compartment syndrome.

- Ganglion cysts are firm mobile nodules over the wrist that transilluminate.

- A hard, nonpainful, nonmobile mass is suggestive of an osteochondroma or other bone tumor.

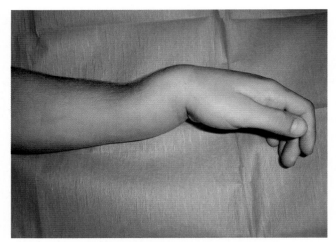

Figure 41-1 Colles fracture. Wrist swelling with obvious deformity.
(Courtesy of William Phillips, MD.)

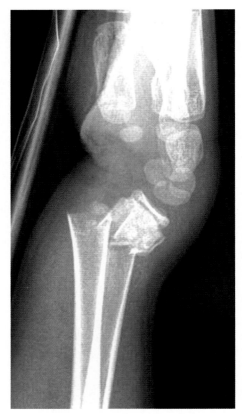

Figure 41-2 Colles fracture. Distal radial fracture with dorsal angulation.
(Courtesy of William Phillips, MD.)

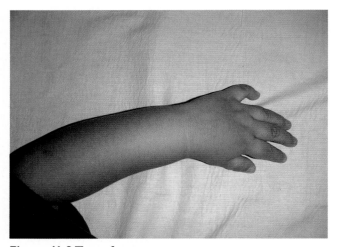

Figure 41-3 Torus fracture.
(Courtesy of Michael C. Distefano, MD.)

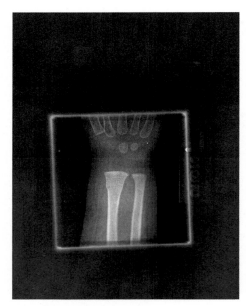

Figure 41-4 Torus fracture.
(Courtesy of Michael C. Distefano, MD.)

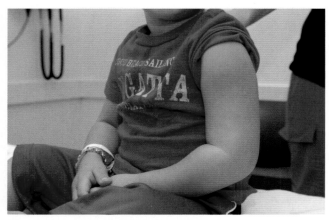

Figure 41-5 Supracondylar fracture. Note the swelling of the left elbow.
(Courtesy of Michael C. Distefano, MD.)

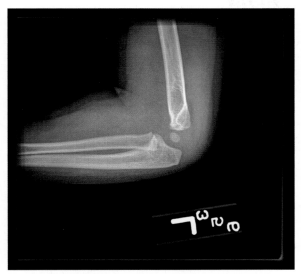

Figure 41-6 Supracondylar fracture. Left Grade I supracondylar fracture (nondisplaced) with associated posterior fat pad. No other radiographic evidence of fracture. (Courtesy of Michael C. Distefano, MD.)

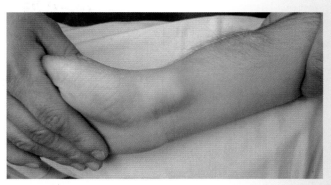

Figure 41-7 Ganglion cyst. Localized swelling over the volar surface of the wrist of a school-aged child. (Courtesy of Mary L. Brandt, MD.)

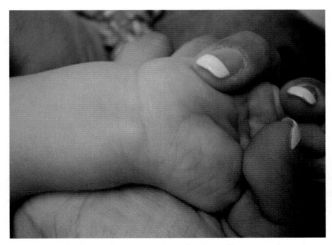

Figure 41-8 Ganglion cyst. Localized swelling over the volar surface of the wrist of an infant. (Courtesy of Mary L. Brandt, MD.)

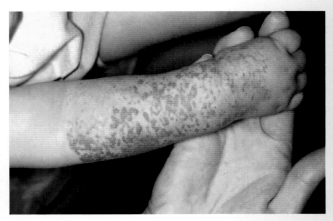

Figure 41-9 Large hemangioma of right forearm of an infant. Swelling with raised areas of vascular prominence are present. (Courtesy of Moise L. Levy, MD.)

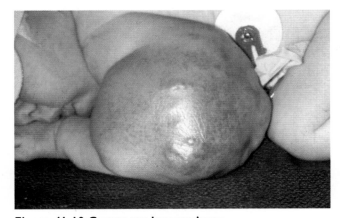

Figure 41-10 Cavernous hemangioma. (Courtesy of Jan Edwin Drutz, MD.)

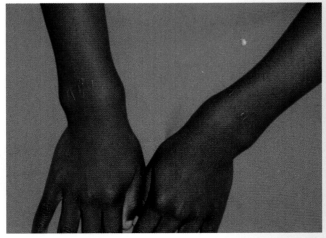

Figure 41-11 Rickets. Bilateral wrist swelling secondary to vitamin D deficiency rickets. (Courtesy of Tom Thacher, MD.)

DIFFERENTIAL DIAGNOSIS

DIAGNOSIS	ICD-9	DISTINGUISHING CHARACTERISTICS	DISTRIBUTION	COMPLICATIONS	TREATMENT GUIDELINES
Wrist Sprain	842.00	Minimal swelling over the wrist with tenderness over involved tendons	Wrist	None	Rest Ice NSAIDs Range of motion exercises
Colles Fracture	813.41 (closed) 813.51 (open)	Distal radial fracture with or without angulation	Distal forearm	Neurovascular damage (rare)	Sugar-tong splint should be applied. Referral to an orthopedic surgeon in 5–7 days or sooner for angulated or displaced fractures
Buckle Fracture (Torus Fracture)	813.45	Distal radial fracture with only minor irregularity in the contour of the cortex	Distal forearm	None	Volar splint for 3 weeks Orthopedic consultation is not required. Serial radiographs to document fracture healing are not needed.
Supracondylar Fracture	812.41 (closed) 812.51 (open)	Swelling of the elbow Grade 1: no or minimal displacement Grade 2: Anterior disruption of the cortex Grade 3: Anterior and posterior disruption of the cortex	Swelling of the entire elbow Fracture of the distal humerus	Median nerve damage Radial nerve damage Vascular compromise—the brachial artery is usually involved. Majority of vascular compromise is due to spasm rather than vascular injury. Compartment syndrome—Volkmann contracture	Nondisplaced or minimally displaced fractures may be immobilized in a long-arm posterior splint with orthopedic follow-up in 5–7 days All nonminimally displaced fractures should be splinted in the position in which they lay (no more than 20 degrees) and have immediate orthopedic evaluation
Ganglion Cyst	727.43	Fixed firm mass over the wrist Transilluminates	Volar wrist Dorsal wrist	None	Often resolves in 12 months Aspiration or surgical excision is only recommended for functional impairment or cosmetic concern (20% recurrence rate).
Hemangioma	228.00	Soft, boggy Bright red (superficial), blue (deep)	Varies	Infection Bleeding	Majority involute by age 7 Erosion, infection, and cosmetic disfigurement should be referred to a dermatologist.
Osteochondroma	213.4 (upper extremity long bone) 213.5 (upper extremity short bone)	Hard, nonpainful, nonmobile mass	Usually proximal humerus	Malignant degeneration to a chondrosarcoma (rare)	Surgical excision for painful or rapidly growing

OTHER DIAGNOSES TO CONSIDER

- Juvenile idiopathic arthritis

- Systemic lupus erythematosus

- Osteomyelitis

- Septic arthritis

- Rickets

WHEN TO CONSIDER FURTHER EVALUATION OR TREATMENT

- Torus fractures can be managed by primary care doctors. There is no need to repeat radiographs in asymptomatic patients after immobilization.

- Angulated Colles fractures should be splinted and referred to an orthopedic surgeon for reduction.

- Wrist sprains that do not improve with rest, ice, and range of motion exercises should be evaluated by an orthopedic surgeon or a sports medicine physician.

- Supracondylar fractures should be referred to an orthopedic surgeon. All nonminimally displaced fractures or patients with neurovascular compromise should be evaluated by an orthopedic surgeon immediately.

- A ganglion cyst causing significant pain, decrease in function, or a cosmetic concern may be referred to a surgeon for aspiration or excision.

- Hemangiomas with significant bleeding, ulceration, or frequent infections should be referred to a dermatologist for treatment, which may include steroids, interferon, laser therapy, or excision.

SUGGESTED READINGS

Bachman D, Santoria S. *Textbook of pediatric emergency medicine.* 5th ed. Philadelphia, PA: Lippincott Williams & Wilkins; 2006:1538–1547.

Copley L, Dormans JP. Benign pediatric bone tumors. Evaluation and treatment. *Pediatr Clin North Am.* 1996;43(4):949–966.

Huurman WW, Ginsburg GM. Musculoskeletal injury in children. *Pediatr Rev.* 1997;18(12):429–440.

Plint AC, Perry JJ, Correll R, et al. A randomized, controlled trial of removable splinting versus casting for wrist buckle fractures in children. *Pediatrics.* 2006;117(3):691–697.

Weston W, Lane A, Moreli J. *Color textbook of pediatric dermatology.* 3rd ed. St. Louis, MO: Mosby; 2002:187–201.

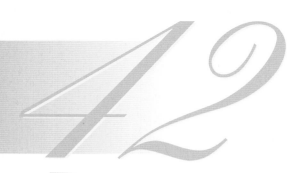

Hand Swelling

APPROACH TO THE PROBLEM

The differential diagnoses of hand swelling may be divided into infectious and noninfectious etiologies. Infections from various organisms may manifest as arthritis, synovitis, osteomyelitis, and cellulitis. Hand swelling may result from viral, bacterial, or fungal infections. Noninfectious causes of hand swelling include reactive arthritis, arthritis as part of a systemic vasculitis, metabolic joint disease, sickle cell disease, trauma, and malignancy.

KEY POINTS IN THE HISTORY

- Viral arthritis commonly presents in a polyarticular fashion, while bacterial arthritis frequently is monoarticular.

- When septic (or pyogenic) arthritis is suspected, the bacteria responsible for the infection vary by the age of the child. *Staphylococcus aureus* is the most common causative agent in all age groups. Disseminated gonococcal infection (DGI) and subsequent arthritis may occur in newborns, adolescent females, particularly during menstruation or pregnancy, and more rarely in males. The most common cause of gram-negative arthritis in children aged 2 months to 5 years is *kingella kingae*.

- Osteomyelitis is most often caused by hematogenous spread. Nonhematogenous osteomyelitis occurs through direct inoculation, such as from a puncture wound, or from a contiguous focus of infection.

- A history of chronic arthritis is seen with infection resulting from mycobacteria or fungi.

- A history of migratory or recurrent arthritis is seen in juvenile idiopathic arthritis (JIA, formerly known as juvenile rheumatoid arthritis).

- A boxer's fracture, or a fracture at the neck of the fifth metacarpal, is usually the result of a closed fist striking against a hard, immobile object.

KEY POINTS IN THE PHYSICAL EXAMINATION

- Septic arthritis in older children is often monoarticular; however, in infancy it commonly presents in multiple joints.

- Viral arthritis often involves the interphalangeal-metacarpal joints with other commonly affected joints being the knee, wrist, ankle, and elbow.

- Blistering distal dactylitis characteristically appears on the distal volar fat pad of a finger as a medium-to-large, tender blister with an erythematous base.

● Dactylitis, a sausage-shaped swelling of the fingers resulting from synovitis of interphalangeal joints and tenosynovium, may be the presenting sign of sickle cell disease. Dactylitis may also be seen with psoriatic JIA or certain infections.

● Among the seven subtypes of JIA, systemic-onset, polyarticular, and psoriatic JIA are more likely to have hand joint involvement.

● Induration of the hands, accompanied by palmar erythema, is one of the principal diagnostic criteria for Kawasaki disease.

DIFFERENTIAL DIAGNOSIS

DIAGNOSIS	ICD-9	DISTINGUISHING CHARACTERISTICS	DISTRIBUTION
Kawasaki Disease	446.1	Classic clinical criteria: Fever for at least 5 days, plus four of five of the following—Edema, erythema, and tenderness of hands, feet; conjunctival injection; changes in oropharyngeal mucosae; rash; cervical lymphadenopathy (>1.5 cm)	Initially in hands and feet, but transient symmetric arthritis can occur in large and small joints
Dactylitis (Hand-Foot Syndrome)	282.61	The first manifestation of sickle cell disease that occurs during infancy Painful, warm, nonerythematous, nonpitting, symmetric swelling	Metacarpals, metatarsals, and proximal phalanges of hands and/or feet
Blistering Distal Dactylitis	681.00	Superficial tender blisters on an erythematous base on the distal volar fat pad Usually caused by group A beta-hemolytic streptococcus or *S. aureus*	Usually affects the distal volar fat pad of a finger
Septic Arthritis	711.00	*S. aureus*—most common cause of septic arthritis in children of all age groups Fever and pain with movement	Usually lower extremities, rarely wrist and small joints
		Neisseria gonorrhoeae—DGI occurs in 1%–3% of all gonococcal infections and most commonly presents as acute polyarthralgias with fever, not genitourinary symptoms. DGI presents as tenosynovitis-dermatitis syndrome or suppurative arthritis syndrome	Tenosynovitis-dermatitis syndrome: polyarthralgias in the wrists, hands, and fingers Suppurative arthritis syndrome: monoarticular in the knee, shoulder, or wrist
Viral Arthritis	711.54	Rubella—retroauricular, posterior cervical and occipital adenopathy	Interphalangeal-metacarpal joints
		Hepatitis B—joint involvement can precede jaundice by days to weeks	Interphalangeal-metacarpal joints
Osteomyelitis	730.24	Mainly caused by *S. aureus* and streptococcus via hematogenous route In young infants, infection spreads rapidly through cortex and periosteum, into adjacent joint cavity and muscle, resulting in edematous fingers In older children, the infection is very focal, rarely affecting surrounding soft tissues because of the thick bony cortex.	Most commonly found in tubular bones—femur, tibia, humerus, phalanges
Juvenile Idiopathic Arthritis	714.30	This term includes all forms of arthritis lasting at least 6 weeks, with onset before 16 years of age, and having excluded all other causes of arthritis Associated with stiffness and flexion contractures Disuse of hand from arthritis leads to forearm muscle wasting	Oligoarticular: usually lower extremity large joints; if wrist/hand, risk for long-term disease increases Polyarticular and systemic-onset: wrist, fingers Psoriatic: dactylitis, small and large joints of hands and feet
Boxer's Fracture	815.04	Fracture of neck of the fifth or fourth metacarpal associated with striking hard immobile object with closed fist Depression of knuckle(s) with proximal edema and discoloration	Lateral aspect of hand

ASSOCIATED FINDINGS	PREDISPOSING FACTORS	TREATMENT GUIDELINES
Acute phase (day 1–11): carditis, meningitis, sterile pyuria Subacute phase (day 11–21): coronary aneurysm, desquamation	All racial groups may be affected, but patients of Japanese descent appear to be particularly at risk.	Treatment with intravenous immunoglobulin (IVIG) may be started on day 4 of fever if four of five classic criteria are met. If coronary abnormalities exist even in the absence of full criteria, treatment may be started.
Splenic infarcts leading to "autosplenectomy" and increased susceptibility to pneumococci, *H. influenzae*, and salmonella Acute splenic sequestration Acute chest syndrome	African Americans (incidence 1:600)	Transfusions for anemia, acute chest syndrome, and during surgical procedures Vaso-occlusive pain events may be managed by adequate hydration and pain medications ranging from NSAIDs to parenteral narcotics depending on the pain severity.
Not associated with poststreptococcal glomerulonephritis	Usually affects children ages 2–16 years old	Incision and drainage plus an antibiotic to which wound organism is sensitive
N/A	Bacterial upper respiratory infection Trauma or puncture wound	An orthopedic surgeon should be consulted to assist with joint aspiration. Initial empiric antibiotic therapy is based on clinical status, age, and local antibiotic resistance patterns. Antibiotic regimen may be narrowed if organism is isolated by culture.
Dermatitis Acute endocarditis Meningitis Osteomyelitis	Neonates Adolescent females, particularly during menstruation or second-third trimester of pregnancy	Initial antibiotic therapy is based on clinical status, age, and local antibiotic resistance patterns. Antibiotic regimen may be narrowed if organism is isolated by culture.
Low-grade fevers, rash, conjunctival injection	Postpubertal females with inadequate rubella vaccination history	Relief of symptoms with NSAIDs
Urticaria Angioedema	Perinatal exposure Contaminated IV drugs or blood products Sexual contact	Relief of symptoms with NSAIDs
Deep venous thrombophlebitis Periosteal abscess Inadequate treatment of acute osteomyelitis may result in chronic osteomyelitis and draining sinuses.	Sickle cell disease Immunocompromised patients Puncture wounds Trauma Surgery	An orthopedic surgeon should be consulted for diagnostic bone aspiration, especially if abscess is present. Initial empiric antibiotic therapy is based on clinical status, age, and local antibiotic resistance patterns.
Oligoarticular: iridocyclitis Polyarticular: Boutonnière and swan neck hand deformities, iridocyclitis Systemic-onset: fevers, rash, hepatosplenomegaly, pericarditis, macrophage activation syndrome Psoriatic: psoriatic rash, nail pitting	Oligoarticular and polyarticular occur more commonly in girls than in boys	Control of pain/inflammation with NSAIDs as first-line therapy, glucocorticoids, and disease-modifying anti-rheumatic agents Physical and occupational therapy Monitor for malnutrition, growth failure, delayed puberty Provide psychosocial support
Other injuries	Aggressive behavior	Closed reduction and external fixation with brace, cast, or taping if fracture is not severely displaced or angulated

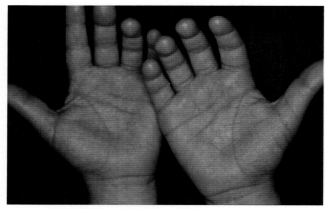

Figure 42-1 Kawasaki disease. Swelling, erythema, and tenderness develop in the hands of this 4-year-old a few days after onset of high fever.
(Courtesy of Mark A. Ward, MD.)

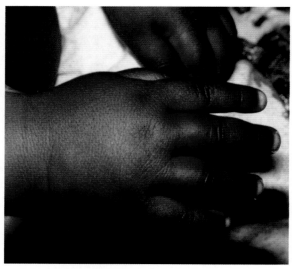

Figure 42-2 Dactylitis. This infant with sickle cell disease presents with painful, nonerythematous, nonpitting, symmetric swelling of his hands.
(Courtesy of Tom Thacher, MD.)

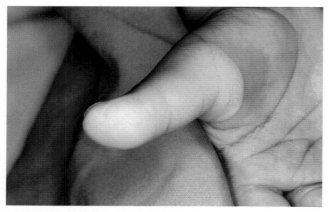

Figure 42-3 Blistering distal dactylitis. A 5-year-old presents with a superficial, tender blister on an erythematous base overlying the distal volar fat pad of his right thumb.
(Courtesy of Mark A. Ward, MD.)

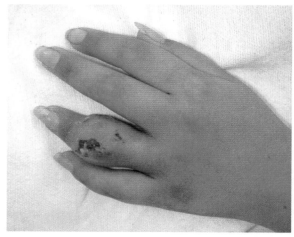

Figure 42-4 Osteomyelitis. In this 12-year-old female with finger osteomyelitis, the infection has also affected the soft tissue surrounding the joint.
(Courtesy of Mary L. Brandt, MD.)

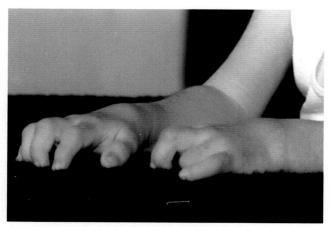

Figure 42-5 Juvenile rheumatoid arthritis. This 5-year-old child with polyarticular JRA has swelling in his wrists and fingers bilaterally. Also, note the flexion contractures at his proximal and distal interphalangeal joints.
(Courtesy of Shriners Hospitals for Children, Houston, Texas.)

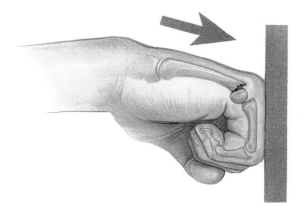

Figure 42-6 Boxer's fracture. A teenager presents with depression of his right fourth and fifth knuckles and proximal edema and discoloration after striking a hard immobile object with a closed fist.
(Used with permission from the Anatomical Chart Company. ACC Systems and Structures Chart Images, p. 2.)

OTHER
DIAGNOSES
TO CONSIDER

- Systemic lupus erythematosus (SLE)

- Serum sickness

- Henoch-Schönlein purpura

- Farber disease (ceramidase deficiency; lysosomal storage disease)

- Soft-tissue tumors

- Leukemia

WHEN TO
CONSIDER
FURTHER
EVALUATION
OR TREATMENT

- Infection resulting in edema and increased pressure within the compartments of the hand may result in compartment syndrome—characterized by the five P's: **p**ain, **p**allor, **p**aralysis, **p**aresthesias, and **p**ulselessness—which is an orthopedic emergency.

- Treatment for Kawasaki disease may be started on day 4 of fever, if four out of five classic criteria—edema/erythema of hands, feet, conjunctival injection, changes in oropharyngeal mucosae, rash, and cervical lymphadenopathy—are met.

- If the skin integrity has been compromised near a hand fracture, consider the fracture open and contaminated and seek urgent surgical consultation.

- Hand fractures that are nondisplaced or minimally displaced, nonarticular (i.e., Salter-Harris type I and II), and not associated with neurovascular compromise, may be splinted and referred for nonurgent outpatient orthopedic consultation.

SUGGESTED READINGS

Ablove RH, Moy OJ, Peimer CA. Pediatric hand disease. Diagnosis and treatment. *Pediatr Clin North Am.* 1998;45(6):1507–1524.

Fixler J, Styles L. Sickle cell disease. *Pediatr Clin North Am.* 2002;49(6):1193–1210.

Gutierrez K. Bone and joint infections in children. *Pediatr Clin North Am.* 2005;52(3):779–794.

Newburger JW, Takahashi M, Gerber MA, et al. Diagnosis, treatment, and long-term management of Kawasaki disease: a statement of the Council on Cardiovascular Disease in the Young, American Heart Association. *Pediatrics.* 2004;114(6):1708–1733. Erratum in: *Pediatrics.* 2005;115(4):1118.

Rhody C. Bacterial infections of the skin. *Prim Care.* 2000;27(2):459–473.

Weiss JE, Ilowite NT. Juvenile idiopathic arthritis. *Rheum Dis Clin North Am.* 2007;33(3):441–470.

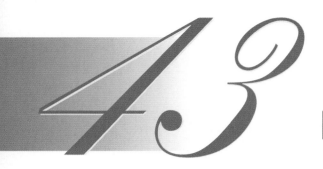

PATRICK D. COLE
AND LARRY H. HOLLIER, Jr.

Finger Abnormalities

APPROACH TO THE PROBLEM

Congenital finger anomalies affect 1% to 2% of newborns. Although many of these anomalies occur in isolation, it is important for the physician to be aware that these anomalies may be associated with systemic conditions. The deformity should never be dismissed as isolated, and a thorough evaluation of these patients is essential. The most widely accepted classification of congenital digit anomalies defines anomalies according to the etiology of developmental failure. The most common finger abnormalities primarily involve (1) failure of differentiation—syndactyly, (2) duplication—polydactyly, (3) skeletal contracture—clinodactyly, (4) soft tissue contracture—camptodactyly, (5) overgrowth—macrodactyly, and (6) undergrowth—brachydactyly. Of these defects, by far the most frequently encountered are isolated syndactyly and polydactyly.

KEY POINTS IN THE HISTORY

- Syndactyly may be either spontaneous or inherited as an autosomal dominant trait. Complex presentations may be linked to a syndrome, most notably Poland syndrome—symbrachydactyly, Apert syndrome—acrocephalosyndactyly, or Pfeiffer's syndrome—simple syndactyly.

- Preaxial (radial side) polydactyly is more common in Caucasians, and postaxial (ulnar side) polydactyly is more common in African Americans.

- Whereas preaxial polydactyly is typically unilateral, sporadic, and isolated, postaxial polydactyly is frequently inherited in an autosomal dominant pattern with variable penetrance.

- Clinodactyly can be inherited and is considered to be an autosomal dominant trait with variable expressivity and incomplete penetrance. This defect may be associated with many chromosomal abnormalities and genetic syndromes, most notably Down syndrome (Trisomy 21), in which the prevalence is between 35% and 79%.

- Thumb clinodactyly is a prominent feature of Apert syndrome, Rubinstein-Taybi syndrome, diastrophic dwarfism, and triphalangeal thumbs.

- Camptodactyly, a painless flexion deformity, is progressive with patient age. Although most presentations are sporadic, syndromic camptodactyly may occur in conjunction with craniofacial disorders, short stature, and chromosomal abnormalities.

- Macrodactyly is usually an isolated abnormality, but it may occur with neurofibromatosis or Klippel-Trenaunay-Weber syndrome (limb hypertrophy, hemangiomas, and varicose veins).

- Brachydactyly, shortened digit(s), is a frequent feature of syndromic presentations, most commonly Down syndrome. Maternal thalidomide exposure has also been linked to this defect.

KEY POINTS IN THE PHYSICAL EXAMINATION

- Syndactyly may present as a simple skin connection between digits, or may involve complex underlying bone deformities. The interconnection may encompass the entire length of both digits in complete syndactyly or it may discontinue proximal to the fingertip in partial syndactyly.

- Polydactyly may occur on the preaxial (radial) and the postaxial (ulnar) side of the limb. Postaxial polydactyly may be well-developed (type A) or rudimentary or pedunculated (type B).

- Clinodactyly typically affects the middle phalanx of the fifth digit and produces an angulation of the distal interphalangeal joint. The deviation is usually in a radial direction.

- Camptodactyly also most commonly affects the fifth digit and occurs at the proximal interphalangeal (PIP) joint. There is no intra-articular or periarticular swelling, and the metacarpophalangeal and distal interphalangeal joints are not affected. Camptodactyly is bilateral in approximately two thirds of patients.

- Macrodactyly represents overgrowth of all structures of the involved digit(s) and is different from an isolated enlargement of the bone as with an enchondroma or enlargement of the blood vessels as with a hemangioma.

- Brachydactyly appears as a short, stubby finger and multiple digits of both the hand and foot may be involved.

PHOTOGRAPHS OF SELECTED DIAGNOSES

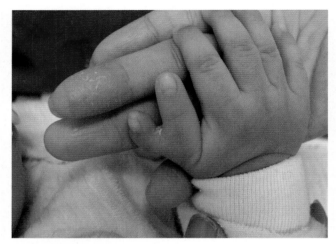

Figure 43-1 Polydactyly. An infant with a preaxial thumb duplication.
(Courtesy of Esther K. Chung, MD, MPH.)

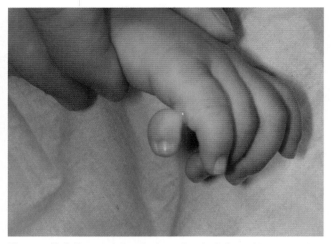

Figure 43-2 Postaxial polydactyly. An infant with postaxial fifth finger duplication on the right hand.
(Courtesy of Paul S. Matz, MD.)

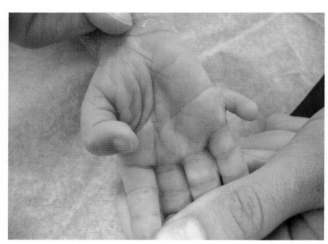

Figure 43-3 Postaxial polydactyly. A newborn with postaxial fifth finger duplication of the right hand.
(Courtesy of Paul S. Matz, MD.)

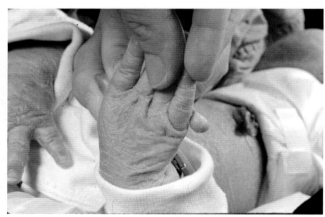

Figure 43-4 Postaxial polydactyly. A newborn with right fifth finger duplication. Note the partially formed digit is conceded by a thin band of tissue.
(Courtesy of Kenneth Rosenbaum, MD.)

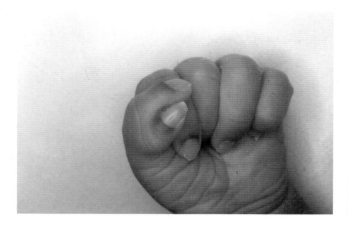

Figure 43-5 Preaxial polydactyly. A newborn with left preaxial duplication of the thumb.
(Courtesy of Gerardo Cabrera-Meza, MD.)

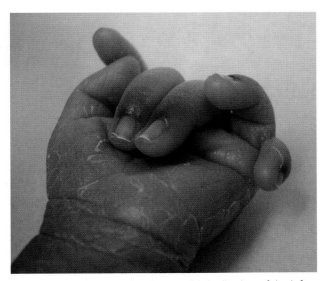

Figure 43-6 Polydactyly. A postaxial duplication of the left fifth finger in an African-American Infant.
(Courtesy of Mary L. Brandt, MD.)

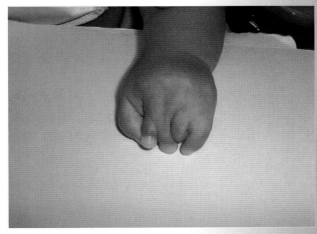

Figure 43-7 Syndactyly/brachydactyly. An infant with syndactyly and brachydactyly of the second, third, fourth, and fifth left fingers in a child with Poland syndrome.
(Courtesy of Robert L. Zarr, MD, MPH, FAAP.)

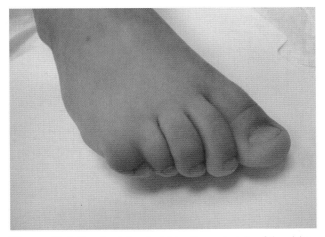

Figure 43-8 Syndactyly. A child with syndactyly of the right fourth and fifth toes.
(Courtesy of Robert L. Zarr, MD, MPH, FAAP.)

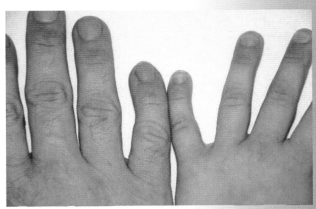

Figure 43-9 Clinodactyly. Inherited clinodactyly in a father (**left**) and son (**right**).
(Courtesy of Julie A. Bloom, MD.)

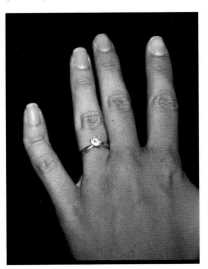

Figure 43-10 Clinodactyly.
(Courtesy of George A. Datto, III, MD.)

DIAGNOSIS	ICD-9	DISTINGUISHING CHARACTERISTICS	DISTRIBUTION
Syndactyly	755.2	Soft tissue of osseous webbing between fingers	Most commonly between third and fourth fingers
Polydactyly/ Supernumerary Digit(s)	755.1	Duplication of fingers	*Preaxial*—radial side (thumb) *Central*—second, third, fourth digits *Postaxial*—ulnar side (fifth digit)
Camptodactly	755.3	Flexion contracture of digit(s)	Most commonly involves PIP joint of fifth digit
Clinodactyly	755.59	Deviation of finger along the radio-ulnar plane.	Usually involves middle phalanx of fifth digit
Macrodactyly	755.65	Overgrowth of all digital structures	More commonly involves radial fingers, but may affect any digit
Brachydactyly	755.5	Shortened digit	May affect any digit on both hands and feet

ASSOCIATED FINDINGS	COMPLICATIONS	PRECIPITATING FACTORS	TREATMENT GUIDELINES
Apert syndrome (high broad forehead, flattened occiput, wide-set eyes, prominent lower jaw) Poland syndrome (absence of pectoralis major, hypoplasia/aplasia of breast/nipple, abnormalities of rib cage) Carpenter syndrome (acrocephaly, syndactyly, polydactyly, congenital heart disease, mental retardation)	May prevent full extension May prevent normal development of digital length and function	Autosomal dominant inheritance; may occur sporadically	Referral to a pediatric hand surgeon
Commonly sporadic Preaxial polydactyly more common in Caucasians Postaxial polydactyly more common in African Americans Familial polydactyly (inherited trait) Ellis-van Creveld syndrome (chondroectodermal dysplasia) Carpenter syndrome Down syndrome (Trisomy 21)	With suture ligation, there is the possibility of infection or a poor cosmetic result.	Preaxial is typically sporadic. Postaxial is frequently autosomal dominant with variable penetrance.	Single digit polydactyly with soft tissue involvement only may be ligated with suture material in the newborn nursery following parental consent if there is a narrow base or stalk If bone is present, referral to a pediatric hand surgeon is indicated.
May be associated with craniofacial disorders, short stature, and chromosomal abnormalities	May prevent full digital extension	Commonly sporadic but can occur in association with a syndrome	Referral to a pediatric hand surgeon
Down syndrome (Trisomy 21) Klinefelters syndrome Trisomy 18 Holt Oram syndrome Turner syndrome	None	Autosomal dominant with variable expression and incomplete penetrance	Usually none required
Neurofibromatosis Klippel-Trenaunay-Weber syndrome	Decreased functionality secondary to bulk and progressive stiffness	None	Referral to a pediatric hand surgeon
Turner syndrome Pseudohypoparathyroidism Poland syndrome VATER syndrome	Decreased functionality	Often syndromic	Referral to a pediatric hand surgeon

OTHER
DIAGNOSES
TO CONSIDER

- Synostosis

- Congenital trigger thumb

- Thumb hypoplasia

- Amniotic disruption sequence

WHEN TO
CONSIDER
FURTHER
EVALUATION
OR TREATMENT

- Radiographs of finger abnormalities are important to determine the presence and position of bony tissue.

- More complex disorders, such as syndactyly, should be referred to a pediatric hand surgeon for evaluation and treatment to assure maximal hand functionality.

- Single digit polydactyly with soft tissue involvement only may be ligated with suture material in the newborn nursery following parental consent. If there is a broad stalk or base and/or bone is present in the extra digit, referral to a pediatric hand surgeon is indicated.

SUGGESTED READINGS

Dobyns JH, Doyle JR, Von Gillern TL, et al. Congenital anomalies of the upper extremity. *Hand Clin.* 1989;5(3):321–342.

McCarroll HR. Congenital anomalies: a 25-year overview. *J Hand Surg [Am].* 2000;25(6):1007–1037.

Netscher DT. Congenital hand problems. Terminology, etiology, and management. *Clin Plast Surg.* 1998;25(4):537–552.

Netscher DT, Baumholtz MA. Treatment of congenital upper extremity problems. *Plast Reconstr Surg.* 2007;119(5):101e–129e.

Van Heest AE. Congenital disorders of the hand and upper extremity. *Pediatr Clin North Am.* 1996;43(5):1113–1133.

Watson S. The principles of management of congenital anomalies of the upper limb. *Arch Dis Child.* 2000;83(1):10–17.

44 Fingertip Swelling

APPROACH TO THE PROBLEM

The majority of cases of fingertip swelling in pediatrics result from traumatic or infectious causes. Trauma to the hand, specifically the fingertip, is the most frequent injury among boys and girls under the age of 5 years. These injuries can cause damage to the soft tissue, nail bed, and distal phalanx. Trauma to the fingertip provides a portal of entry for pathogens, which may result in infection of any component of the nail complex or distal pulp of the fingertip.

KEY POINTS IN THE HISTORY

- Crush injuries, such as those from shutting doors, are the most common causes of fingertip trauma.

- Common penetrating injuries that may lead to an abscess of the distal finger pulp, or a felon, include splinters, shards of glass, abrasions, and minor puncture wounds.

- Children at high risk for fingertip swelling from an infectious etiology are those who bite their nails or suck their thumb.

- Herpetic whitlow occurs as a complication of primary oral or genital herpes lesions.

KEY POINTS IN THE PHYSICAL EXAMINATION

- Angulation of the fingertip can be detected by comparing the planes of the fingernails of both hands with the fingers flexed.

- The swelling associated with a felon generally will not extend proximally to the distal interphalangeal joint.

- Fluctuance and pain are rare in cases of chronic paronychia compared to acute paronychia.

- With herpetic whitlow, the pain may be out of proportion to the physical examination findings.

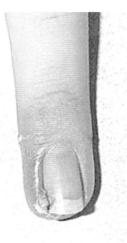

Figure 44-1 Acute paronychia.
Visible swelling, erythema, and discharge along the nail fold, yet the nail itself is intact.
(Courtesy of Mary L. Brandt, MD.)

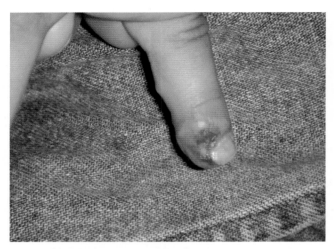

Figure 44-2 Acute paronychia. Swelling, erythema, and discharge along the lateral nail edge.
(Courtesy of Larry H. Hollier, Jr, MD, FACS.)

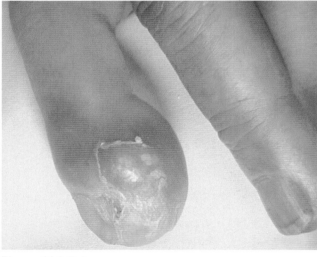

Figure 44-3 Felon.
(Used with permission from Greenberg MI. *Greenberg's atlas of emergency medicine.* Philadelphia, PA: Lippincott Williams & Wilkins; 2005:458.)

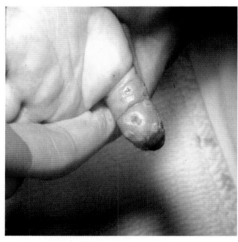

Figure 44-4 Herpetic whitlow. Ulcers where previously there were vesicles along the ventral thumb.
(Courtesy of Mark A. Ward, MD.)

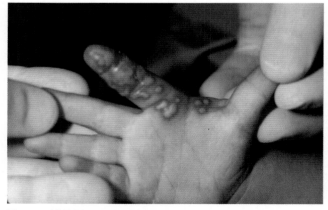

Figure 44-5 Herpetic whitlow. Grouped vesicles on an erythematous base along the ventral surface of the finger.
(Courtesy of Mark A. Ward, MD.)

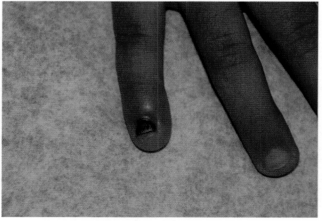

Figure 44-6 Subungal hematoma. A 2-year-old child with a subungual hematoma that resulted from a fall with a plate in his hand.
(Courtesy of Julie A. Boom, MD.)

DIFFERENTIAL DIAGNOSIS

DIAGNOSIS	ICD-9	DISTINGUISHING CHARACTERISTICS	DURATION	ASSOCIATED FINDINGS	PRECIPITATING FACTORS	TREATMENT GUIDELINES
Acute Paronychia	681.02	Swelling, erythema, and pain along nail fold	Onset within 2–5 days after cuticle trauma; resolution often requires antibiotics	Abscess along nail fold	Bacterial invasion from trauma to the cuticle	Oral antibiotics. Elevation and warm water soaks may accelerate healing.
Chronic Paronychia	112.3	Swelling and boggy-appearance along nail fold. Tenderness is mild or absent.	Longer than 6 weeks duration. Resolution often requires antifungal agent.	Fingernail dystrophy	Chronic dermatitis or frequent exposure to water leading to candidal infection	Oral antifungal agents
Felon	681.01	Throbbing pain with redness and swelling of the distal pulp of the finger	Onset within 2–5 days after trauma. Resolution requires antibiotics and/or incision and drainage	May be associated with osteomyelitis or a foreign body	Bacterial invasion from penetrating trauma to fingertip	Radiograph to help rule out a foreign body or osteomyelitis. Oral antibiotics. Prompt incision and drainage by a general surgeon
Herpetic Whitlow	054.6	Grouped, painful vesicles on an erythematous base	Abrupt onset with resolution in 2–3 weeks without medications	Fever, malaise, and regional lymphadenopathy	Primary infection with herpes simplex virus type I	Antiviral agents may be used if the infection is present for <48–72 hrs.
Fracture	816.0	Swelling, tenderness, and often angulation	Abrupt onset	May be associated with nail avulsion or nail bed laceration	Acute trauma to the fingertip, usually from a crush injury	Radiograph to confirm fracture and rule out a foreign body. Anesthetize digit and cleanse nail bed. Splint nondisplaced fractures. Displaced fractures require reduction.
Subungual Hematoma	923.3	Brown, black, or purplish discoloration under the nail bed	Abrupt onset. Resolution often requires drainage.	May be associated with a fracture of the distal phalanx	Acute trauma to nail bed, usually from a crush injury	Drainage of hematoma

OTHER DIAGNOSES TO CONSIDER

- Sprain of the distal interphalangeal joint

- Osler nodes (embolic infectious lesions in the finger pulp)

- Subungual melanoma

WHEN TO CONSIDER FURTHER EVALUATION OR TREATMENT

- If there is no improvement in an acute paronychia 1 to 2 days after starting an oral antibiotic, look for a developing abscess that may require incision and drainage.

- A felon may be associated with osteomyelitis or a foreign body; therefore radiographs are recommended.

- If a felon does not respond to an oral antibiotic in 1 to 2 days, consider referral to a general surgeon for prompt incision and drainage.

- Displaced fingertip fractures require a referral to an orthopedic specialist for surgical reduction of the fracture.

SUGGESTED READINGS

Clark DC. Common acute hand infections. *Am Fam Physician.* 2003;68(11):2167–2176.

Doraiswamy NV, Baig H. Isolated finger injuries in children-incidence and aetiology. *Injury.* 2000;31(8):571–573.

Hart RG, Kleinert HE. Fingertip and nail bed injuries. *Emerg Med Clin North Am.* 1993;11(3):755–765.

Ljungberg E, Rosberg HE, Dahlin LB. Hand injuries in young children. *J Hand Surg.* 2003;28B(4):376–380.

Rockwell PG. Acute and chronic paronychia. *Am Fam Physician.* 2001;63(6):1113–1116.

Shmerling RH. Finger pain. *Prim Care.* 1988;15(4):751–766.

Zitelli BJ, Davis HW. *Atlas of pediatric physical diagnosis,* 4th ed. Philadelphia, PA: Mosby; 2002.

JEOFFREY K. WOLENS
AND AMI D. DHARIA

Leg Asymmetry

APPROACH TO THE PROBLEM

Asymmetry between the lower extremities has a broad differential diagnosis. Discrepancies in length may be caused by structural bone abnormalities or by alterations in rates of bone growth. Variations in the overall size of the lower extremities may be caused by neurological disorders, vascular or lymphatic abnormalities, or processes that restrict growth. Understanding the etiology of the discrepancy is important not only for treatment purposes but because a few of the conditions need to be followed closely for associated disease.

KEY POINTS IN THE HISTORY

- A birth history of oligohydramnios, constriction bands, or peripheral perinatal infection suggests an isolated problem, whereas prematurity, birth trauma, or a central perinatal infection may be associated with systemic disease.

- First-born breech girls are at an increased risk of having developmental dysplasia of the hip.

- Congenital leg length discrepancy may be the result of aplasia, hypoplasia, or hyperplasia but also may be from conditions that change normal anatomic relationships, such as clubfoot or hip dysplasia.

- Acquired leg length discrepancy may be the result of previous trauma, infection, inflammation, or neurological disease.

- Physeal injury may lead to the shortening of a limb, while injuries to other areas of the bone may cause overgrowth.

- Neurological etiologies of leg length discrepancy tend to cause an overall small-sized limb because of disuse and joint contractures.

- Vascular ischemia can lead to shortening of a limb, while vascular malformations may lead to overgrowth.

- Infections and tumors may lead to either shortening or overgrowth of bones.

- Family history is important to consider for hemihypertrophy, developmental dysplasia of the hip, clubfoot, and bone dysplasias.

KEY POINTS IN THE PHYSICAL EXAMINATION

- Leg length discrepancies are considered significant when the difference is more than 2 cm as measured from the iliac crest to the lateral malleolus.

- When a leg length discrepancy is suspected, a lift should be placed under the shorter leg in order to level the pelvis and allow for accurate examination.

- A positive Galeazzi sign—knee height discrepancy when hips are flexed 90 degrees—indicates pathology above the knee such as developmental dysplasia of the hip.

- Children compensate for leg length differences by flexing the hip and knee on the long side or walking on the toes of the short side.

- Hemihypertrophy associated with café-au-lait (CAL) spots suggests neurofibromatosis type I, while hemihypertrophy associated with macroglossia and an omphalocele is seen in Beckwith-Wiedemann syndrome.

- Hemihypertrophy with cutaneous lesions is likely due to a vascular malformation such as Klippel-Trenaunay-Weber syndrome or Parkes-Weber syndrome.

- When examining a patient with lower leg asymmetry, inspection of the back, looking for a midline cutaneous lesion, is essential as hemiatrophy or other asymmetries may be associated with spinal dysraphism and a tethered cord.

- The presence of an abdominal mass in a patient with hemihypertrophy should raise suspicion for a tumor, particularly adrenal carcinoma, Wilms tumor, or hepatoblastoma.

- Localized edema caused by surgery, burns, infection, allergic reactions, trauma, or lymphatic obstruction may result in leg asymmetry.

- Growth restriction may be caused by burns or scarring of the dermis.

- Findings of increased cutaneous warmth, dilated veins around an erythematous macule or red stain, pulsations on palpation, or an audible bruit indicate an arteriovenous malformation.

- The presence of an anterior skin dimple is a sign of an underlying congenital hypoplasia or hemimelia.

PHOTOGRAPHS OF SELECTED DIAGNOSES

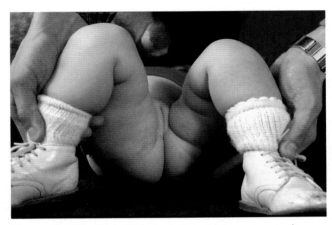

Figure 45-1 Positive Galeazzi sign. Note asymmetry in femoral heights.
(Courtesy of Douglas A. Barnes, MD.)

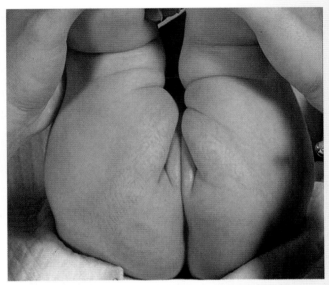

Figure 45-2 Developmental dysplasia of the hip. Note the asymmetry of this infant's thigh folds.
(Courtesy of Texas Scottish Rite Hospital for Children, Dallas, Texas.)

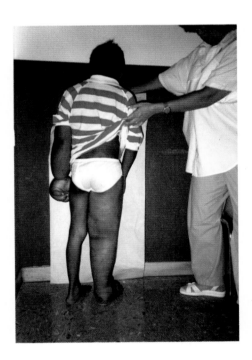

Figure 45-3 Hemihypertrophy secondary to Proteus syndrome. Note the hypertrophy of the right lower extremity and left upper extremity.
(Courtesy of Shriners Hospitals for Children, Houston, Texas.)

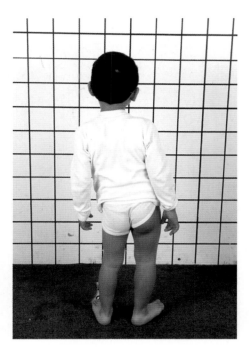

Figure 45-4 Isolated hemihypertrophy. Note the hypertrophy of the right lower extremity.
(Courtesy of Shriners Hospitals for Children, Houston, Texas.)

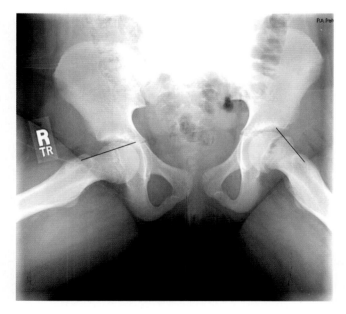

Figure 45-5 Slipped capital femoral epiphysis. Note how Klein's line (drawn as an extension of a line drawn along the top border of the femoral neck) does not intersect any part of the femoral head of the abnormal left side.
(Courtesy of Texas Scottish Rite Hospital for Children, Dallas, Texas.)

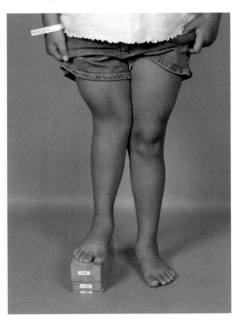

Figure 45-6 Proximal femoral focal deficiency. Note how the diagnosis of this child's congenital leg length discrepancy can be delineated to the right femur by having this child stand on blocks.
(Courtesy of Texas Scottish Rite Hospital for Children, Dallas, Texas.)

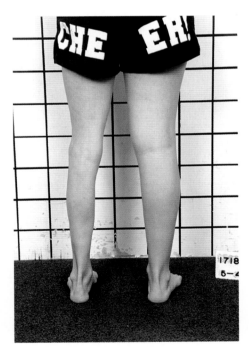

Figure 45-7 Hemiatrophy from linear scleroderma. Note normal appearing size, muscle mass, and overall bulk of the normal right leg.
(Courtesy of Shriners Hospitals for Children, Houston, Texas.)

DIAGNOSIS	ICD-9	DISTINGUISHING CHARACTERISTICS	DISTRIBUTION
Developmental Dysplasia of the Hip	754.30	Leg(s) adducted and externally rotated Limited abduction of the hip Involved side appears shorter Positive Barlow or Ortolani maneuvers in neonatal period	Hip joint
Legg-Calves-Perthes Disease	732.1	Antalgic gait with mild to no pain initially Limited internal rotation and abduction of the hip Unable to maintain pelvis level when standing on involved side Due to avascular necrosis caused by impairment of blood supply to the femoral head	Hip joint
Slipped Capital Femoral Epiphysis	732.2	Painful limp Knee pain referred from hip often present No history of significant trauma Limb held externally rotated	Hip joint
Hemihypertrophy	759.89	May be isolated or associated with overgrowth syndromes like Beckwith-Wiedemann or Proteus syndrome	Isolated or systemic depending on etiology
Vascular Malformations	747.6 or by specific syndrome	May be lymphatic, venous, or arteriovenous in origin Cutaneous lesions often present	Klippel-Trenaunay-Weber syndrome: lymphatic, venous Parkes-Weber syndrome: arteriovenous Servelle-Martorelli syndrome: lymphatic, venous
Hemiatrophy from Neuromuscular Disease	728.2	Abnormal neurological exam	Poliomyelitis Spinal cord injury Cerebral palsy Myelomeningocele or other spinal dysraphism
Trauma/Infection	736.81	History of trauma or infection Unilateral in most cases Not present at birth	Varies by site of injury

ASSOCIATED FINDINGS	COMPLICATIONS	PRECIPITATING FACTORS	TREATMENT GUIDELINES
Positive Galeazzi sign Asymmetric thigh and buttock folds when unilateral	Recurrent dislocation Avascular necrosis of femoral head Early degenerative hip joint disease with pain and stiffness in hip Shortening of affected limb	Positive family history History of breech birth More common in girls than boys	Referral to an orthopedic surgeon Pavlik harness Surgery
May have flexion contracture of affected hip and limb	Hip dislocation Early degenerative hip joint disease	Typical age at onset: 4–11 years More common in boys	Rest Referral to an orthopedic surgeon
May have flexion contracture of affected hip, and limb may appear shorter than other side Endocrinopathies may be found in patients with bilateral involvement.	Avascular necrosis of femoral head Early degenerative hip joint disease	Occurs around puberty typically in obese males	Discontinue any weight bearing Immediate referral to an orthopedic surgeon
Skin and hair are thicker on the affected side. Ipsilateral organs may also be affected. Cutaneous and vascular lesions may be present.	Compensatory scoliosis may develop. Increased incidence of Wilms tumor, hepatoblastoma, or adrenal carcinoma	Unknown	Monitor neonates with Beckwith-Wiedemann syndrome for episodes of hypoglycemia. Routine screening for abdominal tumors is recommended, but controversial.
Varies by anomaly	Verrucous hypertrophy of skin Recurrent infections Fracture	Trauma	Ultrasound with doppler/MRI Referral to an orthopedic surgeon or neurosurgeon
Cutaneous findings overlying the spine—pit, tag, asymmetric gluteal cleft Flaccid paralysis of involved leg Abnormal reflexes	Varies	Varies	Treatment of medical condition Referral to an orthopedic surgeon
With infection: Fever Ill-appearance Pain	Growth plate injury may lead to growth restriction. Hyperemia from trauma/infection can lead to overgrowth.	Trauma/Infection	Referral to an orthopedic surgeon If infection: Culture fluid or tissue when available Antibiotic therapy

OTHER
DIAGNOSES
TO CONSIDER

- Congenital absence or shortening of the tibia, fibula, or femur

- Burns or dermal scarring

- Local swelling because of envenomation or allergic reaction

- Tumors: osteochondroma, those associated with neurofibromatosis

- Silver-Russell syndrome

- Radiation therapy

- Inflammation as in juvenile rheumatoid arthritis

- Hemarthrosis as in hemophilia

- Skeletal dysplasia (Ollier disease, fibrous dysplasia, multiple hereditary exostoses)

- McCune-Albright syndrome

WHEN TO
CONSIDER
FURTHER
EVALUATION
OR TREATMENT

- Any leg length discrepancy of more than 2 cm should be referred to an orthopedic surgeon.

- All girl infants born breech should have a screening hip ultrasound at approximately age 6 weeks.

- Radiographs are essential in the workup of leg length discrepancy.

- Patients with slipped capital femoral epiphysis should avoid weight bearing, and immediate referral to an orthopedic surgeon for surgical pinning is indicated. These patients should also be evaluated for endocrine disorders like hypothyroidism or panhypopituitarism.

- Leg length discrepancies of less than 2 cm are treated supportively with shoe lifts whereas greater differences may require surgical intervention.

- Periodic screening for abdominal tumors with ultrasound in patients with Beckwith-Wiedemann syndrome or non-syndromic hemihypertrophy is recommended, but controversial.

SUGGESTED READINGS

Ballock RT, Wiesner GL, Myers MT, Thompson GH. Hemihypertrophy concepts and controversies. *J Bone Joint Surg Am.* 1997;79(11):1731–1738.

Enjolras O, Chapot R, Merland JJ. Vascular anomalies and the growth of limbs: a review. *J Pediatr Orthop B.* 2004;13(6):349–357.

Finch GD, Dawe CJ. Hemiatrophy. *J Pediatr Orthop.* 2003;23(1):99–101.

Guidera K. Leg length inequality. In: Cramer CE, Scherl SA, eds. *Pediatrics: orthopedic surgery essentials.* Philadelphia, PA: Lippincott Williams & Wilkins; 2004:74–80.

Scherl SA. Common lower extremity problems in children. *Pediatr Rev.* 2004;25(2):52–62.

Storer SK, Skaggs DL. Developmental dysplasia of the hip. *Am Fam Physician.* 2006;74(8):1310–1316.

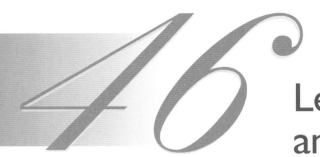

Leg Bowing and Knock Knees

APPROACH TO THE PROBLEM

Leg bowing (genu varum) and knock knees (genu valgum) are two common orthopedic complaints seen by the general pediatrician. Although most often physiological, it is important to be able to identify pathology and the need for further workup and treatment.

During normal growth, the alignment of the knee is initially varum, which becomes more prominent in the second year of life. By 2 years of age, the knee assumes valgus positioning, which peaks between 3 and 5 years. It is not until 7 to 8 years of age that the knees assume the normal adult, slightly valgus, position. Deviation from normal development, rapid progression, or asymmetric findings should prompt further investigation.

KEY POINTS IN THE HISTORY

- Unilateral or progressive deformity should alert the physician to the possibility of pathological disease.

- Angular deformities presenting before the age of 1 year often occur in children with skeletal dysplasias.

- Angular deformities occurring after the age of 5 years are often secondary to previous trauma, infection, or other systemic disease.

- Infantile tibia vara is more common in children who are African American, female, obese, and who started walking at an early age.

- Adolescent tibia vara, which often presents with knee pain, is usually seen in morbidly obese, African-American adolescent males.

- A family history of bowed legs could suggest hypophosphatemic rickets given its X-linked dominant inheritance.

- A family history of short stature or bone deformity suggests possible skeletal dysplasia.

- Poor dietary habits and limited sun exposure may indicate vitamin D deficiency rickets.

- A history of previous trauma or infection causing focal growth arrest could explain asymmetric findings.

KEY POINTS IN THE PHYSICAL EXAMINATION

- A height less than the tenth percentile should alert the physician to possible abnormality such as skeletal dysplasia or rickets.

- The presence of a lateral "thrust" to the knee during the stance phase of gait is a sign of disease, most commonly infantile tibia vara.

- Asymmetric physical examination findings suggest a pathological etiology.

- Bilateral symmetric bowing with varum alignment that is within 2 standard deviations of the mean in an otherwise healthy child less than 2 years of age indicates physiological genu varum.

- Bilateral symmetric knock knees with valgum alignment that is within 2 standard deviations of the mean in an otherwise healthy child 2 to 8 years of age is most consistent with physiological genu valgum.

PHOTOGRAPHS OF SELECTED DIAGNOSES

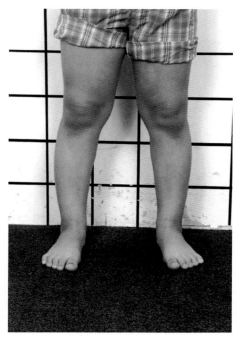

Figure 46-1 Genu varum. Outward angulation of the knees in a child. (Courtesy of Shriners Hospitals for Children, Houston, Texas.)

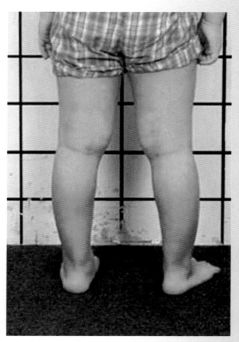

Figure 46-2 Genu varum. Posterior view of a child with genu varum. (Courtesy of Shriners Hospitals for Children, Houston, Texas.)

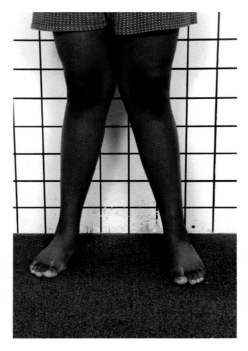

Figure 46-3 Genu valgum. Inward angulation of the knees seen in this child. (Courtesy of Shriners Hospitals for Children, Houston, Texas.)

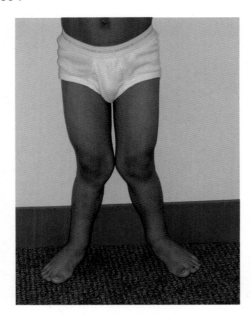

Figure 46-4 Genu valgum. A toddler with notable inward angulation of the knees.
(Courtesy of Bettina Gyr, MD.)

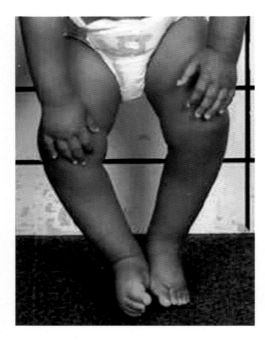

Figure 46-5 Infantile tibial bowing. Outward angulation of the tibia bilaterally in an infant.
(Courtesy of Shriners Hospitals for Children, Houston, Texas.)

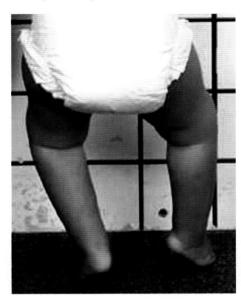

Figure 46-6 Infantile tibial bowing. Outward angulation of the tibia is also notable in the posterior view of the infant with tibial bowing.
(Courtesy of Shriners Hospitals for Children, Houston, Texas.)

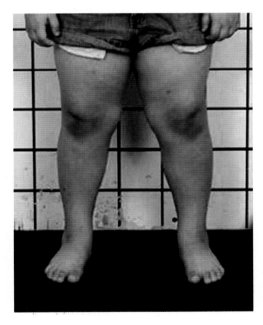

Figure 46-7 Blount disease. Genu varum deformity is seen in this obese male with Blount disease.
(Courtesy of Shriners Hospitals for Children, Houston, Texas.)

Knock Knees (Genu Valgum)

DIAGNOSIS	ICD-9	DISTINGUISHING CHARACTERISTICS	ASSOCIATED FINDINGS
Physiologic	736.41	Symmetric and bilateral Starts at 2 years, maximal between 3–5 years, resolves by 8 years	N/A
Renal Osteodystrophy	268.1	Height <10th percentile Widening of the physis on x-ray	Abnormal serum calcium and phosphate
Trauma	736.41	History of trauma: 1. Metaphyseal fracture of proximal tibia (Cozen fracture) 2. Physeal fracture 3. Fracture malunion	N/A
Infection	736.41	Unilateral involvement at the site of previous infection	N/A
Bone Dysplasias	Varies	Height <10th percentile Systemic involvement Distinctive x-ray findings depending on specific dysplasia	Varies depending on specific dysplasia

Leg Bowing (Genu Varum)

DIAGNOSIS	ICD-9	DISTINGUISHING CHARACTERISTICS	ASSOCIATED FINDINGS
Physiologic	736.42	Bilateral and symmetric Maximal varum at 6 months, resolves by age 2 Entire lower extremity is bowed. Normal physis on x-ray	Often internal tibial torsion
Infantile Tibia Vara (Blount Disease)	732.4	Symmetric and bilateral Pathological continuation of physiological bowlegs Greater deformity of proximal tibia Lateral thrust to the knee with weight bearing Four characteristic x-ray findings 1. Varus angulation at epiphyseal-metaphyseal junction 2. Widened and irregular physeal line medially 3. Medially sloped and irregularly ossified epiphysis 4. Prominent beaking of the medial metaphysis with lucent cartilage islands with beak	Persistent internal tibial torsion
Adolescent Tibia Vara (Blount Disease)	732.4	Usually unilateral Presents at age 8–14 years Presents with knee pain Tenderness along medial joint line of the knee Proximal medial tibial physis widening on x-ray	Varus deformity of distal medial femur Leg length discrepancy in unilateral cases Slipped capital femoral epiphysis
Rickets	268.1	Height <10th percentile Poor dietary history in nutritional rickets Positive family history in X-linked hypophosphatemic rickets Widening of physis and cupping of metaphyseal area as well as decreased bone density on x-ray	Abnormal calcium, phosphate and alkaline phosphatase levels
Skeletal Dysplasias	Varies	Height <10th percentile Distinctive x-ray findings depending on specific dysplasia	Normal blood chemistries
Focal Fibrocartilaginous Dysplasia	733.29	Unilateral Focal indentation at the medial metaphyseal-diaphyseal junction of tibia not involving the physis on x-ray	Hyperextension of the knee
Post Trauma/Post Infection	736.42	Unilateral History of trauma/infection	N/A

COMPLICATIONS	PRECIPITATING FACTORS	TREATMENT GUIDELINES
Lateral patellar subluxation	N/A	None usually required
Short stature Renal failure Anemia	Long standing renal disease in the physiological valgus age group (2–8 years)	Medical management of renal disease Referral to orthopedic surgeon
Lateral compartment arthritis Leg length discrepancy	History of trauma in the physiological valgus age group (2–8 years) Maximal risk 1 year after fracture	Referral to orthopedic surgeon None usually required
Premature degenerative changes in the patellofemoral joint and in the lateral compartment of the knee Leg length discrepancy	History of infection in the physiological valgus age group (2–8 years)	Referral to orthopedic surgeon May require surgery
Varies	N/A	Referral to orthopedic surgeon May require surgery

COMPLICATIONS	PRECIPITATING FACTORS	TREATMENT GUIDELINES
N/A	Early walking	None required
Osteochondrosis (avascular necrosis) Physeal bar formation (growth arrest)	Obesity Early walking	Referral to orthopedic surgeon Bracing and/or surgery
Early closure of all lower extremity physis Strain of lateral collateral ligament of knee	Morbid obesity More common in African Americans	Referral to orthopedic surgeon May require surgery
Skeletal deformity Fracture Growth restriction	Poor nutrition and limited sun exposure, but most commonly due to X-linked dominant hypophosphatemia in developed countries	Referral to metabolic bone disease specialist Medical management depending on etiology
Varies with specific dysplasia	N/A	Referral to orthopedic surgeon May require surgery
N/A	Unknown	Usually self-resolving
Leg length discrepancy	Previous trauma or infection in the physiological varum age group (0–2 years)	Referral to orthopedic surgeon May require surgery

OTHER
DIAGNOSES
TO CONSIDER

- Lead or fluoride intoxication
- Neurofibromatosis
- Congenital bowing
- Osteogenesis imperfecta
- Osteomalacia
- Arthritis of knee—rheumatoid or hemophilia
- Congenital genu valgus
- Iliotibial band contracture

WHEN TO
CONSIDER
FURTHER
EVALUATION
OR TREATMENT

- Genu valgum that is severe enough to produce mechanical axis (line from center of hip to center of ankle when knees placed forward) deviation beyond the lateral margin of the tibia is pathological and should be corrected.
- If medial foot, knee, or leg pain is present with physiological genu valgum, orthotics may help to alleviate symptoms, but do not change the overall course of disease.
- Radiographs should be obtained in the presence of short stature, history of trauma or infection, metabolic bone disease, asymmetry, deviation from normal angular development, or atypical progressive deformity. Referral to orthopedics should also be considered.
- Concern for metabolic bone disease should be referred to an endocrinologist or nephrologist.

SUGGESTED READINGS

Do TT. Clinical and radiographic evaluation of bowlegs. *Curr Opin Pediatr.* 2001;13(1):42–46.
Greene WB. Genu varum and genu valgum in children: differential diagnosis and guidelines for evaluation. *Compr Ther.* 1996;22(1):22–29.
Herring JA. *Tachdjian's pediatric orthopedics.* Philadelphia, PA: NB Saunders Company; 2002:839–863.
Kling TF Jr. Angular deformities of the lower limbs in children. *Orthop Clin North Am.* 1987;18(4):513–527.
Tachdjian MO. *Clinical pediatric orthopedics: the art of diagnosis and principle of management.* Stamford, CT: Appleton & Lange; 1997:118–132.

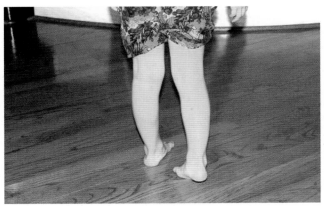

Figure 47-1 Foot progression angle. A 4-year-old child with a negative foot progression angle.
(Courtesy of Julie A. Boom, MD.)

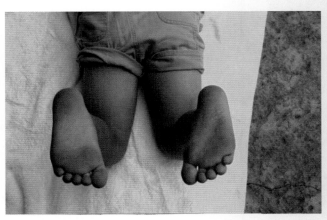

Figure 47-2 Tibial torsion. A 4-year-old child with a negative thigh foot angle.
(Courtesy of Julie A. Boom, MD.)

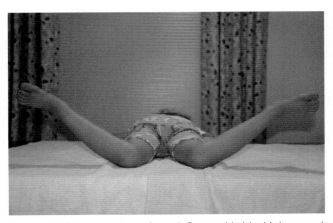

Figure 47-3 Femoral torsion. A 5-year-old girl with increased medial rotation of the hips because of femoral torsion.
(Courtesy of Julie A. Boom, MD.)

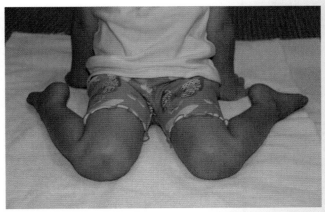

Figure 47-4 Femoral torsion. A 5-year-old girl comfortably "W" sitting.
(Courtesy of Julie A. Boom, MD.)

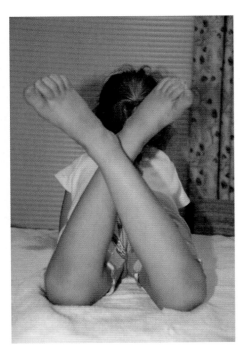

Figure 47-5 Femoral torsion. Limited lateral hip rotation in a 5-year-old girl with femoral torsion.
(Courtesy of Julie A. Boom, MD.)

DIFFERENTIAL DIAGNOSIS

DIAGNOSIS	ICD-9	DISTINGUISHING CHARACTERISTICS	DURATION/CHRONICITY
Metatarsus Adductus	754.53	Medial deviation of forefoot Deep medial crease Medial border of the foot is concave or "C" shaped. Heel bisector lateral to third toe	Usually resolves by 3–4 years of age
Tibial Torsion	736.89	A negative thigh foot angle	Present at birth Usually resolves by school age
Femoral Anteversion	755.63	Decreased hip abduction to approximately 15 degrees Increased adduction of approximately 80 degrees Patient comfortable in reverse tailor or "W" sitting position	Slowly corrects by 8–10 years of age
Clubfoot	754.7	Adduction of midfoot and forefoot Varus deformity of hindfoot Cavus deformity of midfoot	May be diagnosed in utero Chronic unless treated

ASSOCIATED FINDINGS	COMPLICATIONS	PREDISPOSING FACTORS	TREATMENT GUIDELINES

Typically none
If persistent, an abnormally shaped cuneiform may be present
	Typically none
	Occasionally, difficulty fitting shoes
		Intrauterine molding
		Increased incidence in twins
		Increased incidence if positive family history
			Depends on severity:
			  Mild—none indicated as it resolves spontaneously
			  Moderate—stretching exercises
			  Severe—serial manipulation and casting

May enhance ability to sprint by improving push-off	None	Related to positioning in utero	Treatment is seldomly indicated; corrects as the child grows
None	None	Possible genetic inheritance with increased occurrence in siblings and offspring of individuals with femoral anteversion	Resolves without treatment Discouraging sitting in the "W" position is controversial.
Multiple associated syndromes	If untreated, significant gait abnormalities If treated, gastrocsoleus weakness and difficulty with push-off may occur.	First-degree relatives have 17 times higher occurrence Maternal smoking may increase risk. Multiple genetic models proposed Boys more commonly affected than girls	Referral to an orthopedic surgeon for bracing, casting and possible surgical correction

OTHER DIAGNOSES TO CONSIDER

- Metatarsus primus varus
- Neuromuscular disorders such as cerebral palsy
- Genu valgum or knock knees

WHEN TO CONSIDER FURTHER EVALUATION OR TREATMENT

- Severe cases of metatarsus adductus resembling a clubfoot deformity should be evaluated early to optimize treatment options.
- Metatarsus adductus is associated with hip dysplasia in 2% to 10% of cases and a careful hip evaluation is essential.
- Intoeing associated with pain, swelling, or a limp should not be attributed to metatarsus adductus, tibial torsion, or femoral anteversion.
- Severe tibial torsion in a child greater than 8 to 10 years that causes significant problems with walking is an indication for further evaluation.
- Severe femoral anteversion in children greater than 9 to 10 years that causes tripping and/or unsightly gait should be referred for further evaluation.

SUGGESTED READINGS

Common Disorders. In-toeing (rotational deformities) Morgan Stanley Children's Hospital of New York – Presbyterian Columbia University Medical Center website http://www.childrensorthopaedics.com/intoeing.html. Accessed June 17, 2008.

Kasser JR. The foot. In Morrissy RT, Weinstein SL, eds. Lovell and Winter's pediatric orthopaedics. 6th ed. Philadelphia, PA: Lippincott Williams & Wilkins; 2006:1258–1328.

Roye BD, Hyman J, Roye DR Jr. Congenital idiopathic talipes equinovarus. Pediatr Rev. 2004;25(4):124–130.

Scherl SA. Common lower extremity problems in children. Pediatr Rev. 2004;25(2):52–62.

Staheli LT. Fundamentals of pediatric orthopedics. 4th ed. Philadelphia, PA: Lippincott Williams & Wilkins; 2008.

Zitelli BJ, Davis HW, eds. Atlas of pediatric physical diagnosis. 5th ed. Philadelphia, PA: Mosby; 2007.

JULIE A. BOOM
AND LISA E. DE YBARRONDO

Knee Swelling

APPROACH TO THE PROBLEM

Knee swelling in the pediatric patient suggests a broad differential diagnosis including musculoskeletal, rheumatic, and infectious processes. Knees are large joints commonly involved in juvenile idiopathic arthritis (JIA) (also known as juvenile rheumatoid arthritis). Because there are many soft tissue structures within it, the knee may be injured in almost every type of sport. The knee is involved in approximately 90% of cases of joint swelling associated with Lyme disease. As a swollen knee on physical examination may be nonspecific in appearance, a history of trauma or symptoms of systemic disease is key to identifying the correct etiology.

KEY POINTS IN THE HISTORY

- An acute onset of knee swelling suggests trauma, septic arthritis, rheumatic fever, or Lyme disease. Chronic knee swelling suggests JIA or malignancy.

- The mechanism of trauma may provide clues to the most likely structures injured. For example, a history of knee hyperextension may suggest an anterior cruciate ligament (ACL) injury.

- An audible (pop) may be concerning for a serious ligamentous injury or fracture.

- Knee instability or "giving way" may indicate a ruptured ACL or patellar instability.

- Knee locking with limited extension may indicate a torn meniscus, avulsed cruciate ligament, or bony fragment.

- Extremely painful migratory polyarthritis involving the knees, elbows, wrists, and ankles and prior group A streptococcal infection warrant the consideration of rheumatic fever.

- Pain in septic arthritis is constant, and it generally worsens over time.

- Fever may be suggestive of an infectious or rheumatologic process; high intermittent fevers (≥39.5°C) that occur once or twice daily may indicate systemic-onset JIA.

- An evanescent rash (small, pale red macules with central clearing) that occurs during periods of temperature elevation is suggestive of systemic-onset JIA.

- Consider Lyme disease when knee arthritis with an erythema chronicum migrans rash follows a tick bite or exposure to a Lyme-endemic area.

KEY POINTS IN THE PHYSICAL EXAMINATION

- The site of bruising may provide a clue to the direction of force that caused the swelling.

- An effusion, indicated by asymmetry of the suprapatellar pouches, may indicate synovitis—the hallmark of late Lyme disease.

- Effusion immediately following trauma may suggest acute bleeding into the knee.

- Fluid palpated over the center of the patella suggests a prepatellar bursitis.

- Pain with palpation over the tibial tuberosities suggests Osgood-Schlatter disease.

- A mass palpated in the popliteal area suggests the presence of a popliteal cyst.

- The discovery of a new heart murmur, especially one consistent with mitral or aortic insufficiency, may suggest acute rheumatic fever.

- Excruciating knee pain with bright erythema or dramatic warmth is characteristic of acute rheumatic fever or septic arthritis.

- Knee swelling accompanied by urticarial wheals, erythematous maculopapules, or purpura involving primarily the lower extremities with gastrointestinal symptoms suggests Henoch-Schönlein purpura.

- The presence of a mass with severe pain, refusal to use a limb, or abnormal hematologic findings may suggest malignancy.

PHOTOGRAPHS OF SELECTED DIAGNOSES

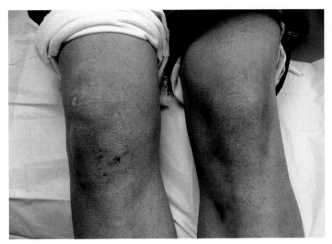

Figure 48-1 Knee effusion. Clinically obvious effusion of the right knee.
(Used with permission from Fuchs MA. Hemarthrosis. In: Greenberg MI, ed. *Greenberg's atlas of emergency medicine.* Philadelphia, PA: Lippincott Williams & Wilkins; 2005:525.)

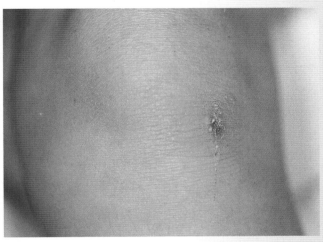

Figure 48-2 Knee cellulitis. Localized erythema suggestive of cellulitis overlying the knee.
(Used with permission from Fleisher GR, Ludwig S, Baskin MN, eds. *Atlas of pediatric emergency medicine.* Philadelphia, PA: Lippincott Williams & Wilkins; 2004:202.)

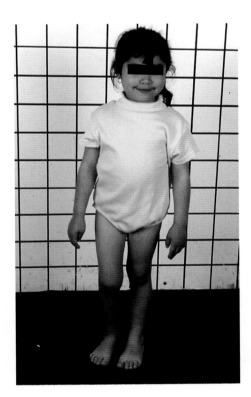

Figure 48-3 Juvenile idiopathic arthritis. Unilateral swelling of the right knee in a young girl with JIA.
(Courtesy of Shriners Hospitals for Children, Houston, Texas.)

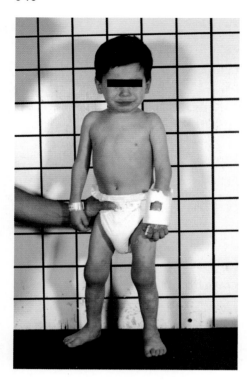

Figure 48-4 Juvenile idiopathic arthritis. A toddler with bilateral knee swelling due to JIA.
(Courtesy of Shriners Hospitals for Children, Houston, Texas.)

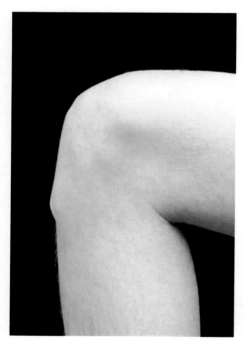

Figure 48-5 Osgood-Schlatter disease. Lateral view demonstrating prominence of the tibial tuberosity.
(Courtesy of Julie A. Boom, MD.)

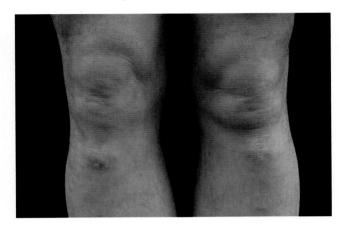

Figure 48-6 Osgood-Schlatter disease. Pain with palpation over the tibial tuberosity is suggestive of Osgood-Schlatter disease. (Courtesy of Julie A. Boom, MD.)

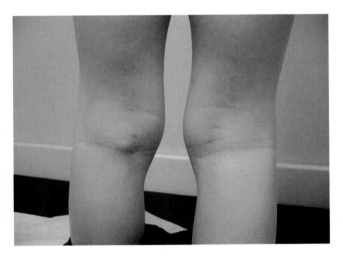

Figure 48-7 Baker cyst. Discrete swelling in the left popliteal fossa without overlying erythema. (Courtesy of Mary L. Brandt, MD.)

DIAGNOSIS	ICD-9	DISTINGUISHING CHARACTERISTICS	DISTRIBUTION	ASSOCIATED FINDINGS
Trauma	959.7	Asymmetry with bruising and point tenderness Decreased ROM depending on location of trauma	Unilateral	Usually none
Septic Arthritis	711.06	Warmth, swelling, tenderness, or an effusion with decreased ROM in all directions Swelling after several days of decreased movement Limp or refusal to walk in a previously ambulatory child	Usually monoarticular	Irritability Poor oral intake Fever in children >12–18 months Crying with passive movement Voluntary splinting to prevent movement
Rheumatic Fever	390	Painful polyarthritis Arthritis presents early and lasts <4 weeks	Polyarticular (elbows, wrists, and ankles)	Carditis Erythema marginatum Subcutaneous nodules Sydenham chorea
Juvenile Idiopathic Arthritis (JIA)	714.30	Joint swelling lasting ≥6 weeks May limp or may refuse to walk	Ankle, wrist, and elbow swelling Polyarticular >5 joints Pauciarticular <4 joints	Fatigue High regularly spiking fevers Pleuritis Pericarditis Anemia Leukocytosis Rash Lymphadenopathy Uveitis
Lyme Disease	088.81	Migratory, painful arthritis of sudden onset	Monoarticular or oligoarticular Usually large joints, but any may be affected	Most commonly, expanding skin rash, erythema chronicum migrans Malaise Fatigue Neck stiffness Arthralgia Low grade fevers

COMPLICATIONS	PREDISPOSING FACTORS	TREATMENT GUIDELINES
Intra-articular fractures, injury to more than one ligament, or neurovascular compromise require(s) immediate orthopedic or vascular surgical consultation	Fall or blow to the knee Hyperextension or twisting injury	Initiate PRICE within 24 hrs of injury P—protection R—rest I—ice C—compression E—elevation Nonsteroidal anti-inflammatory medication for analgesia If a fracture is suspected or if there is a gross deformity (knee dislocation), immobilization and transfer to an emergency department for orthopedic consultation
Permanent decreased range of motion because of tissue destruction, scarring or necrosis Impaired growth if epiphysis involved	Penetrating trauma causing direct inoculation Hematogenous spread from another location	Joint aspiration and examination of the synovial fluid; cell count, Gram stain and culture IV antibiotics to cover methicillin-resistant *Staphylococcus aureus* and streptococcal infections, until culture results are obtained In sexually active adolescents consider treatment for gonococcal infection. Orthopedic consultation for possible open drainage and lavage
Carditis Valvulitis (especially mitral) leading to vascular insufficiency Recurrence can occur unless secondary prophylaxis is instituted	History of recent streptococcal infection	Anti-inflammatory agents until all symptoms are absent and the erythrocyte sedimentation rate and C-reactive protein are normal Evaluation by a cardiologist; consider corticosteroids for severe carditis. Antibiotic therapy during the acute illness; long-term antibiotic prophylaxis every 4 weeks until age 18–20 years, if no relapse
Joint degeneration Contractures Leg length discrepancies Loss of vision because of chronic uveitis	HLA-B27 positivity ANA positivity	Nonsteroidal anti-inflammatory medications Corticosteroids Disease-modifying antirheumatic drugs
Cardiovascular abnormalities including AV block, pericarditis, cardiomegaly and left ventricular dysfunction Neurologic abnormalities including meningitis, cranial neuropathy and peripheral radiculopathy	Tick bite of the Ixodes genus, the deer tick that is infected with the spirochete, *Borrelia burgdorferi* Lyme endemic areas in the United States include: the Northeast, Mid-Atlantic region, upper North-Central region, and northwestern California 92% of cases occur in the following states: CT, RI, NJ, NY, PA, DE, MD, MA, and WI	Disseminated disease treatment: oral or IV antibiotics depending on age of patient Lyme arthritis (joint swelling) treatment; initially oral antibiotics; if no improvement after 28 days consider IV antibiotics.

- Osteochondritis dissecans

- Serum sickness

- Systemic lupus erythematosus

- Osteomyelitis

- Viral arthritis because of parvovirus, rubella, mumps, varicella, adenovirus, hepatitis B

- Malignancy including leukemia, neuroblastoma, lymphoma, Hodgkin disease, malignant histiocytosis, rhabdomyosarcoma, osteogenic sarcoma, and Ewing sarcoma

- Neurovascular injury to the popliteal artery and peroneal nerve occurs most commonly in knee dislocations and displaced fractures. Immediate vascular surgery consultation is warranted if popliteal artery compromise is suspected.

- According to the Ottawa Knee Rules, radiographs of the knee should be obtained after an acute injury in children who meet one of the following criteria: isolated tenderness of the patella, tenderness at the head of the fibula, inability to flex the knee to 90 degrees, inability to bear weight immediately and in the emergency department for four steps, regardless of limp.

- The most serious complication of pauciarticular JIA is the development of uveitis or iridocyclitis, which occurs most commonly in the subgroup of children below 6 years of age who are ANA positive. A prompt ophthalmology evaluation and routine screening are necessary.

- Bleeding disorders should be considered when hemarthrosis of the knee occurs with minimal or no recollected trauma. Initial laboratory tests include a complete blood count, prothrombin time, and activated partial thromboplastin time. Joint bleeding is typically seen in deficiencies in coagulation factors such as hemophilia.

- Recurrent painful monoarticular hemarthrosis of the knee may be caused by a synovial hemangioma, which occurs more commonly in children. MRI is the preferred mode for imaging the lesion. Refer to orthopedic surgery for treatment, which includes embolization, local steroid injection, and surgical excision.

SUGGESTED READINGS
Baskin MN. Injury knee. In Fleisher GR, Ludwig S, Henretig FM, eds. *Textbook of pediatric emergency medicine*. 5th ed. Philadelphia, PA: Lippincott Williams & Wilkins; 2006:383–391.
Fleisher GR, Ludwig S, Baskin MN, eds. *Atlas of pediatric emergency medicine*. Philadelphia, PA: Lippincott Williams & Wilkins; 2004:202.
Greenberg MI, ed. *Greenberg's atlas of emergency medicine*. Philadelphia, PA: Lippincott Williams & Wilkins; 2005:525.
Mirkinson L. The diagnosis of rheumatic fever. *Pediatr Rev.* 1998;19:310–311.
Schaller JG. Juvenile rheumatoid arthritis. *Pediatr Rev.* 1997;18:337–349.
Schwartz MW, Bell LM, Bingham P, et al, eds. *The 5-minute pediatric consult*. 5th ed. Philadelphia, PA: Lippincott Williams & Wilkins; 2008:58–59, 724–725, 760–761.

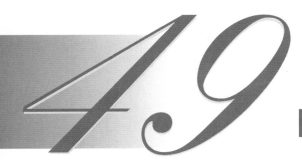

PATRICK D. COLE
AND LARRY H. HOLLIER, Jr.

Foot Deformities

APPROACH TO THE PROBLEM

An understanding of the natural history, a careful physical examination, a torsional profile, and serial measurements allow proper diagnosis for most pedal deformities. Most importantly, the timing of presentation is critical. Pes planus (flatfeet) may be either of the soft or rigid variety, and both are typically noticed as the child begins to ambulate. Flat feet are common in children because arch development occurs primarily before 4 years of age, and because the development has a wide variation in the rate or onset in any given child. The treatment of these defects is overwhelmingly conservative, and surgery is reserved for older children with severe deformities that will not improve over time.

KEY POINTS IN THE HISTORY

- Congenital pedal deformities include metatarsus adductus and clubfoot.

- In-toeing and out-toeing may result from more proximal, tibial, femoral or hip defects, such as long bone torsion, bowlegs, or knock-knees.

- While the majority of clubfoot and pes planus deformities are sporadic, these deformities have also been linked to inherited defects.

- The timing of ambulation in children with metatarsus adductus and pes planus is not generally delayed.

- Metatarsus adductus typically improves with time.

- Whereas metatarsus adductus, clubfoot, and flexible pes planus are infrequently associated with pain, rigid pes planus may be associated with significant discomfort.

- Metatarsus adductus is the most common congenital foot deformity. It occurs more frequently in women, and is more common on the left side than the right side.

- Trauma, occult infection, a foreign body, tarsal coalition, bone tumors, or osteochondrosis of the tarsal navicular bone may cause a stiff and painful flat foot.

- The presence of systemic symptoms, such as fever, may be suggestive of more serious foot disorders such as infection or malignancy.

- When metatarsus adductus is also associated with hindfoot inversion, plantar flexion, a hypoplastic ipsilateral calf or a slightly shortened tibia, a diagnosis of clubfoot should be considered.

- With a clubfoot defect, the foot does not plantar flex beyond normal. The heel is in varum (medial deviation), and the sole is kidney shaped when viewed from the bottom. Also, callous and hyperpigmentation may be present on the dorsolateral clubfoot.

- Flexible pes planus (flatfoot) is identified by appearance of the pedal arch when the child stands on his or her toes. Upon standing, however, the arch disappears.

- In evaluation of metatarsus adductus, the forefoot has a convex lateral border and a crease over the medial midfoot is visible. Also, the forefoot easily corrects to midline with gentle pressure.

- Rigid pes planus (flatfoot) is indicated by the lack of pedal arching while both standing normally and standing on one's toes.

- A compensatory flatfoot may occur as the result of a tight heel cord.

- Substantial pain upon gentle palpation, erythema, or localized firmness may be suggestive of more significant underlying pathology, such as cellulitis, osteomyelitis, joint infection, or malignancy.

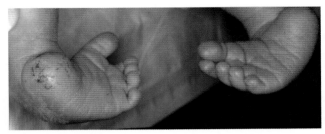

Figure 49-1 Clubfeet. Bilateral clubfeet in an infant with notable metatarsus adductus.
(Courtesy of Gerardo Cabrera-Meza, MD.)

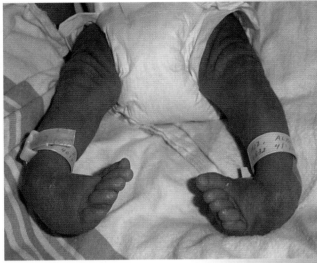

Figure 49-2 Clubfeet. Dorsal view of clubfeet in an infant with plantar flexion and foot inversion.
(Courtesy of Gerardo Cabrera-Meza, MD.)

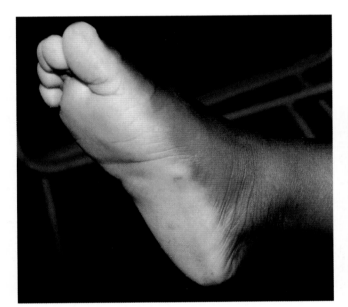

Figure 49-3 Pes planus. Arch absent in nonweight-bearing position in this child with rigid pes planus.
(Courtesy of Tom Thacher, MD.)

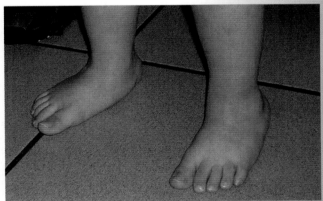

Figure 49-4 Pes planus. Mild pronation noted in this child with pes planus.
(Courtesy of Sujata R. Tipnis, MD.)

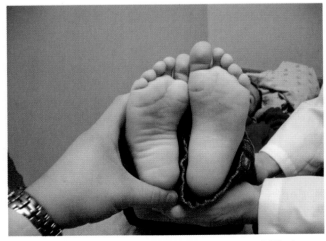

Figure 49-5 Metatarsus adductus. The convex ("C") shape of the child's right foot suggests metatarsus adductus.
(Courtesy of Paul S. Matz, MD.)

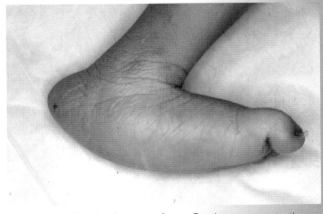

Figure 49-6 Rockerbottom feet. Gentle curvature to the bottom of this infant's feet is typical of rockerbottom feet and may be associated with Patau syndrome or Edward syndrome.
(Courtesy of Gerardo Cabrera-Meza, MD.)

DIAGNOSIS	ICD-9	DISTINGUISHING CHARACTERISTICS	DISTRIBUTION	DURATION CHRONICITY
Clubfoot	754.7	Adduction of midfoot and forefoot Varus deformity of hindfoot Cavus deformity of midfoot	May be bilateral in approximately 50% of cases	May be diagnosed in utero Chronic unless treated
Flexible Pes Planus	734	Arch present in sitting (nonweight bearing) and in toe standing positions Arch absent when standing (weight bearing)	Typically bilateral	Ubiquitous in newborns Usually resolves by school age without therapy
Rigid Pes Planus	734	Arch absent in weight-bearing and nonweight-bearing positions Subtalar joint rigid	May be bilateral in approximately 50% of cases	Persists into school age and adolescence
Metatarsus Adductus	754.53	Medial deviation of forefoot Deep medial crease Prominent proximal fifth metatarsal	Typically bilateral	Usually resolves by 3–4 years of age

ASSOCIATED FINDINGS	COMPLICATIONS	PRECIPITATING FACTORS	TREATMENT GUIDELINES

Associated syndromes:
  Prune belly
  Mobius syndrome
  Arthrogryposis
  Constriction bands
  Pierre Robin sequence
  Diastrophic dwarfism
  Larson syndrome
  Opitz syndrome
  Meningomyelocele
	If untreated, significant gait abnormalities may result
	
	If treated, gastrocsoleus weakness and difficulty with push-off may occur
		Multiple genetic models proposed
		First-degree relatives have 17 times higher occurrence.
		Maternal smoking may increase risk.
		Boys more commonly affected than girls
			Referral to an orthopedic surgeon for bracing, casting and possible surgical correction

Occasionally associated with a tight Achilles tendon	If fails to resolve with age, foot pain and lower extremity stress injuries may occur.	Incidence decreases with increasing age May be more common in boys Valgus knees, joint laxity, and obesity may increase incidence.	None indicated
Tarsal coalition Heel cord contracture	Pain Abnormal gait	Cerebral palsy Bone abnormalities	Referral to an orthopedic surgeon
Intoeing	None	Increased incidence if positive family history Increased incidence in twins	Mild forms resolve spontaneously over time.

- Trauma (sprains, strains or fractures)
- Infection
- Cavus foot (high-arched foot)
- Neoplasia

- Clubfoot deformity should be referred to an orthopedic surgeon for bracing, casting, and possible surgical correction.
- Flexible pes planus and metatarsus adductus should be simply observed as treatment is not indicated.
- A stiff or painful flat foot should be referred to an orthopedic surgeon.
- A tight heel cord should be further evaluated by an orthopedic surgeon or by a neurologist if hypertonicity is present.

SUGGESTED READINGS

Dietz FR. Intoeing – fact, fiction and opinion. Am Fam Physician. 1994;50(6):1249–1259.

Kasser JR. The foot. In: Morrissy RT, Weinstein SL, eds. Lovell and Winter's pediatric orthopaedics. 6th ed. Philadelphia, PA: Lippincott Wiliiams & Wilkins; 2006:1258–1328.

McCrea, JD. Pediatric orthopedics of the lower extremity: an instructional handbook. Mount Kisco, NY: Futura Publishing Company, Inc.; 1985.

Roye BD, Hyman J, Roye DP Jr. Congenital idiopathic talipes equinovarus. Pediatr Rev. 2004;25(4):124–130.

Sass P, Hassan G. Lower extremity abnormalities in children. Am Fam Physician. 2003;68(3):461–468.

Scherl SA. Common lower extremity problems in children. Pediatr Rev. 2004;25(2):52–62.

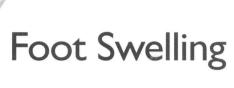

LISA E. DE YBARRONDO

Foot Swelling

APPROACH TO THE PROBLEM

Foot swelling or edema is a common manifestation of many disease states. It may be part of a localized or generalized process. Unilateral foot swelling may develop from a variety of causes including trauma, infection, allergic reactions, vasculitis, insect bites, snake bites with envenomation, soft tissue, or bone tumors. Pain may be a significant complaint with all of these etiologies except for allergic reactions. Skin changes will also help determine the etiology of the swelling. Bilateral painless foot swelling is more likely due to an underlying systemic condition such as nephrotic syndrome (NS), heart failure, cardiomyopathy, cirrhosis, malnutrition, hypoproteinemia, renal failure, or pregnancy. Medications such as calcium channel blockers and vasodilators may also cause peripheral edema.

KEY POINTS IN THE HISTORY

- The typical ankle sprain is an inversion injury that occurs in the plantar-flexed position. The lateral stabilizing ligaments are most commonly injured in this type of injury.

- Ankle sprains in children are less common than fractures because the ligaments of a preadolescent are much stronger than the growth plate or bone. Associated avulsion fractures are typically present if a ligamentous injury occurs.

- Most foot fractures in children result from direct trauma, such as crush injuries from a falling object or the child falling from a height.

- Acute traumatic compartment syndrome of the foot is the result of a serious injury such as a fracture, dislocation, and/or crush injury. Vascular injuries and coagulopathies are risk factors for the development of this condition.

- Acute, painful, unilateral foot swelling is often associated with infection or trauma. Chronic unilateral painful foot swelling over a period of weeks to months may indicate a benign or a malignant neoplasm of the soft or bony tissue.

- Recurring paroxysms of subcutaneous angioedema in the extremities, face, trunk, genitals, or the intestinal and laryngeal submucosae are characteristic of hereditary angioneurotic edema. Family history is positive in 75% of patients.

- Unilateral or bilateral, neonatal pedal edema suggests a diagnostic evaluation for Turner syndrome or Milroy disease (hereditary congenital lymphedema).

- Kwashiorkor (protein malnutrition) is rare in the United States but can occur in cases of child abuse and severe neglect. The symptoms include failure to thrive, fatigue, lethargy, edema, and abdominal distention.

- Findings associated with severe ankle sprains include swelling, bruising, pain on palpation, and a positive anterior drawer test of the ankle. Patients with all four of these findings are likely to have a lateral ligament rupture.

- Angioedema secondary to cutaneous vessel damage in Henoch-Schölein purpura may be significant. It may precede the palpable purpura and it is most prominent over the dorsal hands and feet, and the periorbital regions.

- Peripheral edema may occur in the later stages of cirrhosis.

- Subcutaneous angioedema in hereditary angioedema is nonpruritic, noneythematous, and well circumscribed. It is not accompanied by urticaria and is most commonly seen on the extremities.

- Edema is the major clinical manifestation of NS. It is more noticeable in the face in the morning upon arising and predominately in the lower extremities later in the day. It is generally pitting in nature.

- Infants with beriberi have muscle wasting, upper and lower extremity edema, pallor, restlessness, and diarrhea. Infants who are breast-fed by a thiamine-deficient mother are at risk for developing beriberi.

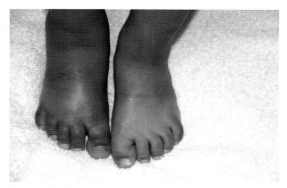

Figure 50-1 Insect bite. A 2-year-old child with swelling and erythema of the right foot and ankle because of an insect bite. A pustule and vesicles are noted over the dorsum of the foot. (Courtesy of Julie A. Boom, MD.)

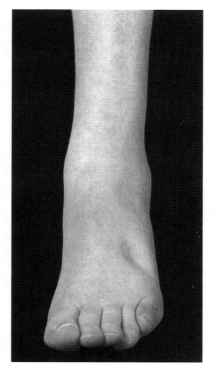

Figure 50-3 Pitting edema of the foot. An edematous foot with evidence of pitting following firm pressure.
(Used with permission from Bickley LS, Szilagyi P, eds. *Bates guide to physical examination and history taking.* 8th ed. Philadelphia, PA: Lippincott Williams & Wilkins; 2003:455.)

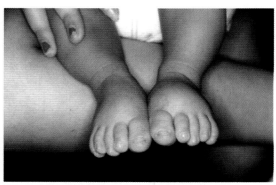

Figure 50-5 Congenital Lymphedema. Bilateral foot swelling noted by the mother of a newborn, 4 days following hospital discharge.
(Courtesy of Jan Edwin Drutz, MD.)

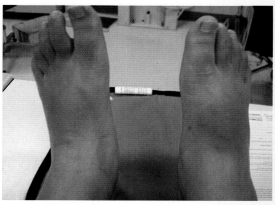

Figure 50-2 Traumatic foot swelling. This 9-year-old boy presents with swelling, bruising, and pain in the right foot 30 minutes after falling during a basketball game at school. This picture shows a comparison of the injured right foot with the normal left foot. Bruising and swelling are visible on the dorsum of the right foot. (Courtesy of Aida Z. Khanum, MD.)

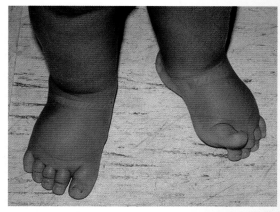

Figure 50-4 Lower extremity and foot edema. Clinical picture of lower extremities showing marked edema.
(Used with permission from Gold DH, Weingeist TA. *Color atlas of the eye in systemic disease.* Baltimore, MD: Lippincott Williams & Wilkins; 2001:643.)

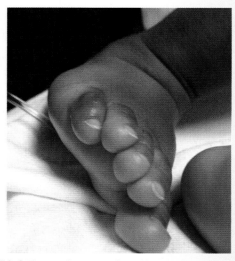

Figure 50-6 Foot edema and erythema in a child with Kawasaki disease.
(Courtesy of Esther K. Chung, MD, MPH.)

361

DIAGNOSIS	ICD-9	DISTINGUISHING CHARACTERISTICS	DISTRIBUTION	DURATION/CHRONICITY
Insect Bite	919.4	Pruritic, erythematous, urticarial papules, central punctum	Unilateral or bilateral local reaction May have multiple lesions on exposed areas of skin	Swelling may not be apparent until the next day.
Ankle or Foot Sprain	845.0	Acute onset Inversion injury, most common Minimal to severe pain Swelling Ecchymosis	Unilateral swelling localized to the injured ligaments	Swelling subsides within 48–72 hrs. Recovery depends on severity and location: mild ankle sprain, within 2 weeks; severe sprain, 6 weeks
Ankle Fracture	824.8	Acute onset Inversion injury, in the preadolescent most commonly causes a Salter Type I fracture of the distal fibula	Unilateral swelling localized to the injured bone or more diffuse swelling	Depends on the type of fracture, usually between 3–6 weeks
Foot Fracture	825.2	Acute onset Metatarsal fractures are the most common in children. Most frequently fractured metatarsal in older children is the fifth. Stress fractures present with progressive worsening of pain.	Unilateral swelling can be diffuse or localized.	Depends on the fracture location, usually between 3–6 weeks
Cellulitis and/or Abscess	682.7 (foot) 682.6 (ankle)	Acute onset Pain Erythema Warmth Induration	Unilateral Localized or diffuse Swelling	Symptomatic improvement within 24–48 hrs after initiating antimicrobial therapy Visible improvement within 72 hrs
Dactylitis	282.62	Acute onset Painful swelling of the hands and feet Occurs typically between 6 months–3 years	Bilateral	Lasts 1–2 weeks Rarely occurs after age 5
Angioedema	995.1	Rapid onset over minutes to hours Skin may be normal in color or erythematous Painful Warm to palpation	Asymmetrical pattern Face, genitalia, bowel wall, and mucosal tissues commonly involved	Resolves in 24–48 hrs
Orthostatic Edema	782.3	Painless, pitting edema in postpubertal females	Bilateral, primarily in lower legs, ankle, and feet	Duration variable, weeks to months after therapy initiated
Nephrotic Syndrome (NS)	581.9	Painless, progressive swelling Pitting edema Male-to-female ratio 2:1 Peak incidence 2–3 years Minimal change nephritic syndrome is most common.	Bilateral	Duration variable Edema improves after initiation of treatment: 90% of steroid-sensitive NS respond to steroids with 4 weeks. Few develop renal failure or renal insufficiency.

ASSOCIATED FINDINGS	COMPLICATIONS	PREDISPOSING FACTORS	TREATMENT GUIDELINES
Pain associated with hymenoptera stings, spider bites, and biting flies	Infection: impetigo, cellulitis, abscess Central necrosis/eschar (Brown recluse spider)	Warm months of the year, moist environment	Oral antihistamines Topical corticosteroids Insect control measures including repellants
Loss of functional ability Difficulty bearing weight with moderate to severe sprains Point tenderness over the affected ligaments	Chronic ankle instability Residual pain Recurrent sprains Stiffness Recurrent swelling	History of previous ankle sprain Sports such as basketball, ice skating, and soccer have highest prevalence of ankle injuries. Limited dorsiflexion may increase risk	Initiate **PRICE** within 24 hrs of injury: **P**—protection **R**—rest (up to 72 hrs) **I**—ice **C**—compression **E**—elevation Exercises to restore motion and strength within 48–72 hrs Lace-up or semi-rigid supports are more effective than tape or elastic bandages. Nonsteroidal anti-inflammatory medication
Pain, swelling, and ecchymosis observed over the lateral malleolus with the Salter type I distal fibula injury Inability to bear weight immediately after injury	Compartment syndrome Arthritis Chronic pain Gait disturbances Infection, if open fracture Chronic instability Nonunion Stiffness	Sports injury Crush injury Motor vehicle and auto-pedestrian accidents Bone tumors may predispose to pathological fractures.	Depends on the type of fracture: Salter type I distal fibula fracture—a below-the-knee walking cast is applied for 3 weeks. Salter type II requires closed reduction and a long leg cast. Salter-Harris type III (Tillaux fracture) requires open reduction with internal fixation.
Pain, swelling, ecchymosis, point tenderness over the affected bone Difficulty bearing weight Fifth metatarsal fractures often difficult to differentiate from an ankle injury because of swelling at the lateral malleolus	Compartment syndrome Arthritis Nonunion Reflex sympathetic dystrophy Chronic pain Malunion	Falls from a height or at a level surface Sports injury Crush injury Stress fractures from repetitive stress: high incidence in military recruits but also common in ballet dancers, gymnasts, and athletes.	Stress fractures require rest for 3–4 weeks, use of crutches or a walking boot, physical therapy Metatarsal shaft fractures are treated with a short leg nonweight-bearing cast for 4–12 weeks. Jones fractures of the fifth metatarsal may need closed reduction and internal fixation, if severe
For puncture wounds on the plantar surface of the foot, look for evidence of a foreign body Systemic symptoms; fever, chills, malaise, headache	Lymphangitis Osteomyelitis Septic arthritis Tissue necrosis Septic emboli	Diabetes mellitus Immunocompromise Burns Trauma Penetrating injuries Foreign bodies Lacerations Crush injuries Degloving injuries Tinea pedis/onychomycosis, lymphedema, venous insufficiency	Depends on the type of infection Cellulitis (mild/superficial): oral antibiotics directed toward *S. aureus* and group A streptococci, 7–10 days, rest, elevation Treatment for *P. aeruginosa* if puncture wound occurs through sneakers or tennis shoes. Surgical I&D or debridement for abscesses or deep infections
Low grade fever Leukocytosis Warmth and tenderness around the affected bones Infarction of bone marrow in the metacarpals, metatarsals, and proximal phalanges	Permanent shortening of the involved digits Osteomyelitis Septic arthritis	Sickle cell disease Sickle cell/hemoglobin C disease Sickle cell/beta thalassemia disease More common during colder months	Hydration Analgesics for pain relief Nonsteroidal anti-inflammatory medications Hot packs Hydroxyuria
Urticaria with intense pruritus Respiratory compromise; dyspnea, wheeze, stridor, chest or throat tightness Hypotension, tachycardia, syncope Gastrointestinal symptoms	Life threatening if laryngeal edema with anaphylaxis or hereditary angioedema Secondary to asphyxia and respiratory compromise Cardiovascular collapse	Mast-cell mediated: exposure to common allergens from food, drugs, stinging insects, latex, inhalants, and food additives Hereditary angioedema: following trauma, infection, emotional stress, puberty	Immediate stabilization of anaphylaxis using: Epinephrine IM Antihistamines Corticosteroids H_2 antihistamines Bronchodilators Hereditary angioedema: Intravenous C1-inhibitor if severe laryngeal attacks or severe abdominal attacks
Weight gain during the day May present with fatigue, dizziness, syncope, headache, abdominal swelling, breast swelling, breast discomfort, pruritus Symptoms worse in hot weather	Susceptible to bacterial infections and poor healing if trauma Associated psychological symptoms	Postpubertal females Genetic predisposition	Sodium intake reduction Avoidance of excessive fluid intake unless orthostatic hypotension is present Exercise Compression stockings Dextroamphetamine, ephedrine, and pseudoephedrine are agents that have been used.
Edema usually appears first in the periorbital, scrotal, and labial regions. Weight gain Hypertension Hypoalbuminemia/hypoproteinemia Hyperlipidemia Proteinuria Ascites Hematuria	Chronic renal failure Infections Atherosclerosis, thrombotic complications Congestive heart failure Malnutrition Long term immunosuppression may cause osteoporosis, nephrolithiasis, obesity, diabetes mellitus	Congenital nephrotic syndrome Infection Collagen vascular disease Sickle cell disease Toxins Medications Diabetes mellitus Henoch-Schönlein purpura	Glucocorticoid therapy, high dose then maintenance Diuretics Antihypertensives Ambulatory monitoring and home monitoring of urine protein/albumin Dietary salt restriction Alkylating agents

OTHER
DIAGNOSES
TO CONSIDER

- Juvenile idiopathic arthritis
- Deep venous thrombosis
- Glomerulonephritis, renal failure
- Burns
- Myxedema
- Kawasaki disease
- Primary lymphedema (Turner syndrome, Milroy disease)
- Secondary lymphedema (filariasis, lymphatic obstruction)
- Köhler disease (avascular necrosis of the navicular bone)
- Acute hemorrhagic edema of infancy

WHEN TO
CONSIDER
FURTHER
EVALUATION
OR TREATMENT

- It is important to re-examine an ankle sprain 3 to 5 days following the injury to assess the extent of ligamentous injury (partial tear vs. rupture). Consider referral to orthopedic surgery for a severe sprain that includes a ligament rupture.
- If there is a suspicion of compartment syndrome, then a prompt surgical evaluation is required with intracompartmental pressure monitoring.
- Indications for referral to an orthopedic surgeon include fracture, dislocation, subluxation, tendon rupture, wound penetrating into the joint, or bone tumors (benign or malignant).
- If cellulitis has not visibly improved within 72 hours and/or symptomatic improvement has not occurred within 24 to 48 hours after starting oral antibiotics, consider resistant pathogens or alternative diagnoses (i.e., abscess, etc.).
- Evaluation for a deeper soft tissue infection should be considered in patients with underlying conditions such as diabetes or lymphedema, and in patients who are systemically ill.
- Close medical follow-up and supportive counseling are needed for adolescents with orthostatic edema.

SUGGESTED READINGS

Bachman D, Santora S. Orthopedic trauma. In: Fleisher GR, Ludwig S, eds. *Textbook of pediatric emergency medicine*. 3rd ed. Baltimore, MD: Williams & Wilkins; 1993:1236–1287.

Barillas-Arias L, Adams A, Lehman A. Pediatric vasculitic syndrome: Henoch-Schönlein purpura. *Consultant for Pediatricians*. 2008;7(9):361–367.

Bibbo C, Lin SS, Cunningham FJ. Acute traumatic compartment syndrome of the foot in children. *Pediatr Emerg Care*. 2000;16(4):244–248.

Braun KR, Zevel JA. Visual diagnosis: an adolescent who has swelling of the foot. *Pediatr Rev*. 2001;22(9):316–320.

Ciarallo L. Edema. In: Fleisher GR, Ludwig S, eds. *Textbook of pediatric emergency medicine*. 5th ed. Baltimore, MD: Williams & Wilkins; 2005:259–262.

Farkas H, Varga L, Szeplaki G, et al. Management of hereditary angioedema in pediatric patients. *Pediatrics*. 2007;120(3):e713–e722.

Ivins D. Acute ankle sprain: an update. *Am Fam Physicians*. 2006;74(10):1714–1720.

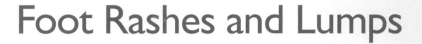

DENISE W. METRY

Foot Rashes and Lumps

APPROACH TO THE PROBLEM

Dermatologic conditions of the feet are common and often result from the extreme amount of stress and trauma constantly inflicted by everyday footwear and activities. Some conditions are related to the weight-bearing function of the feet, while others are associated with the warm, moist environment of the shoe-enclosed foot. Feet are also a site of several common dermatologic conditions. Because the feet are so heavily depended on, correct diagnosis and successful treatment of such ailments are important.

KEY POINTS IN THE HISTORY

- Tinea pedis and dyshidrotic eczema are more common in the warm, summer months, while juvenile plantar dermatosis is more common during the fall and winter months.

- A correlation with new footwear may support the diagnosis of a corn or callus.

- The use of communal showers, baths, and pools has been associated with infections, including tinea pedis and plantar warts.

- Tinea pedis and plantar warts are more common in adolescents, while juvenile plantar dermatosis is more common among prepubertal children.

- Tinea pedis is less common in children younger than 10 years old, but it may occur particularly when other family members are affected.

KEY POINTS IN THE PHYSICAL EXAMINATION

- After paring, plantar warts will often show pinpoint black dots, which are thrombosed capillaries. Calluses will have a smooth, glassy, homogenous surface.

- Plantar corns are more sensitive to direct pressure, whereas plantar warts are more sensitive to lateral compression or pinching.

- The diagnosis of a scaly, pruritic foot dermatitis may be determined based on the distribution.

- Juvenile plantar dermatosis tends to affect the balls of the feet bilaterally with a shiny, smooth, "glazed doughnut" appearance. The involvement of the interdigital spaces is more often seen in tinea pedis.

- Allergic contact dermatitis usually affects the dorsum of the feet sparing the toe webs and soles.

- Dyshidrotic eczema tends to favor the lateral fingers and toes, palms, and soles.

- Plantar warts usually disrupt skin lines, while skin lines usually are maintained in calluses.

DIFFERENTIAL DIAGNOSIS

DIAGNOSIS	ICD-9	DISTINGUISHING CHARACTERISTICS	DISTRIBUTION
Corn or Callus	726.91 (bone)	Corn: • Hard—well-circumscribed, hyperkeratotic lesion with central conical core and a glassy, homogenous surface after paring • Soft—macerated appearance of hyperkeratosis after absorbing an extreme amount of moisture from perspiration Callus: • Broad-based hyperkeratotic plaque of relatively even thickness • Skin lines usually maintained • May be painful	Corn: • Hard type—most common on the dorsum of the fifth toe, but any toe may be affected • Soft type—generally occurs between toes, most commonly between fourth and fifth Callus: • Usually found on the ball of the foot and margins of the heel, under the metatarsal heads
Plantar Wart	078.19	Round, firm, often callused papule, nodule, or plaque with a rough surface; disrupts skin lines and often occurs in multiples Often has "black dot" pattern because of thrombosed capillaries Common in both younger children and adolescents	Especially common over weight-bearing areas of soles
Tinea Pedis	110.4	Interdigital (most common)—peeling, maceration, and fissuring with erythema Moccasin—dry, fine scaly patches or hyperkeratotic papules with mild erythema, more chronic Vesicular—vesicles and pustules Uncommon before puberty Common in adolescents (M > F)	Generally affects toe webs and soles on one or both feet Often, sharp border between the involved and uninvolved skin Interdigital pattern involves web spaces (especially fourth digit space), may spread to dorsal foot and undersurface of toes Moccasin pattern is diffuse and involves plantar and lateral foot surfaces. Vesicular usually involves instep.
Dyshidrotic Eczema (Pompholyx)	705.81	Two stages: • Vesicular stage—multiple deep-set, tiny, clear vesicles (may coalesce to form bullae) with intense pruritus lasting a few days to weeks, which progresses to the next stage • Dry, desquamating stage—skin peels, cracks, or crusts over 2–3 weeks Recurrent episodes with disease-free periods Uncommon before school age Most common in ages 20–40 years (F > M)	Along lateral edges of fingers, toes, palms, and soles Usually bilateral and symmetric
Juvenile Plantar Dermatosis	709.9 (Unspecified disorder of skin and subcutaneous tissue)	Chapped, fissured feet with shiny, smooth "glazed doughnut" appearance, erythema, and scaling Pruritus Pain associated with fissuring Mainly in prepubertal children	Bilateral and symmetrical, favors the anterior third of the soles, heels, and toes (especially great toes), with sparing of interdigital spaces

ASSOCIATED FINDINGS	PREDISPOSING FACTORS	TREATMENT GUIDELINES
Corn: • Hammer toe deformity	High levels of activity/friction, irritation, and pressure or abnormal foot mechanics Mechanical stress—intrinsic, including bony prominences, or extrinsic, including tight shoes	Careful paring Abrasive reduction after soaking Regular application of salicylic acid plasters
May be painful, especially with application of lateral pressure	Direct contact from person-to-person spread, or auto-inoculation, or indirect by contact with contaminated surfaces or objects (barefoot activities) Trauma may facilitate spread through minor skin abrasions.	Most commonly repeated paring followed by the application of salicylic acid
Onychomycosis and tinea manuum ("one hand, two feet")	Use of communal showers, pools Activities that cause feet to sweat; occlusive and/or damp shoes (including not allowing athletic shoes to dry in between activities) Warm weather Household members with tinea pedis	Topical antifungal agents
N/A	Often associated with hyperhidrosis and exacerbated by warm weather, intense emotions Possible association with primary irritants (excessive washing, detergents, chemicals), nickel allergy, or as an "id" reaction to tinea or candidal infections	Topical corticosteroids or immunomodulators, emollients
N/A	Associated with hyperhidrosis and exacerbated by occlusive, synthetic footwear (especially tennis shoes), rapid drying without moisturizing Worse in atopic persons during the winter months	Frequent changing of cotton socks, emollients, topical corticosteroids, or immunomodulators

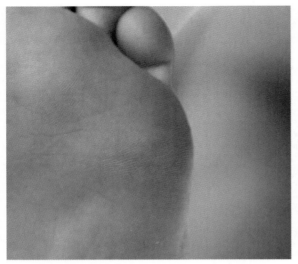

Figure 51-1 Callus. The skin over the head of the fifth metatarsal is thickened and slightly yellow. Skin lines are maintained.
(Courtesy of Julie A. Boom, MD.)

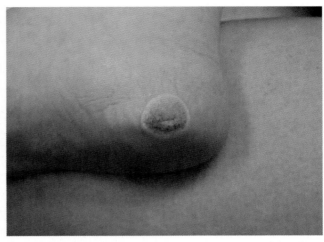

Figure 51-2 Plantar wart. Plantar wart on the medial surface of the heel.
(Courtesy of Denise W. Metry, MD.)

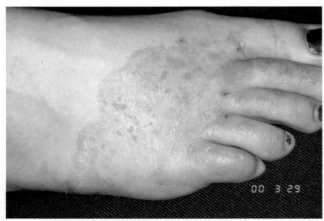

Figure 51-3 Tinea pedis. The interdigital pattern of tinea pedis is common. Note the spread onto the dorsum of the foot.
(Courtesy of Denise W. Metry, MD.)

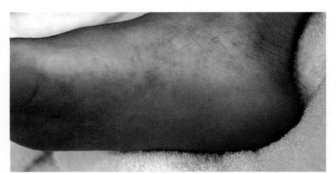

Figure 51-4 Dyshidrotic eczema. A 7-year-old boy with multiple deep-set, clear vesicles over the medical surface of his right foot.
(Courtesy of Julie A. Boom, MD.)

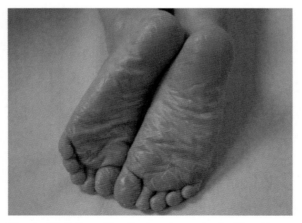

Figure 51-5 Juvenile plantar dermatosis. The skin on the soles has a smooth, shiny appearance with multiple fissures and cracks.
(Courtesy of Denise W. Metry, MD.)

OTHER
DIAGNOSES
TO CONSIDER

- Allergic contact dermatitis

- Pustular psoriasis

- Black heel

- Pitted keratolysis

WHEN TO
CONSIDER
FURTHER
EVALUATION
OR TREATMENT

- Alternative medical or surgical approaches may be considered for painful plantar warts that do not respond to traditional therapies.

- Severe tinea pedis may require treatment with a systemic antifungal agent, especially if secondary onychomycosis occurs.

- Severe dyshidrotic eczema or juvenile plantar dermatosis may rarely require systemic immunosuppressive therapy.

SUGGESTED READINGS

Buescher ES. Infections associated with pediatric sport participation. *Pediatr Clin North Am.* 2002;49(4):743–751.

Freeman DB. Corns and calluses resulting from mechanical hyperkeratosis. *Am Fam Physician.* 2002;65(11):2277–2280.

Guenst BJ. Common pediatric foot dermatoses. *J Pediatr Health Care.* 1999;13(2):68–71.

Omura EF, Rye B. Dermatologic disorders of the foot. *Clin Sports Med.* 1994;13(4):825–841.

Section

THIRTEEN

Genital and Perineal Region

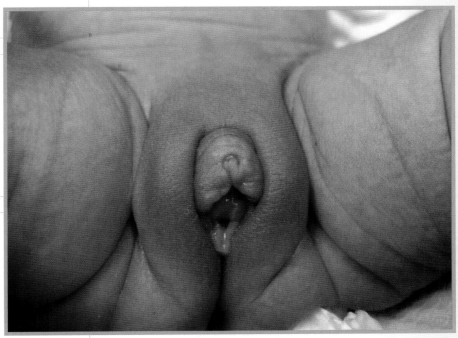

(Courtesy of Philip Siu, MD.)

COLETTE C. MULL

Female Genitalia—Variations

APPROACH TO THE PROBLEM

Variations in the physical appearance of female genitalia encompass findings within the spectrum of normal, ambiguous genitalia, and abnormalities—congenital or acquired. Although most variations represent isolated external findings, some are associated with variations in the structure and/or function of other organ systems. Identifying such variations depends on the physical characteristics, the stage of the child's genital development, the presence of associated symptoms, ongoing parental involvement in the child's genital care, and the primary care provider's consistent inclusion of a careful genital examination at every health maintenance visit. Early detection may be imperative as with ambiguous genitalia, preferred as with imperforate hymen, or inconsequential as with normal hymenal variants. In addition, any complaints of abdominal pain, urinary symptoms, perineal/vaginal symptoms, change in bowel habits, and/or sexual maltreatment should prompt the clinician to carefully examine the perineum.

KEY POINTS IN THE HISTORY

- A patient's age and Tanner stage are key to establishing whether a particular external genital finding is within the limits of normal.

- Imperforate hymen or a vaginal web may present with complaints of abdominal or lower back pain, pain with defecation, diarrhea, extremity pain, urinary retention, and nausea and vomiting.

- There may be a genetic predisposition to imperforate hymen.

- Congenital adrenal hyperplasia (CAH) occurs with higher frequency in Ashkenazi Jewish, Hispanic, Slavic, and Italian populations.

- A family history of neonatal death may represent a missed diagnosis of CAH.

- A family history of ambiguous genitalia, consanguinity, infertility, or amenorrhea suggests a genetic basis for ambiguous genitalia.

- Maternal history of certain ovarian tumors, drug ingestion, or teratogen exposure during pregnancy may contribute to the development of ambiguous genitalia.

- Labial adhesions are common and may result from vulvar exposure to irritants, including residual feces between the labia, bubble baths, harsh soaps, detergents, accidental trauma as with vigorous cleaning, or nonaccidental trauma as with child sexual abuse.

KEY POINTS IN THE PHYSICAL EXAMINATION

- The physiological red coloring of the prepubertal child's genital mucosa may be mistaken for child maltreatment.

- In a newborn with ambiguous genitalia, gonadal material palpable in the inguinal canal or labioscrotal folds is most commonly testicular material and rarely a herniated ovary or ovotestis in a hermaphrodite; its presence eliminates the diagnoses of Turner syndrome and pure gonadal dysgenesis.

- Varying degrees of labial adhesion typically create a fused segment, posteriorly to anteriorly.

- Imperforate hymen may be detected when yellow/white tissue as with mucohydrocolpos, or red/blue tissue, as with hematocolpos, is seen protruding from a child's vagina upon straining or crying.

PHOTOGRAPHS OF SELECTED DIAGNOSES

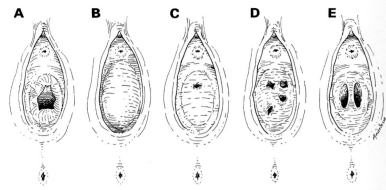

Figure 52-1 Types of hymens: (A) normal, (B) imperforate, (C) microperforate, (D) cribriform, and (E) septate.
(Used with permission from Emans SJ, Laufer MR, Goldstein DP, eds. *Pediatric and adolescent gynecology.* 5th ed. Philadelphia, PA: Lippincott Williams & Wilkins; 2005:10.)

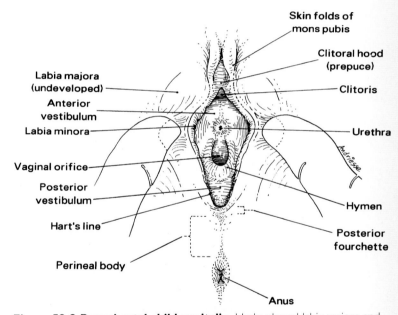

Figure 52-2 Prepubertal child genitalia. Undeveloped labia majora and other external structures are notable.
(Used with permission from Emans SJ, Laufer MR, Goldstein DR, eds. *Pediatric and adolescent gynecology.* 5th ed. Philadelphia, PA: Lippincott Williams & Wilkins; 2005:3.)

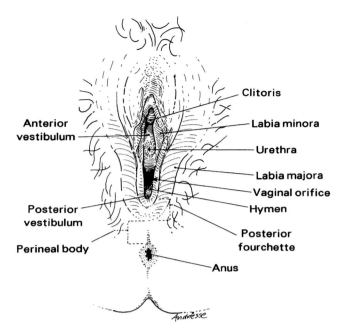

Figure 52-3 Pubertal child genitalia. Evidence of maturation of the external genitalia is prominent.
(Used with permission from Emans SJ, Laufer MR, Goldstein DP, eds. *Pediatric and adolescent gynecology.* 5th ed. Philadelphia, PA: Lippincott Williams & Wilkins; 2005:28.)

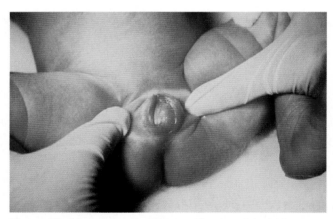

Figure 52-4 Imperforate hymen. Opening of the labia minora is not visualized.
(Used with permission from Emans SJ, Laufer MR, Goldstein DP, eds. *Pediatric and adolescent gynecology.* 5th ed. Philadelphia, PA: Lippincott Williams & Wilkins; 2005:plate 21.)

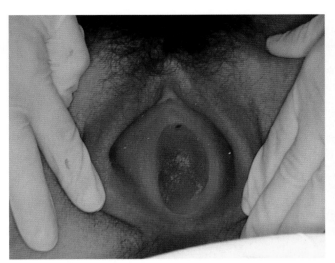

Figure 52-5 Hematocolpos. Bluish bulging membrane in a child with primary amenorrhea and lower abdominal pain.
(Used with permission from Fleisher GR, Ludwig S, Baskin MN, eds. *Atlas of pediatric emergency medicine*. Philadelphia, PA: Lippincott Williams & Wilkins; 2004:145.)

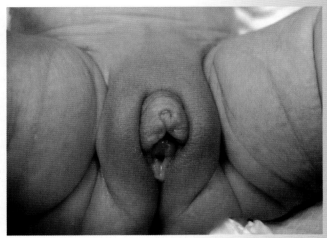

Figure 52-6 Ambiguous genitalia in a child with CAH. Note the prominent clitoris.
(Courtesy of Philip Siu, MD.)

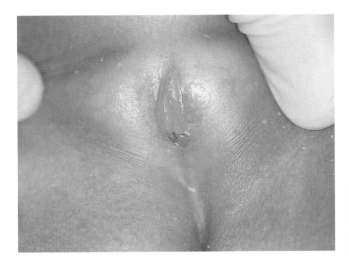

Figure 52-7 Labial adhesions. Fused labia majora in a prepubertal child.
(Used with permission from Fleisher GR, Ludwig S, Baskin MN, eds. *Atlas of pediatric emergency medicine*. Philadelphia, PA: Lippincott Williams & Wilkins; 2004:146.)

DIFFERENTIAL DIAGNOSIS

DIAGNOSIS	ICD-9	DISTINGUISHING CHARACTERISTICS	DURATION/CHRONICITY
Normal Genitalia	V21.9 Newborn Genitalia	Findings are related to maternal estrogen effects: • Prominent labia majora • Thick labia minora • Pale pink and moist mucosa • Annular or redundant hymen May see variations (septate, microperforate, cribriform hymen)	Continuum between newborn and prepubertal periods
	V21.9 Prepubertal Genitalia	Larger labia Labia minora exposed Crescentic or posterior rim hymen is common Mucosa pink-red, less moist Redundant or fimbriated hymen and annular hymen may be seen.	
	V21.1 Pubertal Genitalia	Labia larger Hymen thick, elastic, and redundant Mucosa pale pink and moist	Puberty
Imperforate Hymen	752.42	Shiny membrane between labia Membrane yellow/white or red/blue and bulging	May present in the newborn period Less commonly detected in early infancy as hydrocolpos, mucocolpos, or hematocolpos Often detected in adolescents with menarche as hematocolpos
Ambiguous Genitalia	752.7 Female Pseudohermaphroditism 255.2 Congenital Adrenal Hyperplasia	Variable virilization Ranges from mild clitoral gland enlargement to "male" phallus and scrotum	Diagnosed at birth
	752.7 Male Pseudohermaphroditism 255.2 Congenital Adrenal Hyperplasia	Inadequate virilization Microphallus, variable hypospadias, chordee, bilateral cryptorchidism, female external genitalia	
Labial Adhesions	752.49	Pale, smooth, avascular line of fusion between labia minora	3 months–6 yr

ASSOCIATED FINDINGS	COMPLICATIONS	PRECIPITATING FACTORS	TREATMENT GUIDELINES
Physiological leukorrhea Pseudomenses	N/A	N/A	N/A
N/A	N/A	Onset of puberty with unopposed estrogen production	N/A
Physiological leukorrhea Onset of menses	N/A	N/A	N/A
Primary amenorrhea Lower abdominal mass Soft, tender, fluctuant mass on rectal exam Abdominal distension	Urinary retention Constipation Hydronephrosis	N/A	Surgical repair under anesthesia with membrane incision and drainage, excess tissue excision, and vaginal mucosa repair Best performed during newborn, premenarchal, and postpubertal periods, after tissue has undergone estrogen stimulation
Salt loss Salt retention/hypertension Testicular and ovarian tissue present: true hermaphroditism Salt loss Salt retention, hypertension Hypokalemia	Vascular collapse and death from salt-wasting nephropathy Gender misassignment	N/A	Immediate medical and psychosocial issue stabilization Evaluate and treat as salt-wasting form of CAH until proven otherwise. Careful evaluation of patient and family by a multidisciplinary team including specialists from pediatric endocrinology, genetics, pediatric surgery/urology, and psychology or social work Perform the following laboratory blood tests: electrolytes, adrenal steroid levels, karyotype. Obtain pelvic and abdominal ultrasound. Correct hypovolemia, hypoglycemia, hyponatremia, and hyperkalemia. Administer stress doses of glucocorticoids after adrenal steroid levels obtained. Provide mineralocorticoid replacement therapy. Careful gender identity assignment and consideration for early genital surgery Long-term support for psychosexual issues

N/A	Variable genitourinary outflow obstruction
	Urinary tract infections
		Vulvar inflammation or irritation	Typically self-limited
			When treatment requested or required for symptoms:
			  Estrogen cream to line of fusion twice a day for 2 wks
			  Follow-up with single application before bed for 1 wk
			  May need longer course or larger volume of application
			To maintain labial separation:
			  Single application before bed of barrier cream/ointment to labial edges for 2–3 months
			  Irritant avoidance/removal
			  Meticulous perineal hygiene
			  Manual labial separation discouraged
			  Endocrinology evaluation (gender differentiation or androgen production abnormalities) required in cases of labial fusion present at 1–3 months of age or labial adhesions resistant to outlined treatment

OTHER
DIAGNOSES
TO CONSIDER

- Incomplete hymenal fenestration: microperforate, septate, and cribriform hymens

- Obstructive anomalies of the vagina

- Vulvar lichen sclerosis

- Vulvar hemangioma

- Vulvar trauma

- Urethral prolapse

- Rectal prolapse

- Child sexual abuse

WHEN TO
CONSIDER
FURTHER
EVALUATION
OR TREATMENT

- Surgery for imperforate hymen should be performed immediately in symptomatic patients and during the newborn, premenarchal, or postpubertal periods in asymptomatic patients.

- Evaluate and treat ambiguous genitalia immediately upon detection.

- Treat ambiguous genitalia as the salt-wasting form of CAH until proven otherwise.

- Gender assignment and genital surgery for ambiguous genitalia should be undertaken after careful research and deliberation by family and multidisciplinary team of specialists.

- Medical treatment of labial adhesions should be considered if patient is symptomatic, if process involves a large portion of the labia, if the urinary stream is affected, and/or if the adhesions have not resolved after puberty.

- Surgical treatment of labial adhesions should only be performed if patient is anuric, when parent/patient objects to or is noncompliant with medical treatment, and/or in cases of medical treatment failure.

- Further evaluation by endocrinology should be considered in cases of labial fusion present at 1 to 3 months of age or labial adhesions resistant to outlined treatment.

SUGGESTED READINGS

American Professional Society on the Abuse of Children. *Glossary of terms and the interpretations of findings for child sexual abuse evidentiary examinations.* Chicago, IL: APSAC; 1998.

Bacon, JL. Prepubertal labial adhesions: Evaluation of a referral population. *Am J Obstet Gynecol.* 2002; 187:327–331.

Dickson CA, Saad S, Tesar JD. Imperforate hymen with hematocolpos. *Ann Emerg Med.* 1985;14:467–469.

Schober J, Dulabon L, Martin-Alguacil N, et al. Significance of topical estrogens to labial fusion and vaginal introital integrity. *J Pediatr Adolesc Gynecol.* 2006;19:337–339.

Sultan C, Paris F, Jeandel C, et al. Ambiguous genitalia in the newborn: diagnosis, etiology, and sex assignment. *Endocr Dev.* 2004;7:23–38.

Wall EM, Stone B, Klein BL. Imperforate hymen: a not-so-hidden diagnosis. *Am J Emerg Med.* 2003;21:249–250.

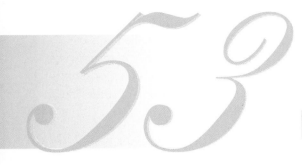

T. ERNESTO FIGUEROA
AND DANIEL T. WALMSLEY

Penile Abnormalities

APPROACH TO THE PROBLEM

Penile abnormalities occur frequently. The recognition and accurate identification of these conditions are important because some carry significant consequences for the patient and his family. Genital anomalies are often isolated problems, although they may occur as part of a congenital syndrome, such as Noonan, Opitz, Prader-Willi, Robinow, Beckwith-Wiedemann, or Trisomy 18 syndrome.

Evaluation for genital anomalies begins in the neonatal period. It starts with a careful examination where the genitalia are inspected. Systematically, the examination of the genitalia should assess the appearance of the prepuce (normal or incomplete), the location of the urethral meatus (if visible), the size and appearance of the penis, the presence of penile chordee or torsion, the appearance of the scrotum, and the location and size of the testes. Important diagnostic maneuvers are palpation of the scrotum or inguinal area to assess for two testes in the male and to check the corporal integrity of the penis.

KEY POINTS IN THE HISTORY

- Phimosis is a condition in which the prepuce cannot be retracted. It is considered a normal condition in infancy and childhood; hence, it is often referred to as physiological phimosis. The timing for natural retraction of the prepuce varies, but most uncircumcised boys have a retractile prepuce by 5 years of age.

- Penile adhesions are extremely common. They are universally present in uncircumcised boys and present in about 60% of circumcised boys at some point. The adhesions occur between the glans and the adjacent inner mucosal surface of the prepuce. These adhesions may separate naturally when given time. The two processes that aid in the natural separation of adhesions are erections and formation of smegma between the inner mucosal surface of the prepuce and the glans.

- A hidden penis is a penis that does not protrude beyond the surface of the abdominal wall. This is mainly due to subcutaneous fat displacing the penile skin away from the shaft. In contrast, a concealed penis is buried by a cicatrix of the prepuce. This can occur following neonatal circumcision in males who have limited penile skin or when an excessive amount of penile skin is removed during the circumcision. If the glans recedes behind the healing preputial wound, then the scar will contract and bury the penis. Concealed penis can be managed nonsurgically by the application of topical corticosteroids, although many patients will require a surgical release with revision of the circumcision.

- Hypospadias is a frequent anomaly, occurring in 1/300 live male births. Elements of hypospadias include a hooded prepuce, a ventral meatus, and chordee. The severity is variable, with most boys (75%) having a distal abnormality—glanular, coronal, or distal shaft. In more severe cases, profound androgenic failure may be evident, with the findings of a microphallus, bifid scrotum, and penoscrotal transposition.

- Chordee, present with or without hypospadias, is a ventral curvature of the penis. Most patients with hypospadias have chordee, partially because of the asymmetry between the normal dorsal penile skin and the hypoplastic ventral penile skin. This is referred to as cutaneous chordee. In more severe cases, as with fibrous chordee, the curvature may involve the ventral surface of the penis including the corpus spongiosum and corpora cavernosa in addition to the cutaneous abnormality.

- Penile torsion is a lateral rotation of the penis in reference to the midline penoscrotal raphe. In approximately 5% to 10% of boys, the raphe may be directed laterally, causing the lateral rotation of the penile shaft.

- A micropenis is a phallus more than 2 standard deviations below the mean length for expected age. These are often visually abnormal penises, appearing small in context to the rest of the child's body habitus. The prepuce is normally formed. If the testes also are abnormally small or if other findings suggest an endocrine disorder, the patient should be evaluated by an endocrinologist.

- Ambiguous genitalia refers to incomplete or abnormal genital development, preventing accurate definition of gender based on the appearance of the genitalia. Awareness of the possibility of sexual and genital ambiguity is critical to its recognition. These children may suffer from extremely variable conditions, ranging from excessive androgen production in the female with congenital adrenal hyperplasia causing virilization of the genitalia to the underdevelopment of the genitalia in a male patient with 5-alpha reductase insufficiency.

KEY POINTS IN THE PHYSICAL EXAMINATION

- Phimosis refers to a conical protrusion of prepuce that cannot be retracted proximally. Contrast this with a secondary phimosis, a cicatrix in a flat distal prepuce that prevents retraction of the prepuce.

- Penile adhesions are soft attachments between inner (mucosal) prepuce and any part of the glans and will eventually separate on their own. Contrast this with skin bridging, where a band of skin becomes fused to the corona or glans following circumcision. The latter requires surgical repair.

- Paraphimosis refers to the condition in which a phimotic prepuce is retracted behind the corona of the glans. Because of the constricting effect of the phimosis, edema and swelling of the glans occur distally to the preputial orifice.

- Hidden penis refers to the appearance of a small penile shaft and excess penile skin. Retracting the prepubic fat pad usually reveals a normal-sized and circumcised penis.

- Micropenis refers to a small but normally formed penis.

- Chordee refers to abnormal ventral curvature, producing a curved penis.

- Hypospadias refers to a hooded prepuce and a ventral meatus in the area of the corona, shaft, or scrotum, accompanied by a chordee.

- Penile torsion refers to clockwise or counterclockwise rotation of the penile shaft and meatus with a laterally displaced penile raphe.

- Ambiguous genitalia refers to the appearance of phallus (penis or clitoris), bifid scrotum or labia, or ventral orifice that could represent hypospadias or a urogenital sinus.

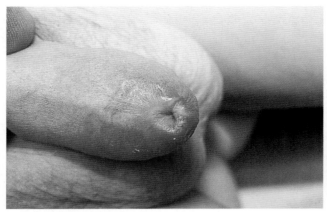

Figure 53-1 Phimosis. Notice the nonretractible prepuce consistent with this diagnosis.
(Courtesy of T. Ernesto Figueroa, MD, FAAP, FACS.)

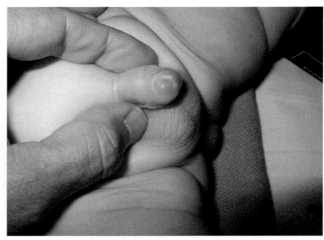

Figure 53-2 Penile adhesion. Whitish yellow mucosal attachments are noted between the prepuce and shaft of the penis.
(Courtesy of T. Ernesto Figueroa, MD, FAAP, FACS.)

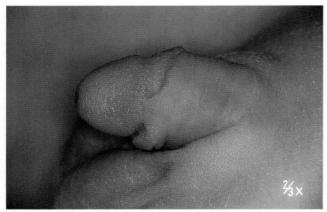

Figure 53-3 Skin bridging. Note the band of skin fused with the glans.
(Courtesy of T. Ernesto Figueroa, MD, FAAP, FACS.)

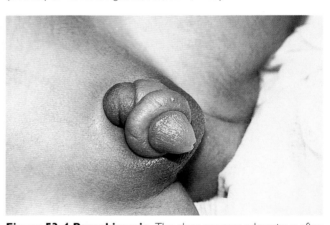

Figure 53-4 Paraphimosis. The glans appears edematous after becoming retracted behind the corona.
(Courtesy of T. Ernesto Figueroa, MD, FAAP, FACS.)

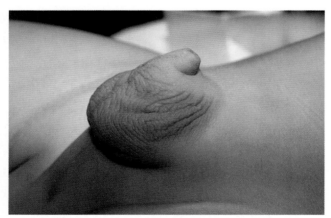

Figure 53-5 Concealed penis. Notice how the penis is buried by part of the prepuce.
(Courtesy of T. Ernesto Figueroa, MD, FAAP, FACS.)

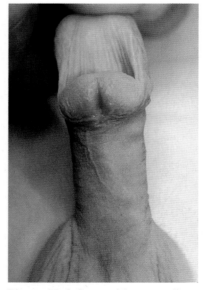

Figure 53-6 Coronal hypospadias. Note the ventral meatus and associated hooded prepuce.
(Courtesy of T. Ernesto Figueroa, MD, FAAP, FACS.)

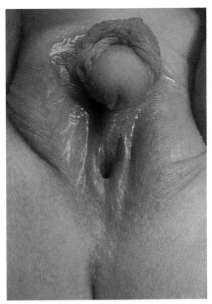

Figure 53-7 Perineal hypospadias.
(Courtesy of T. Ernesto Figueroa, MD, FAAP, FACS.)

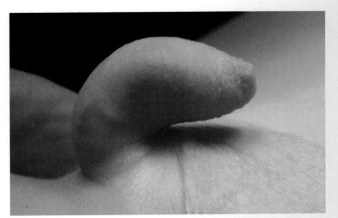

Figure 53-8 Chordee. A ventral curvature of the penis is evident.
(Courtesy of T. Ernesto Figueroa, MD, FAAP, FACS.)

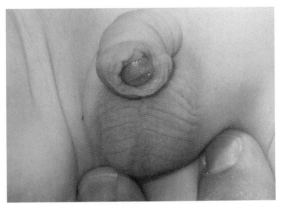

Figure 53-9 Penile torsion. Note the counterclock-wise rotation of the penile meatus and shaft.
(Courtesy of T. Ernesto Figueroa, MD, FAAP, FACS.)

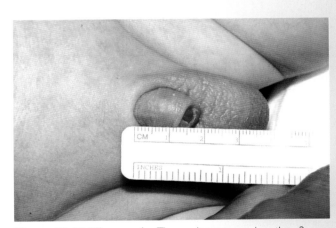

Figure 53-10 Micropenis. The penis measures less than 2 cm.
(Courtesy of T. Ernesto Figueroa, MD, FAAP, FACS.)

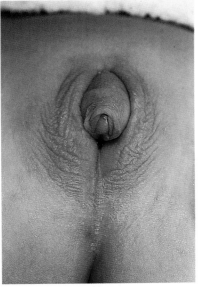

Figure 53-11 Ambiguous genitalia.
The scrotum appears to be absent.
(Courtesy of T. Ernesto Figueroa, MD, FAAP, FACS.)

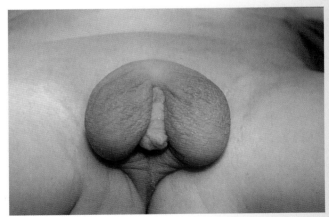

Figure 53-12 Penoscrotal transposition.
(Courtesy of T. Ernesto Figueroa, MD, FAAP, FACS.)

DIFFERENTIAL DIAGNOSIS

DIAGNOSIS	ICD-9	DISTINGUISHING CHARACTERISTICS	DISTRIBUTION	DURATION/ CHRONICITY
Phimosis	605	Nonretractile prepuce	Universal at birth	Resolves by 5 yrs of age
Penile Adhesion	605A	Retractile prepuce with mucosal attachments Distinct from skin bridging	60% of circumcised infants	Resolves by 5 yrs of age
Paraphimosis	605R	Entrapment of the glans by constrictive preputial annulus causing edema of glans and prepuce	Rare	Acute event
Hidden Penis	752.65	Apparently small size, abundant prepubic fat Distinct from concealed penis Normal size penis	Very common in infancy	Resolves by 2–3 yrs of life
Hypospadias	752.61	Ventral meatus, hooded prepuce, ventral penile hypoplasia	1/300 live male births	Lifelong consequences in more severe cases
Chordee	607.89c	Bent penis, or penile curvature because of abnormal skin (cutaneous chordee) Abnormal corporal bodies (fibrous chordee)	Similar to hypospadias	Correctable in most cases
Penile Torsion	607.89	Abnormal axis of meatus and lateral rotation of shaft Most are rotated counter-clockwise.	15% of boys	Correctable in most cases
Micropenis	752.64	Abnormally small penis, must distinguish between primary end organ or secondary hypogonadism	Rare	May be lifelong condition
Ambiguous Genitalia (Disorder of Sexual Differentiation)	752.7 (indeterminate sex)	Abnormal genitalia of uncertain gender	Uncommon	Lifelong condition

ASSOCIATED FINDINGS	COMPLICATIONS	PREDISPOSING FACTORS	TREATMENT GUIDELINES
Normal penis	Inability to retract prepuce, poor hygiene, urinary tract infection (UTI)	Congenital, normal Secondary to injury to preputial annulus either by circumcision or by forceful retraction of prepuce	Reassurance Surgical correction if secondary
Normal penis, either circumcised or uncircumcised	Tearing of adhesions Penile deviation	May occur after circumcisions Common in uncircumcised males	Reassurance as they typically will resolve on their own After circumcisions parents can gently pull the skin covering the head of the penis down and apply some lubricating material like Vaseline, with diaper changes.
Tight proximal preputial ring	Glanular ischemia	Tight preputial annulus, retracting the prepuce proximally without returning the prepuce to its normal position	Attempt at manual decompression of the glans and prepuce to reduce it through the tight band. Severe cases may require surgery where the phimotic band is split open.
Prepubic fat pad	Skin irritation secondary to urine pooling in the area	Obesity, small penis, excessive or incomplete circumcision	Reassurance Penis size is usually normal when measured with the fat pad pressed down.
Chordee, micropenis	If meatus is stenotic, difficulty urinating Abnormal penile appearance	Abnormal production/timing of androgens in utero Genetic predisposition	Surgical repair before age 1 The infant should not be circumcised in the newborn period. Thorough examination to check for other congenital anomalies as further workup, such as a karyotype, may by warranted
Hypoplastic ventral penile surface Possible hypospadias	May interfere with quality of sexual intercourse	Abnormal corpus spongiosum	Surgical correction between 6 and 18 months of age
Abnormal symmetry of penile skin	Deviated urine stream	N/A	Surgical correction
Hypogonadism Prader-Willi syndrome—infant will also have poor feeding and hypotonia Kallmann syndrome—anosmia, hypoglycemia and septic-optic dysplasia	Endocrinopathy Sexual intercourse may be difficult.	Endocrinopathy	Evaluation for a cause with treatment based on the etiology Some labs to obtain are comprehensive metabolic panel, karyotype, FSH, LH, HCG, and testosterone levels
Male pseudohermaphroditism-associated with infertile aunts Congenital adrenal hyperplasia—excessive scrotal pigmentation, growth delay, hyponatremia, and hyperkalemia	Related to etiology Multiple complications, including need for surgery Psychological adjustment Infant may present in shock due to mineralocorticoid deficiency in congenital adrenal hyperplasia	Depends on underlying etiology Congenital adrenal hyperplasia—absence of enzymes needed for cholesterol synthesis 21-alpha hydroxylase deficiency is most common. 5-alpha reductase deficiency in male pseudohermaphroditism	Dependent on etiology Congenital adrenal hyperplasia-treat with mineralocorticoid and glucocorticoid replacement in consultation with a pediatric endocrinologist.

OTHER
DIAGNOSES
TO CONSIDER

- Secondary phimosis

- Concealed penis

- Penile skin bridging

- Idiopathic penile edema

- Epispadias

WHEN TO
CONSIDER
FURTHER
EVALUATION
OR TREATMENT

- A micropenis, which is defined as a penis less than 3 cm in length, should prompt endo-crinologic and genetic evaluations.

- In a patient with ambiguous genitalia, a family history of infertile aunts should raise suspicion for male pseudohermaphroditism (testicular feminization syndrome).

- Features of Beckwith-Wiedemann syndrome include hypospadias, macroglossia, mac-rosmia, and hypoglycemia.

- Hypospadias with undescended testes warrants a genetic workup, including a karyo-type.

- A boy with poor feeding, hypotonia, and micropenis raises suspicion for Prader-Willi syndrome.

- Evaluation of sex hormones and a karyotype are required prior to assigning gender in cases of ambiguous genitalia.

SUGGESTED READINGS

Elder JS. Abnormalities of the genitalia in boys and their surgical management. In: Walsh, ed. *Campbell's urology*. 8th ed. Philadelphia, PA: WB Saunders; 2002:2334–2352.

Figueroa TE. Congenital adrenal hyperplasia. In: Siedmon EJ, Hanno PM, Kaufman JJ, eds. *Current urological therapy*. 3rd ed. Philadelphia, PA: WB Saunders; 1994:2–6.

Figueroa TE, Casale P. Circumcision. In: Mattel, ed. *Surgical directives: pediatric surgery*. New York, NY: Lippincott Williams & Wilkins; 2002:709–712.

Kennedy AP, Figueroa TE. Common urological problems in the fetus and neonate. In: Spitzer A, ed. *Intensive care of the neonate and fetus*. 2nd ed. Philadelphia, PA: Hanley & Belfus Press; 2003:1369–1383.

Perovic S. *Atlas of congenital anomalies of the external genitalia*. Yugoslavia: Refot-Arka; 1999:15–33.

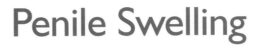

DAVID M. PRESSEL

Penile Swelling

APPROACH TO THE PROBLEM

Penile swelling is a frightening experience for both boys and their families. Heightened anxiety related to urination or sexual functioning may accompany the encounter. Embarrassment regarding this area of the body may delay disclosure of the problem by older children or lead to an incomplete or inaccurate description by the caregiver. The causes of penile swelling are relatively straightforward and may be distinguished by a thorough history and physical examination. Laboratory tests and/or radiological studies are rarely necessary to evaluate penile swelling. With careful assessment and implementation of appropriate treatment, the physician caring for a child with penile swelling can rapidly affect clinical improvement and emotional reassurance for the child and family.

The causes of penile swelling may be primary and localized to the genitalia or due to a secondary, systemic process. Secondary causes of penile swelling whether due to an allergic reaction, cardiac, renal, or hepatic disease generally should be recognized as such and, after assuring that the patient is able to pass urine, care should focus on the underlying cause of swelling. Primary causes of penile edema may be congenital—congenital lymphedema if apparent as a neonate, or lymphedema praecox, if swelling becomes apparent with age. Acquired causes of penile swelling, whether from infection, inflammation, or trauma, are more likely to be diagnostically challenging and anxiety-provoking to the family. Certain types of penile swelling may only occur in the uncircumcised male. The assessment of symptom duration, pain, erythema, and, importantly, the ability to pass urine are the first steps in the assessment of penile swelling.

KEY POINTS IN THE HISTORY

- In the infant or toddler, there may not be a clear history of trauma.
- Insect bites in the genitalia may not be recognized at the time of presentation.
- Boys hurrying to zip their pants may get the skin of the penis caught in the zipper.
- Traumatic penile injuries are likely to be painful.
- Traumatic injury may compromise the ability to urinate.
- Surgery in the pelvic area may result in painless dependent edema.

- Paraphimosis and phimosis are problems related to the foreskin. Paraphimosis occurs when the foreskin is retracted behind the glans, becomes edematous, and the swelling of the foreskin prevents it from being returned to the normal position. This leads to further venous congestion, exacerbating the condition. Phimosis occurs when the foreskin cannot be retracted due to scarred adhesions and excessive foreskin tightness. If the phimosis is severe enough to make the foreskin opening stenotic, the foreskin may balloon during urination.

- Posthitis or balanoposthitis, infection and inflammation of the foreskin and foreskin/glans, respectively, does not occur in the circumcised male.

- Balanitis, infection of the glans, may occur in a circumcised or uncircumcised male.

- The presence of a prolonged, painful erection should raise the suspicion for priapism due to a vasocclusive crisis of the penis seen in sickle cell disease. There have also been reports of priapism in boys who have accidentally ingested medication for erectile dysfunction.

KEY POINTS IN THE PHYSICAL EXAMINATION

- Dependent edema that is nonerythematous and nontender may occur after pelvic surgery, in allergic reactions, and with systemic disease processes associated with hypoalbuminemia and other conditions characterized by low oncotic pressure.

- A distended bladder by palpation and percussion may be evidence of urinary retention. A constricting ring of hair or thread may be concealed in the edematous penis; therefore, it is important to do careful inspection of the penis.

- Any child with a traumatic genital injury that is not readily apparent as accidental (e.g., recent history of bicycle or playground straddle injury) may be a victim of child sexual abuse. A further examination is warranted to look for other evidence of abuse.

- An infection of the penis will present with swelling, erythema, and possibly discharge or drainage. These findings may extend up the shaft to the perineum.

- Posthitis may be associated with phimosis.

PHOTOGRAPHS OF SELECTED DIAGNOSES

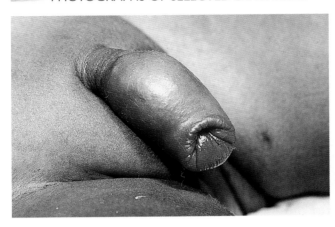

Figure 54-1 Penile edema after reduction of paraphimosis.
(Courtesy of T. Ernesto Figueroa, MD, FAAP, FACS.)

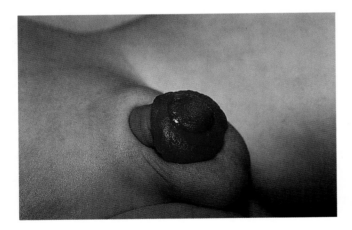

Figure 54-2 Idiopathic penile edema.
(Courtesy of T. Ernesto Figueroa, MD, FAAP, FACS.)

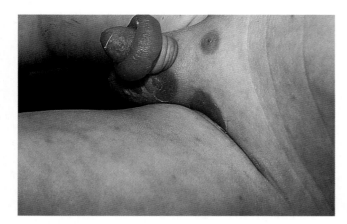

Figure 54-3 Penile edema in association with varicella.
(Courtesy of T. Ernesto Figueroa, MD, FAAP, FACS.)

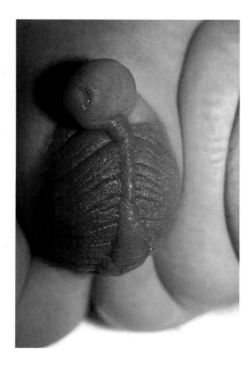

Figure 54-4 Lymphedema.
(Courtesy of T. Ernesto Figueroa, MD, FAAP, FACS.)

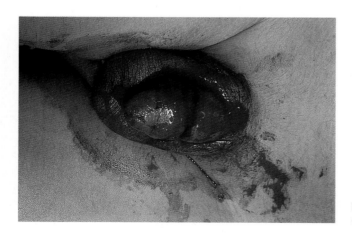

Figure 54-5 Penile trauma.
(Courtesy of T. Ernesto Figueroa, MD, FAAP, FACS.)

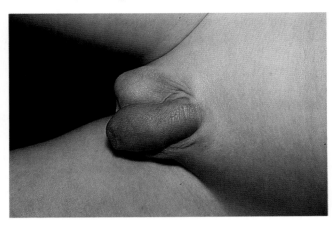

Figure 54-6 Balanoposthitis.
(Courtesy of T. Ernesto Figueroa, MD, FAAP, FACS.)

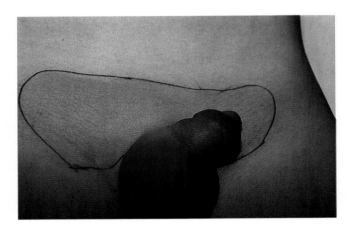

Figure 54-7 Balanoposthitis with cellulitis.
(Courtesy of T. Ernesto Figueroa, MD, FAAP, FACS.)

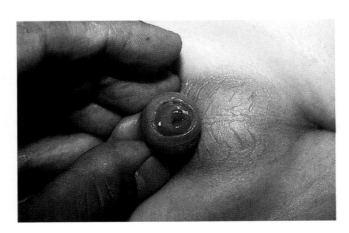

Figure 54-8 Acute posthitis.
(Courtesy of T. Ernesto Figueroa, MD, FAAP, FACS.)

DIAGNOSIS	ICD-9	DISTINGUISHING CHARACTERISTICS	DURATION/CHRONICITY
Penile Edema	607.83	Painless and without erythema Dependent edema may be seen in other body parts	Acute or chronic in congenital lymphedema or lymphedema praecox
Penile Trauma **Tourniquet** **Zipper** **Straddle Injury** **Sexual Abuse** **Insect Bite**	959.14 E918 E918 E888.1 995.53 919	History of trauma Bleeding Bruising Bite mark	Acute
Paraphimosis	605	Swollen, retracted foreskin Painful	Acute condition, worsens without treatment
Infection **Balanitis** **Balanoposthitis** **Posthitis** **Fournier's Gangrene**	607.2 607.1 607.1 608.83	Red, swollen, tender May have discharge if foreskin present (posthitis)	Acute
Priapism	607.3	Persistent erection May be painless or painful	Acute

ASSOCIATED FINDINGS	COMPLICATIONS	PRECIPITATING FACTORS	TREATMENT GUIDELINES
Related to primary cause of edema	Voiding difficulties	Surgery Allergic reaction Heart, liver, kidney disease	Catheterization, if voiding difficulties Urologic referral if lymphatic drainage obstruction
Pain	Voiding difficulties Scar formation Urologic injury Penile necrosis	Child sexual abuse	Consider urology referral and Child Protective Service referral
Pain	Necrosis to the tip of the penis	Phimosis	Local anesthetic to aid traction and reduction Circumcision, in some instances
May extend up shaft to perineum May be associated with yeast or bacteria	Fournier's gangrene associated with circumcision and systemic illness Voiding difficulties Phimosis	Phimosis Diabetes Poor hygiene	Antibiotics Antifungal agents when indicated Warm soaks Urologic referral for severe infection
Systemic symptoms if associated with sickle cell crisis or leukemia	Impotence Urinary retention	Sickle cell disease Sildenafil ingestion Leukemia	Urology and hematology referrals

- Scrotal swelling (see Chapter 58)

- Nephrotic syndrome

- Paraphimosis is painful and requires emergency treatment, which includes application of ice and manual pressure to reduce the swelling. A local anesthetic dorsal penile block may be helpful. Rarely surgical division of the foreskin may be necessary to permit reduction.

- Priapism warrants emergent consultation with a hematologist if the suspected etiology is sickle cell disease. If the cause of priapism is unclear or suspected ingestion, a urologist and the local Poison Control Center (http://www.aapcc.org/dnn/Home/tabid/36/Default.aspx) should be contacted.

- Any penile swelling accompanied by urinary obstruction requires emergent urologic evaluation and bladder decompression.

SUGGESTED READINGS
Klauber GT, Sant GR. Disorders of the male and external genitalia. In: Kelalis, King, Belman eds. *Pediatric urology*. 2nd ed. Philadelphia, PA: WB Saunders; 1985.
Leslie JA, Cain MP. Pediatric urologic emergencies and urgencies. *Pediatr Clin North Am*. 2006:53:513–527.
Synder HM. Urologic emergencies. In: Fleisher, Ludwig, eds. *Textbook of pediatric emergency medicine*. 5th ed. Philadelphia, PA: Williams & Wilkins; 2008.

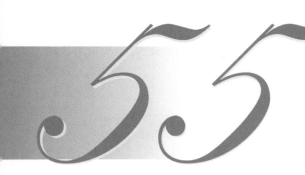

KATHLEEN CRONAN

Perineal Red Rashes

APPROACH TO THE PROBLEM

Diaper dermatoses, some of the most common skin disorders in infants and toddlers, peak at age 9 to 12 months. A variety of acute inflammatory skin reactions in the diaper area may occur. Chafing or frictional dermatitis is the most prevalent cause of diaper rash, followed in frequency by irritant contact dermatitis. Older children and adolescents with groin rashes present with lesions predominantly caused by fungal infections, such as vulvovaginitis and tinea cruris. In most cases, frequent diaper changes and the application of topical barrier agents are the mainstays of therapy. Groin rashes that indicate the presence of infection require topical antifungal or antibiotic agents. It is crucial to perform an entire body examination when evaluating rashes in the perineal area.

KEY POINTS IN THE HISTORY

- A rash elsewhere on the skin suggests the possibility of seborrhea, psoriasis, or, less likely, Langerhans histiocytosis.

- A history of recent antibiotic use often precedes a *Candida albicans* diaper rash or vulvovaginitis in an adolescent female.

- Extremes of moisture or heat in the groin area may lead to contact dermatitis, candidal diaper dermatitis, or tinea cruris.

- Seborrheic, atopic, and contact dermatitis disrupt the integrity of the skin and place the patient at risk for infection with *Candida albicans*.

- A family history of psoriasis may provide a clue regarding the etiology of a persistent diaper rash.

- Chafing diaper dermatitis waxes and wanes quickly.

- Persistent diarrhea may contribute to contact diaper dermatitis.

- Genital herpes presenting in prepubertal children should warrant an investigation for child sexual abuse.

KEY POINTS IN THE PHYSICAL EXAMINATION

- Seborrhea, psoriasis, scarlet fever, and Langerhans histiocytosis are associated with rashes outside of the diaper region.

- The distribution of the diaper rash provides clues to the diagnosis: a red rash in the intertriginous areas indicates seborrhea, intertrigo, *Candida albicans*, or tinea cruris, while a rash on the exposed convex surfaces is suggestive of contact dermatitis.

- Evaluation of the margins of the rash assists in making the diagnosis. Satellite lesions are seen with candidal dermatitis, and sharp borders are seen with tinea cruris.

- The color may help to distinguish one rash from another. Red beefy lesions indicate candidal diaper dermatitis, salmon yellow lesions suggest seborrhea, silvery scales over-lying red bases indicate psoriasis, and yellow to reddish brown papules may suggest Langerhans histiocytosis.

- Henoch-Schönlein purpura may present with palpable purpura in the buttocks and thighs of young children.

- An ulcerative rash in the perineal area of an adolescent suggests herpes simplex virus.

- Pustules and bullae formation is indicative of impetigo due to staphylococcus or streptococcus.

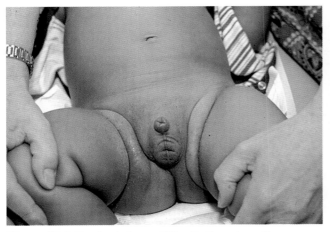

Figure 55-1 Contact dermatitis. Erythematous diaper dermatitis distributed primarily on convex surfaces with sparing of the intertriginous folds in an infant.
(Courtesy of George A. Datto, III, MD.)

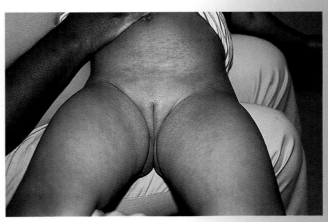

Figure 55-2 Contact dermatitis. Older child with contact dermatitis from a bathing suit.
(Courtesy of George A. Datto, III, MD.)

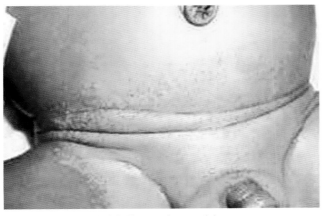

Figure 55-3 Candidal diaper dermatitis.
(Courtesy of Moise L. Levy, MD.)

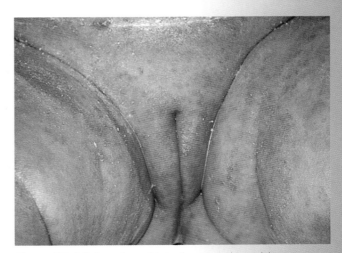

Figure 55-4 Seborrhea. Note the greasy intertriginous dermatitis with yellowish scale.
(Used with permission from the Benjamin Barankin Dermatology Collection.)

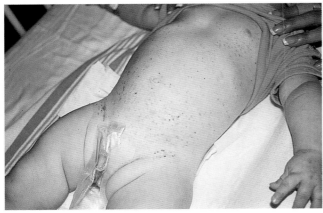

Figure 55-5 Histiocytosis. Clusters of hemorrhagic papules in groin and on abdomen.
(Courtesy of George A. Datto, III, MD.)

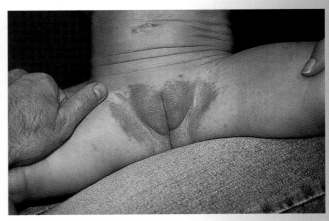

Figure 55-6 Psoriasis. Erythematous plaque with scale in diaper area; also note smaller lesions on abdomen.
(Courtesy of George A. Datto, III, MD.)

DIFFERENTIAL DIAGNOSIS

DIAGNOSIS	ICD-9	DISTINGUISHING CHARACTERISTICS	DISTRIBUTION
Chafing Dermatitis	691.0	Due to friction Mild redness and scaling Waxes and wanes quickly	Inner thighs Genitalia Buttocks Lower abdomen
Irritant Contact Dermatitis	692.9	Spares intertriginous areas Located on convex surfaces Erosions occur occasionally	Buttocks Vulva Perineum Lower abdomen Upper thighs
Candidal Infection	112.2	Vivid beefy red color Raised edges with sharp margination White scales at the border Pinpoint satellite lesions	Buttocks Lower abdomen Inner thighs Intertriginous areas Occasionally generalized with an "id" reaction
Impetigo	684	Pustules filled with exudate and bullae with straw-colored fluid	Can occur in any location, often not limited by diaper margin
Genital Herpes Virus Infection	054.10	Vesicles and ulcerated lesions involving the skin and mucous membranes	Usually clustered around vaginal area or penis
Intertrigo	695.89	Typical in hot weather Intense erythema in skin folds Often with white or yellow exudate	Inguinal creases Intergluteal area Thigh creases
Seborrhea	690.12	Salmon-colored, greasy lesions—yellowish scale	Intertriginous areas Spares convex areas
Tinea Cruris	110.3	Symmetrical, scaly, erythematous plaques Sharply demarcated Most common in male adolescents	Intertriginous folds near the scrotum and upper inner thighs Occasionally on buttocks, perineum Spares penis
Cutaneous Candidiasis (in Adolescent Female)	112.1	Redness and swelling White patches on red bases on mucosal surfaces Cheesy exudate Itching, burning, dysuria	Labia Perineum Perianal area Gluteal folds
Langerhans Histiocytosis	202.56	Clusters of yellow-to-reddish brown papules with purpuric qualities Hemorrhagic, seborrhea-like eruption	Groin Axilla Retroauricular areas Palms and soles
Psoriasis	696.1	Erythematous plaques with a scaling eruption Remissions and exacerbations typical Fails to respond to usual diaper dermatitis therapies	Girls—clitoral hood to upper gluteal cleft Boys—base of penis, inner thighs, gluteal cleft

ASSOCIATED FINDINGS	COMPLICATIONS	PREDISPOSING FACTORS	TREATMENT GUIDELINES
N/A	None	Friction	Frequent diaper changes and careful diaper hygiene
N/A	Bacterial superinfection	Contact with proteolytic enzymes and irritant chemicals Alkaline pH Excessive heat and moisture Moderate to severe diarrhea Infrequent diaper changes	Frequent diaper changes
Oral thrush	None	Systemic antibiotic therapy Warm, moist, occluded skin	Topical antifungal agent Avoid topical steroids, which are likely to make the rash worse. If severe, oral fluconazole
	Can progress to systemic infection in immunocompromised or in young infants	Break in skin integrity	Topical antibacterial agent If severe, oral or parenteral antibacterial
	Bacterial superinfection Pain	Exposure to herpes simplex virus	Acyclovir begun in the first 72 hrs may shorten duration of outbreak.
Same findings in neck folds and axillae	Candidal superinfection	Hot weather Overdressing of infant	Open wet compresses Cautious use of dusting powders
Involvement of the scalp, face, neck, postauricular areas, and flexural areas	Secondary candidal or bacterial infection	High sebaceous gland density	Low-dose topical steroids Antifungal agents or antibiotics if superinfected
Leukorrhea Itching Burning Painful urination	Bacterial superinfection	*Epidermophyton floccosum* *Trichophyton rubrum* Hot, humid weather Vigorous exercise Tight-fitting clothing	Topical antifungal agents for 3–4 wks Avoid tight clothes Thorough drying of area
Pruritus	None	Antibiotics Diabetes mellitus Pregnancy Oral contraceptives	Antifungal vaginal tablets, cream, or suppositories
Bone lesions, particularly skull Mucosal involvement Premature tooth eruption Lymphadenopathy	Varies with extent of disease	Abnormal proliferation/accumulation of cells of the monocyte-macrophage system	Observation alone if restricted to skin
Dark red plaques with silvery scales on the trunk, face, scalp, axillae Nail involvement	None	Genetic predisposition	Topical corticosteroids

OTHER
DIAGNOSES
TO CONSIDER

- Acrodermatitis enteropathica (disorder due to zinc deficiency)

- Jacquet dermatitis

- Granuloma gluteale infantum

- Scarlet fever

- Henoch-Schönlein purpura

- Herpes simplex virus infection

WHEN TO
CONSIDER
FURTHER
EVALUATION
OR TREATMENT

- Diaper dermatitis is often recurrent, and recurrence does not always indicate treatment failure.

- Prior to initiating therapy, the etiology of the perineal rash must be determined.

- If secondary bacterial infection of the dermatitis is suspected, topical or systemic antibiotics are indicated.

- When a diaper rash is determined to be resistant to standard therapies, consider other diagnoses, such as psoriasis or Langerhans histiocytosis, and seek further evaluation.

- If the infant with a diaper rash is febrile and appears ill, a complete evaluation is warranted.

- Newborns with diffuse impetigo in the groin area should be given systemic (oral or parenteral) antibiotics. Evaluate for a systemic infection if the child presents with symptoms such as fever, ill appearance, or constitutional symptoms.

SUGGESTED READINGS

Boiko S. Making rash decisions in the diaper area. *Pediatr Ann.* 2000;29:50–56.

Cohen B. A baby, a skin lesion—and an efficient approach to recognition and management. *Contemp Pediatr.* 2004;21:28–30.

Hansen RC, Krafchik BR, Lane AT, et al. Dealing with diaper dermatitis. *Contemp Pediatr.* 1998;(Suppl):5–14.

Paller AS, Mancini AJ. (eds). Diaper dermatitis. In: *Hurwitz clinical pediatric dermatology.* 3rd ed. Philadelphia, PA: WB Saunders; 2006:27–30.

Ward DB, Fleischer AB Jr, Feldman SR, et al. Characterization of diaper dermatitis in the United States. *Arch Pediatr Adoles Med.* 2000;154:943–946.

Zsolway K, Harrison A, Honig P. Diaper rash in a young infant. *Pediatr Case Rev.* 2002;2(4):220–225.

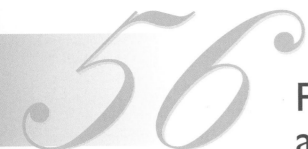

ALLAN R. DE JONG

Perineal Sores and Lesions

APPROACH TO THE PROBLEM

The most common cause of genital irritation and bleeding in a prepubertal girl beyond the neonatal period is vulvovaginitis, and hygiene-related problems are often implicated. Other causes of postneonatal genital bleeding include genital warts, trauma, vaginal foreign body, hemangioma, tumors, and urethral prolapse. Dermatologic conditions—psoriasis; lichen sclerosis; impetigo; and seborrheic, contact, and atopic dermatitis—commonly cause rashes, pain, itching, bleeding, and fissures in the anogenital area. The distribution of the individual lesions is important for differentiating a generalized dermatitis from localized infections, trauma, and congenital lesions. The differential diagnosis of perineal sores and lesions includes child sexual abuse, which must be addressed by an experienced clinician.

KEY POINTS IN THE HISTORY

- When approaching child sexual abuse, most of the medical history, review of systems, and context and content of the child's disclosure can be obtained from adults who accompany the child without the child present. The child should be interviewed without the caretakers' presence, if necessary for medical management. Questioning should be nonleading, open-ended, and carefully documented.

- The key to diagnosis of sexual abuse is the clear history of sexual contact provided by the child, while the diagnosis of straddle injury is supported by a clear history of blunt genital impact particularly during a fall onto an object.

- Midline fusion defects and hemangiomas should be recognized within the first few months of life if not detected at birth.

- The history of painful oral plus genital lesions suggests herpes simplex virus infection or Behçet syndrome.

- The history of dermatologic or allergic conditions involving other body sites should be considered because the anogenital rash, itching, pain, bleeding, or lesions may be the result of the same generalized condition.

- A history of maternal, congenital, or acquired syphilis with inadequate treatment precedes the condyloma lata of secondary syphilis.

- Genital itching typically accompanies candidal dermatitis and/or vaginitis, lichen sclerosis, and genital warts.

● Pain typically accompanies trauma (which may result from rubbing or itching), lesions from viral infections (including herpes, varicella, Epstein-Barr, coxsackie, or influenza), and Behçet syndrome.

KEY POINTS IN THE PHYSICAL EXAMINATION

● The evaluation of a child who presents with a chief complaint of sexual abuse is often done best at a local or regional sexual abuse center. Clinicians should explain the examination in advance to the child who should be reassured that examination of the genital area by a physician is all right and that it will not be painful. A gentle, deliberate manner is appropriate, and physical force should not be used.

● The most common physical findings in cases of sexual abuse are normal or nonspecific anogenital examinations. When sexual abuse injuries are found, they are typically near the posterior midline within the vaginal vestibule and involve the hymen.

● Injuries from straddle trauma are typically unilateral or asymmetrical and anterior or anterolateral in location.

● Lesions associated with bleeding include acute straddle or sexual abuse injuries, hemangiomas, lichen sclerosis, and genital warts. Unlike most of the other lesions, hemangiomas and failure of midline fusion should be completely unchanged when re-examined 2 to 4 weeks later.

● Oral ulcerations with genital ulcerations suggest herpes simplex virus infection or Behçet syndrome.

● Lesions in nongenital areas may be found in some individuals with perineal hemangiomas, genital warts, or both.

● Molluscum contagiosum does not involve mucous membranes or palms and soles, but a rash of the palms and soles may accompany condyloma lata.

● Bilateral, diffuse labial redness usually is from vulvovaginitis, but it may also accompany lichen sclerosis.

● Hemangiomas typically blanch with pressure, but most other lesions do not.

PHOTOGRAPHS OF SELECTED DIAGNOSES

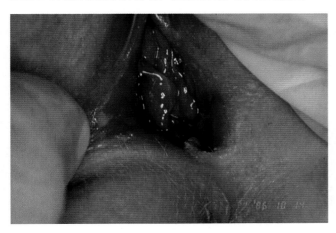

Figure 56-1 Sexual abuse, acute. Tissue edema and hemorrhage in a 19-month-old girl 4 days after penile vaginal penetration. Prominent lacerations to the vaginal wall, hymenal membrane, and posterior commissure are present.
(Used with permission from De Jong AR, Finkel MA. Medical findings in child sexual abuse. In: Reece R, Ludwig S, eds. *Child abuse: medical diagnosis and management* 2nd ed. Philadelphia, PA: Lippincott Williams & Wilkins; 2001:248.)

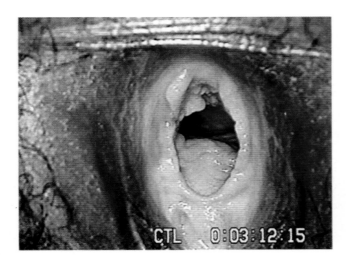

Figure 56-2 Sexual abuse, nonacute. Deep, wide posterior midline hymenal cleft extending to the vaginal wall. Cleft represents healed complete hymenal tear or transection in a 15-year-old female who disclosed multiple acts of penile vaginal penetration.
(Courtesy of Allan R. De Jong, MD.)

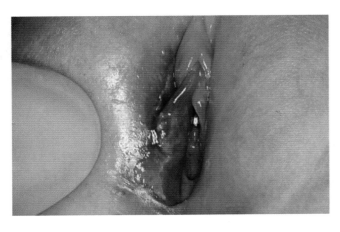

Figure 56-3 Straddle injury. Crush injury to the right labia minor and labia major in a 6-year-old girl who provided a clear history of a fall onto a metal bar of a jungle gym.
(Used with permission from De Jong AR, Finkel MA. Medical findings in child sexual abuse. In: Reece R, Ludwig S, eds. *Child abuse: medical diagnosis and management* 2nd ed. Philadelphia, PA: Lippincott Williams & Wilkins; 2001:249.)

Perineal Sores and Lesions

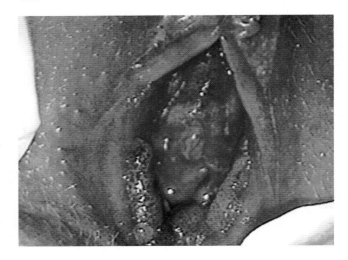

Figure 56-4 Genital warts. Multiple genital warts are seen in vaginal vestibule of 6-year-old girl who disclosed only digital penetration. Blood vessels in the irregular masses create the red stippling of the wart surface.
(Courtesy of Allan R. De Jong, MD.)

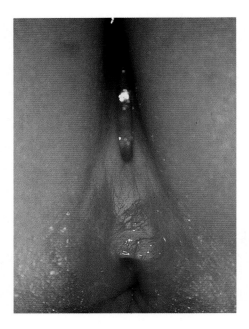

Figure 56-5 Failure of midline fusion. Midline, pale indented defect with prominent vascularity and the appearance of mucosa that was initially mistaken for trauma.
(Used with permission from Bays J. Conditions mistaken for child sexual abuse. In: Reece R, Ludwig S, eds. *Child abuse: medical diagnosis and management.* 2nd ed. Philadelphia, PA: Lippincott Williams & Wilkins; 2001:292.)

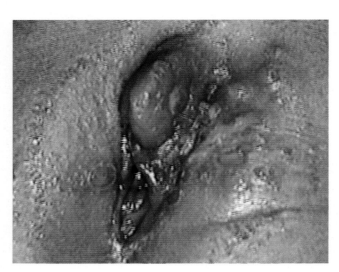

Figure 56-6 Herpes simplex virus infection. Multiple, painful, erythematous ulcerations on the labia of a 4-year-old girl who reported penile genital contact with an adult relative. Culture was positive for herpes simplex virus type II.
(Courtesy of Allan R. De Jong, MD.)

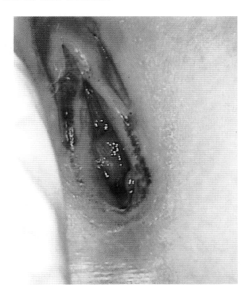

Figure 56-7 Lichen sclerosus et atrophicus. Characteristic subepidermal hemorrhages in a 4-year-old girl with a 3-week history of genital itching and intermittent dysuria. Lesions showed only slight improvement at follow-up weeks later. (Courtesy of Allan R. De Jong, MD.)

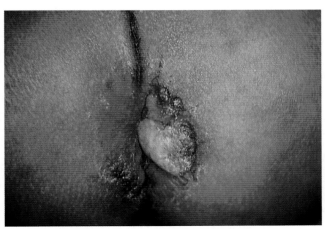

Figure 56-8 Condyloma lata. Pale hypertrophic plaque of condyloma lata in a 2-year-old girl with previously untreated primary syphilis.
(Used with permission from De Jong AR, Finkel MA. Medical findings in child sexual abuse. In: Reece R, Ludwig S, eds. *Child abuse: medical diagnosis and management.* 2nd ed. Philadelphia, PA: Lippincott Williams & Wilkins; 2001:259.)

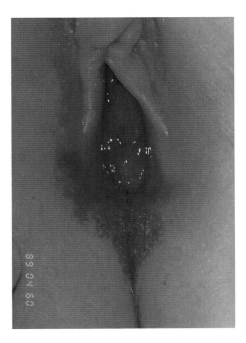

Figure 56-9 Hemangioma. Superficial, red capillary hemangioma of the posterior commissure and perineal body. Initially mistaken as an abrasion, it blanched with pressure.
(Used with permission from Bays J. Conditions mistaken for child sexual abuse. In: Reece R, Ludwig S, eds. *Child abuse: medical diagnosis and management.* 2nd ed. Philadelphia, PA: Lippincott Williams & Wilkins; 2001:290.)

DIFFERENTIAL DIAGNOSIS

DIAGNOSIS	ICD-9	DISTINGUISHING CHARACTERISTICS	DISTRIBUTION
Sexual Abuse	995.53	Acute—laceration or bruising of hymen Nonacute—hymenal transection or healed tear (cleft) extending to the base of hymen or vaginal wall	Injuries when present typically involve posterior one third of hymen and vestibule.
Straddle Injury	926.0	Asymmetrical bruising, swelling, or laceration accompanied by acute pain Has clear history of blunt impact or straddle event	Typically involves anterior two thirds of vulva especially the labia, periclitoral folds, or folds between labia majora and labia minora
Genital Warts	078.11	On mucosal surfaces, flesh-colored to pink, raised lesions with red stippling On moist skin surfaces, usually multiple irregular papules, filiform, and multidigited lesions	Usually multifocal Can involve skin and mucosal surfaces
Molluscum Contagiosum	078.0	Dome-shaped, skin-colored papules on nonerythematous base Often umbilicated with white center	Any body surface except palms and soles
Herpes Simplex Virus Infection	054.1	Multiple vesicular and ulcerative lesions Associated with pain and erythema	Often involves both skin and mucosa May be clustered or scattered individual lesions
Lichen Sclerosus et Atrophicus	701.0	White, wrinkled plaques with fissures producing "parchment-like" skin Subepidermal bruising or bullae and bleeding with minor trauma	Sharp demarcation from normal skin Symmetrical "figure 8" or "hour glass" depigmentation and involvement of vulva and perianal area
Hemangioma	228.0	Reddish-to-bluish flat or elevated lesion that often blanches with pressure Appearance depends on type and size of blood vessels	Often asymmetrical Lesions, multiple or single
Failure of Midline Fusion	759.9 (congenital anomaly NOS)	Painless indented midline lesion Pale tissue centrally at base of lesion with normal vascularity and smooth edges bordering lesion	Midline and symmetrical lesion extending posteriorly from posterior commissure
Condyloma Lata	091.3	Large, moist, pale, hypertrophic plaques	Moist, warm areas including labia and perianal tissues
Behçet Syndrome	136.1	Painful, persisting ulcerations of vagina, vulva, and cervix associated with simultaneous oral ulcers	Genital area but not involving genitocrural folds or interlabial sulci

DURATION/ CHRONICITY	ASSOCIATED FINDINGS	PREDISPOSING FACTORS	TREATMENT GUIDELINES
Acute or nonacute Single episode or multiple episodes (chronic)	Sexually transmitted infections occasionally present Most victims show no specific injuries or infections.	Multiple psychosocial risk factors, such as poor parental attachment, nonbiologically related males in household, parental drug/alcohol abuse, child with unmet emotional needs, adolescent risk-taking	Acute injury treated with proper hygiene, sitz baths, topical emollient or antibiotic ointments Reporting of suspected abuse to police and child protective service agencies is required.
Acute onset Resolving completely in days to weeks	Rarely involves injury to hymen	Activities involving boys' bicycles, monkey bars, balance beams, and falls onto other objects or being kicked in the genital area	Acute injury treated with proper hygiene, sitz baths, topical emollient or antibiotic ointments
Variable duration, can grow very slowly and spontaneously Regress after months or years	Occasionally, warts present on hands or feet or around lips	Sexual contact Autoinoculation Perinatal transmission Vertical transmission	Consider waiting for spontaneous resolution. Patient-applied therapy with topical podofilox or imiquimod can be considered.
Chronic, variable duration	Can appear inflamed or pustular when resolving	Exposure to individual infected with viral agent (5% of all children infected)	Consider waiting for spontaneous resolution Curettage, cryotherapy, or topical catharidin, trichloroacetic acid or imiquimod can be considered.
Acute lesions resolve within 2–3-weeks. Can be recurrent	Primary infection often associated with fever and inguinal adenopathy Pain may precede rash.	Caretaker or child with oral herpes lesions (cold sores) Perinatal transmission Primary herpes gingivostomatitis Sexual contact	Oral or topical acyclovir Alternative treatment with famciclovir, or valacyclovir in adolescents and adults only
Chronic but variable course; many cases improve with puberty	Peak at 6–8 years of age Itching and burning are frequent symptoms.	Predilection for areas of mechanical or thermal skin injury	Proper perineal hygiene practices Avoid tight fitting clothing. Topical mid-to-high potency steriods
Chronic, with typically unchanging appearance	Can ulcerate and bleed or change slowly with involution Other nongenital lesions common	None (congenital)	No treatment required If involuting lesions become ulcerative, consider topical antibiotic ointments.
Chronic (congenital)	Mucosal appearance Often associated with anterior placement of anal opening	None (congenital)	No treatment required
Chronic	Secondary syphilis lesions, including maculopapular or papulosquamous rash, especially on palms, soles	Untreated congenital syphilis or primary syphilis	Single intramuscular dose of penicillin G benzathine (50,000 units per kg, to maximum of 2.4 million units)
Chronic, relapsing pattern	Triad of recurrent oral ulcers, genital ulcers, and eye lesions Skin lesions and positive pathergy test (induration and erythema produced at the site of a sterile needle stick)	None	Topical anesthetics Topical or intralesional steroids In severe disease, systemic treatment with immunosuppressant or immunomodulatory agents

OTHER DIAGNOSES TO CONSIDER

- Poor hygiene

- Seborrheic, psoriatic, atopic, or contact dermatitis

- Impetigo, streptococcal vulvovaginitis

- Labial adhesions or agglutination

- Ulcerations from varicella, herpes zoster, influenza, Epstein-Barr, or coxsackievirus infection

- Stevens-Johnson syndrome

- Crohn disease

WHEN TO CONSIDER FURTHER EVALUATION OR TREATMENT

- Sexual abuse requires a multidisciplinary approach. Medical care providers should initiate medical evaluation and treatment, including counseling, but suspected cases should be reported to the state child protective services agency and to local police departments for further investigation.

- The general treatment of genital injuries, infections, and inflammation include maintaining excellent perineal hygiene, sitz baths with warm water only, and topical lubricant ointments.

- Avoidance of irritants including soaps, application of topical aluminum acetate solution, and several days of low-dose topical steroids are helpful for specific and nonspecific vulvovaginitis.

- The diagnosis of genital warts, genital infections with herpes virus, and genital syphilis should result in evaluation for other sexually transmitted infections and consideration of possible sexual abuse.

SUGGESTED READINGS

Baldwin DD, Landa HM. Common problems in pediatric gynecology. *Urol Clin North Am*. 1995;22:161–176.

Bays J. Conditions mistaken for child sexual abuse. In: Reece R, Ludwig S, eds. *Child abuse: medical diagnosis and management*. 2nd ed. Philadelphia, PA: Lippincott Williams & Wilkins; 2001:287–306.

De Jong AR, Finkel MA. Medical findings in child sexual abuse. In: Reece R, Ludwig S, eds. *Child abuse: medical diagnosis and management*. 2nd ed. Philadelphia, PA: Lippincott Williams & Wilkins; 2001:207–286.

Emans SJH, Laufer MR, Goldstein DP, eds. *Pediatric and adolescent gynecology*. 5th ed. Philadelphia, PA: Lippincott-Raven Publishers; 2005:565–684, 939–975, 1024–1036.

Quint EH, Smith YR. Vulvar disorders in adolescent patients. *Pediatr Clin North Am*. 1999;46:593–606.

57

Vulvar Swelling and Masses

APPROACH TO THE PROBLEM

Swelling and masses found in the female external genitalia include acquired and congenital lesions. Acquired lesions typically present with symptoms including masses, pain, urinary symptoms, and/or bleeding but may be found as incidental findings on examination. Congenital lesions are often recognized as masses in the perinatal period, but they may go unrecognized until later childhood. The presence or absence of symptoms and the location of the mass are essential pieces of information when considering the differential diagnosis. Some benign lesions may require surgical intervention. Malignant tumors are rare in childhood.

KEY POINTS IN THE HISTORY

- Neonatal onset of swelling is common in paraurethral duct cysts, mucocolpos or hematocolpos, and inguinal hernias, but these lesions may also appear later in life. Other masses are rarely present in the neonatal period.

- Painless genital bleeding or spotting is the presenting symptom in most cases of urethral prolapse and in some cases of genital tumors.

- Labial abscesses, incarcerated or strangulated hernias, or secondarily infected cysts are accompanied by acute pain, while other genital masses usually are not.

- Typically, a history of urinary tract infections (UTIs), incontinence, or voiding difficulties accompanies prolapsed ureteroceles, and occasionally accompanies Gartner duct cysts and urethral prolapse. They are rarely associated with other genital masses.

- A history of intermittent swelling, particularly increasing with crying or Valsalva maneuvers, is only typical for masses caused by hernias.

- Abdominal pain, lower abdominal mass or increasing abdominal girth, and amenorrhea are common symptoms of hematocolpos or hematometrocolpos.

- A positive family history is present in 10% of children with hernias.

KEY POINTS IN THE PHYSICAL EXAMINATION

- Masses that originate or are present in the midline include urethral caruncle, urethral prolapse, prolapsed ureterocele, sarcoma botryoides, mucocolpos, and hematocolpos.

- Asymmetrical or nonmidline masses include most inguinal hernias; labial abscesses; and Bartholin, Gartner, and paraurethral duct cysts.

- Paraurethral duct cysts usually displace the urethral opening from the midline; whereas, all other common genital masses do not.

- Urethral prolapse is the only vulvar or urogenital lesion producing a circular mass surrounding the urethral opening.

- Most urogenital masses are nontender to palpation except for labial abscesses, incarcerated or strangulated hernias, or secondarily infected cysts.

- If painful, enlarged inguinal nodes accompany the mass, the mass is either a labial abscess or a secondarily infected cyst.

- The presence of blood with the mass is most indicative of a urethral prolapse, but occasionally blood will accompany a sarcoma botryoides.

- Lower abdominal masses may accompany mucocolpos and hematocolpos because retained mucus and/or blood causes distention of the uterus.

PHOTOGRAPHS OF SELECTED DIAGNOSES

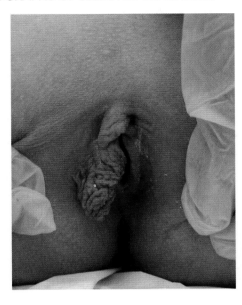

Figure 57-1 Labial hypertrophy.
Unilateral hypertrophy of the right labia minor in an 8-year-old
girl with Down syndrome.
(Courtesy of Joyce Adams, MD.)

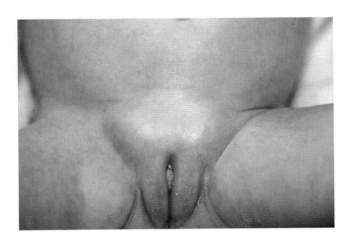

Figure 57-2 Inguinal hernia. 1-month-old girl with bilateral
inguinal hernias. Normal ovaries were found in the hernia sacs.
(Courtesy of Allan R. De Jong, MD.)

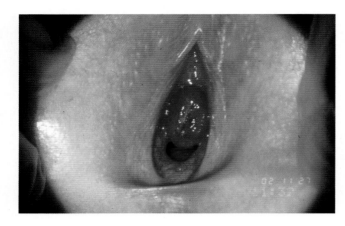

Figure 57-3 Urethral prolapse. Circular, reddish mass in the anterior midline, with the urethral opening in the center of the mass and a portion of the crescentic hymen and hymenal opening seen inferior to the mass. This 4-year-old girl presented with painless genital bleeding.
(Courtesy of Tony Olsen, MD.)

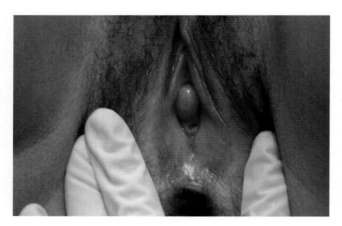

Figure 57-4 Paraurethral duct cyst. Yellowish, smooth mass in a 12-year-old with dysuria. Urethral opening is obscured, but hymenal opening is clearly visible below mass.
(Courtesy of Joyce Adams, MD.)

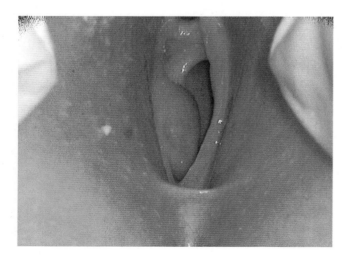

Figure 57-5 Gartner duct cyst. Cystic perihymenal mass in anterolateral wall of vaginal vestibule. Incidental finding in asymptomatic 8-year-old girl evaluated for suspected sexual abuse.
(Courtesy of Jayme Coffman, MD.)

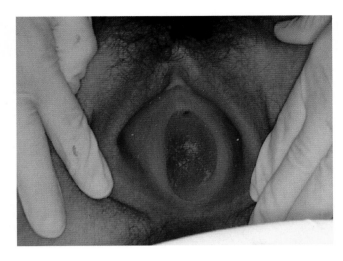

Figure 57-6 Hematocolpos. Bulging midline mass in a
14-year-old girl with imperforate hymen resulting in hematocolpos.
This adolescent presented with amenorrhea and lower abdominal
mass.
(Used with permission from Fleisher GR, Ludwig S, Baskin MN, eds. *Atlas
of pediatric emergency medicine.* Philadelphia, PA: Lippincott, Williams &
Wilkins; 2004:145.)

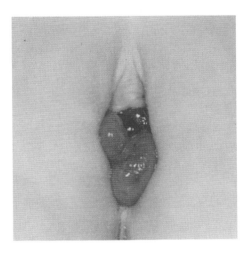

Figure 57-7 Sarcoma botryoides. Grape-like cluster of tissue
protruding between the labia of a prepubertal girl.
(Used with permission from Emans SJH, Laufer MR, Goldstein DP, eds.
Pediatric and adolescent gynecology. 5th ed. Philadelphia, PA: Lippincott–Raven
Publishers; 2005:446–447.)

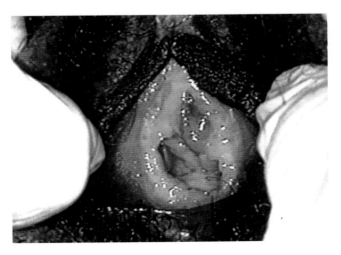

Figure 57-8 Urethral caruncle. Red polypoid mass is seen
protruding from a portion of the urethral opening. Incidental
finding in an asymptomatic 16-year-old girl who reported being
raped 4 months earlier.
(Courtesy of Allan R. De Jong, MD.)

DIFFERENTIAL DIAGNOSIS

DIAGNOSIS	ICD-9	DISTINGUISHING CHARACTERISTICS	ASSOCIATED FINDINGS
Labial Hypertrophy	624.3	Painless enlargement of labia minora in adolescents Usually bilateral, about 10% unilateral	Labia minora measure more than 4 cm in span from medial to most lateral point
Inguinal Hernia	550.9 (unilateral) 550.92 (bilateral)	Bulge or lump in mons pubis or labia majora, usually unilateral Often intermittent, increases with crying or Valsalva maneuver	May include ovary and/or fallopian tube in hernia Discoloration, pain with incarceration/strangulation
Urethral Prolapse	599.5	Circular, doughnut-shaped bright red, purple-to-blue protrusion of the urethral meatus Anterior to hymenal orifice; has urethral meatus in center Usually nontender	Typically presents with painless bleeding or spotting, but may be associated with dysuria or frequency (<25%) May present with urinary retention Predominantly in prepubertal (5- to 8-year-old) black girls (<10% white)
Labial Abscess	616.4	Acute, painful swelling with overlying redness or discoloration	Enlarged, tender, inguinal lymph nodes common
Paraurethral Duct Cyst	599.84	Glistening, tense, bulging, yellowish-white mass Urethral meatus is usually displaced laterally.	May cause dysuria or obstruction May cause deflected urinary stream
Gartner Duct Cyst	752.11	Visible, palpable, nontender, unilateral perihymenal or perivaginal mass, in anterolateral wall of vaginal vestibule Often translucent with retained, pearly white secretions under surface	Usually asymptomatic Visible, normal vaginal and urethral openings Abnormal ureters or kidneys may be present.
Bartholin Duct Cyst	616.2	Visible, palpable, nontender, unilateral mass, medial to labia minora, in posterior part of vaginal vestibule (5 o'clock and 7 o'clock locations) Visible, normal vaginal and urethral openings	Often asymptomatic Infected cysts are accompanied by severe pain and increased swelling.
Prolapsed Ureterocele	753.23	Soft, smooth cystic mass with whitish glistening surface protruding from urethral meatus Commonly presents in infancy or early childhood as UTI	No evidence of bleeding Incontinence, voiding dysfunction common May have bladder outlet obstruction
Hematocolpos	626.8	Presents in neonates as mucocolpos or hydrocolpos with shiny, early grey-to-blue midline mass with hymen stretched over it Presents in adolescence as bulging blue-to-red midline mass covered by hymen	Urethra is superior to mass and hymenal opening is absent. Can present as abdominal pain, lower abdominal mass, or amenorrhea
Sarcoma Botryoides	171.6	Lobulated mass protruding or prolapsing through hymenal opening Moist, grape-like clusters	May present as spotting of blood or vaginal discharge A type of rhabdomyosarcoma
Urethral Caruncle	599.3	Thin, reddish polypoid mass or membrane protruding from a portion of urethral opening Usually asymptomatic	Occasionally associated with dysuria, frequency, urgency, or recurrent UTI

PREDISPOSING FACTORS	COMPLICATIONS	TREATMENT GUIDELINES
None known	Genital pruritus and pain	Improved hygiene, but no other recommended treatment Surgical excisions or reductions may be considered in postpubertal girls
Family history in 10% Male:female prevalence 8:1 Bilateral hernias in girls associated with high risk of testicular feminization	Strangulation Only 2–3% have testes (testicular feminization) and rarely ovotestes (true hermaphroditism) in sac	Surgical repair
Hereditary predisposition UTIs Increased abdominal pressure Constipation Chronic cough Trauma Lack of estrogen	Strangulated prolapse Urinary obstruction Recurrent/persistent prolapse	Topical therapy with estrogen cream for 2 weeks Surgery recommended for complications
Trauma, obesity, excessive shaving, poor hygiene, diabetes, folliculitis, or infected cyst	Sepsis	Incision and drainage accompanied by antibiotics
Most often noted in neonatal period because of congenital obstruction May be result of acquired obstruction from infection	Secondary infection with abscess of cyst	No treatment for asymptomatic cases Excision, if symptomatic
Congenital Vestigial remnants of mesonephric ducts	Secondary infection with abscess of cyst	No treatment for asymptomatic cases Excision, if symptomatic
None with cysts Recurrent infection or abscess of cysts sometimes associated with sexually transmitted infections (STIs)	Secondary infection with abscess of cyst	Surgical intervention ranging from simple drainage to excision or ablation
Mostly associated with abnormal insertion of the ureter, duplicating collection system, and obstructed upper pole	Urinary obstruction, UTI, urosepsis 90% of cases have renal pole duplication	Surgical intervention varies depending on severity of clinical situation, size of ureterocele, and associated abnormalities
Results from imperforated hymen, transverse hymenal septum, or atretic vagina	Often associated with imperforate hymen, but occasionally associated with more significant genital tract malformations	Surgical incision of imperforate hymen in prepubertal girls or excision of portion of hymen in pubertal girls
Peak incidence <2 years, 90% before 5 years of age	Rare spread of tumor beyond vagina	Surgical excision of mass plus chemotherapy
Cause unknown	None	Surgical excision or electrocoagulation

- Labial hematoma

- Lipoma

- Lymphangioma

- Henoch-Schönlein purpura

- Urethral polyps

- Hymenal cysts

- Epithelial inclusion cysts

WHEN TO
CONSIDER
FURTHER
EVALUATION
OR TREATMENT

- Surgical evaluation and intervention are generally not required for labial hypertrophy, urethral prolapse, and asymptomatic cysts.

- Surgical evaluation and intervention are indicated for inguinal hernias, labial abscesses, symptomatic cysts, prolapsed ureteroceles, hematocolpos, sarcoma botryoides, and urethral caruncles.

- Bilateral exploration is recommended up to the age of 5 years for girls with inguinal hernias because bilateral hernias are more common in females than males.

- Evaluation for commonly associated renal and ureteral malformations is needed for all cases of prolapsed ureterocele.

- Primary therapy for urethral prolapse is sitz baths plus topical therapy with estrogen cream two to three times a day for 2 weeks. Some authors recommend supplementing topical estrogen with topical antibiotics and/or corticosteroids. Surgery is recommended for strangulated prolapse, urinary obstruction, or recurrent/persistent prolapse.

- Labial abscesses and infected cysts require antibiotics and surgical intervention. Antibiotic choice should include coverage for group B streptococcus, enterococcus, *Escherichia coli*, Proteus species, and *Staphylococcus aureus* including methicillin resistant *Staphylococcus aureus* (MRSA).

SUGGESTED READINGS

Baldwin DD, Landa HM. Common problems in pediatric gynecology. *Urol Clin North Am*. 1995;22:161–176.

Bays J. Conditions mistaken for child sexual abuse. In: Reece R, Ludwig S, eds. *Child abuse: medical diagnosis and management*. 2nd ed. Philadelphia, PA: Lippincott Williams & Wilkins; 2001:287–306.

Eilber KS, Raz S. Benign cystic lesions of the vagina: a literature review. *J Urol*. 2003;170:717–722.

Emans SJH, Laufer MR, Goldstein DP, eds. *Pediatric and adolescent gynecology*. 5th ed. Philadelphia, PA: Lippincott–Raven Publishers; 2005:446–447.

Fleisher GR, Ludwig 5, Baskin MN, eds. *Atlas of pediatric emergency medicine*. Philadelphia, PA: Lippincott, Williams & Wilkins; 2004:145.

Yerkes, EB. Urologic issues in the pediatric and adolescent gynecology patient. *Obstet Gynecol Clin N Am*. 2009;36:69–84.

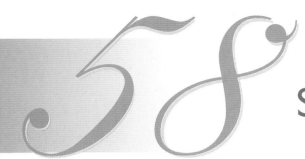

WILLIAM R. GRAESSLE

Scrotal Swelling

APPROACH TO THE PROBLEM

Common causes of scrotal swelling vary by age. Inguinal hernia is a common cause of scrotal swelling at any age. Spermatocele, varicocele, and primary testicular tumors are seen predominantly during adolescence. An acute scrotum may be caused by epididymitis, testicular torsion, or torsion of the testicular appendage (appendix testis torsion). At any age, generalized edema or edema in reaction to local trauma or inflammation may cause scrotal swelling that can be quite significant. To prevent ischemic damage and the need for the removal of the testicle, rapid diagnosis and intervention are essential when testicular torsion is suspected.

KEY POINTS IN THE HISTORY

- A swelling present since birth suggests a hydrocele or hydrocele of the spermatic cord, while the acute onset of scrotal swelling is more suggestive of a reactive hydrocele, testicular torsion, or epididymis.

- Fluctuation in the swelling size with physical activity or Valsalva maneuvers may be seen with a communicating hydrocele or inguinal hernia.

- A history of sexual activity, urethral discharge, or both may be present in patients with epididymitis.

- Pain, especially acute, raises the concern for testicular torsion.

- A history of nausea, vomiting, or abdominal distension in a patient with a suspected inguinal hernia suggests incarceration.

- Recurrent epididymitis may be seen in patients with dysfunctional voiding.

KEY POINTS IN THE PHYSICAL EXAMINATION

- The scrotum of an adolescent male should be examined in the standing position. Varicoceles may be missed when the patient is recumbent.

- Use of a Valsalva maneuver may aid in the detection of hernias, communicating hydroceles and varicoceles.

- Scrotal swelling with fullness at the inguinal ring is consistent with an inguinal hernia or hydrocele of the spermatic cord.

- A smooth mass that transilluminates when a light source is applied directly to the scrotum suggests a hydrocele.

- In testicular torsion, the affected testes may appear to sit higher than the contralateral testes.

- Redness limited to the upper pole of the testis is consistent with torsion of the appendix testis.

- The testicular surface should be smooth; an irregular surface should raise suspicion for a testicular tumor.

- The presence of tenderness, firmness, or discoloration suggests incarceration or strangulation of an inguinal hernia.

- The reduction of an apparent hydrocele is consistent with a communicating hydrocele or an inguinal hernia.

- Edema affecting both sides of the scrotum may occur in patients with generalized edema—for example, in patients with hypoalbuminemia—and in patients with local trauma, including blunt trauma to the perineal area or severe perineal dermatitis.

PHOTOGRAPHS OF SELECTED DIAGNOSES

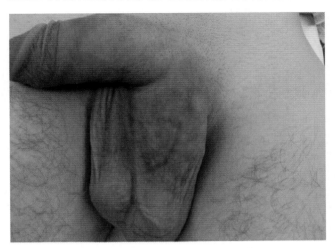

Figure 58-1 Varicocele with "bag of worms" appearance above the testicle.
(Courtesy of T. Ernesto Figueroa, MD, FAAP, FACS.)

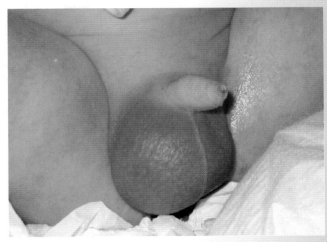

Figure 58-2 Infant with a hydrocele.
(Courtesy of T. Ernesto Figueroa, MD, FAAP, FACS.)

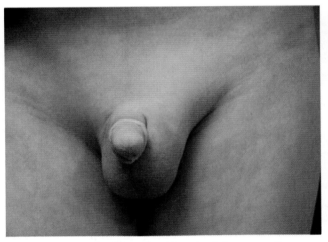

Figure 58-3 Inguinal hernia. Note the fullness near the inguinal ring.
(Courtesy of Philip Siu, MD.)

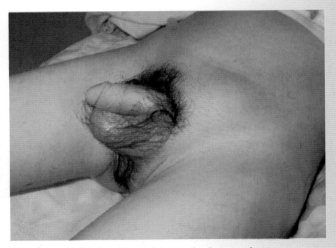

Figure 58-4 Adolescent with testicular torsion.
(Courtesy of T. Ernesto Figueroa, MD, FAAP, FACS.)

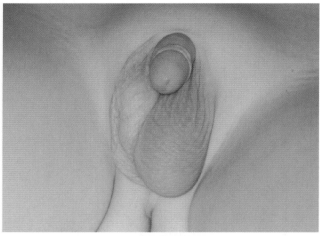

Figure 58-5 Torsion of the appendix testis with reactive hydrocele.
(Courtesy of T. Ernesto Figueroa, MD, FAAP, FACS.)

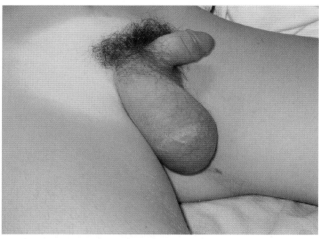

Figure 58-6 Testicular tumor.
(Courtesy of T. Ernesto Figueroa, MD, FAAP, FACS.)

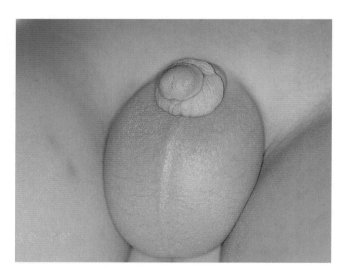

Figure 58-7 Scrotal swelling in a 7-year-old male with nephrotic syndrome.
(Used with permission from Fleisher GR, Ludwig S, Baskin MN. *Atlas of pediatric emergency medicine*. Philadelphia, PA: Lippincott Williams & Wilkins; 2004:304.)

DIAGNOSIS	ICD-9	DISTINGUISHING CHARACTERISTICS	AGE	ASSOCIATED FINDINGS	PREDISPOSING FACTORS	TREATMENT GUIDELINES
Varicocele	456.4	Swelling in upper part of scrotum Feels like a "bag of worms" Usually left-sided	10–15% of postpubertal boys	More pronounced with standing	Acute varicocele may be caused by intra-abdominal venous obstruction.	Treatment is controversial. Referral to urologist to discuss treatment options
Hydrocele	603.9	Swelling around testicle Normal cord palpated above the mass Fluctuation of the fluid around the testis is consistent with a communicating hydrocele.	Common in newborns Seen in 5%, two-thirds are bilateral	Transilluminates If reducible, hernia should be suspected.	Congenital May be reactive to a torsion of an appendix testis	Communicating hydroceles and those that fail to resolve spontaneously require surgical intervention.
Hydrocele of the Spermatic Cord	603.9	Inguinal fluid mass not in communication with peritoneum or scrotum	Infancy	Often associated with hernia and scrotal hydrocele	Congenital	Referral to urologist for elective surgical repair
Hernia Inguinal	550.90 B/L 550.92	Reducible swelling in inguinal area	Any	Inguinal swelling may be accompanied by scrotal mass. Swelling may be fixed when incarcerated.	Increased intra-abdominal pressure Ventriculoperitoneal shunt or dialysis catheter (The extra fluid may make an underlying hernia apparent.)	Incarcerated hernias require emergent evaluation by a urologist or pediatric surgeon. Reducible hernias should be referred for elective correction.
Testicular Torsion	608.2	Enlarged testicle Painful Does not transilluminate	Peak in adolescence with a smaller peak in the neonatal period Can occur at any age	High-riding testicle Nodular cord swelling superior to testis	Some males predisposed because of a high insertion of tunica vaginalis on cord Lack of posterior anchoring of the testis allows free rotation on the spermatic cord (bell clapper deformity).	Emergent ultrasound imaging and surgical intervention Referral to urology or pediatric surgery
Appendix Testis Torsion	608.2	Infarcted appendage may be palpated or visible (blue dot sign) at the upper pole of testis	Most commonly at the onset of puberty	Reactive hydrocele may make differentiation from testicular torsion difficult without imaging	Cause unknown	Evaluation by urologist or pediatric surgeon if testicular torsion suspected Ultrasound to rule out testicular torsion
Epididymitis	604.90	Enlargement and tenderness of epididymis Scrotum may be painful and swollen. Testis should be normal.	Adolescents Younger children with urinary tract abnormalities Older children with voiding dysfunction	Urethral discharge may be present. Pyuria and bacteriuria	Commonly idiopathic Hematogenous spread of viral disease Sexually transmitted diseases	Antibiotics to cover *Chlamydia trachomatis* and *Neisseria gonorrhoeae*
Spermatocele	608.1	Nontender cystic swelling separate from the testis	After onset of puberty	Transilluminates	N/A	Surgical intervention if painful or progressive enlargement Evaluation by urology or pediatric surgery
Meconium Sequestration	608.89 (mass scrotum)	Firm, nodular scrotal mass	Infants and young children	Usually calcifications on ultrasound	History of meconium peritonitis may be present.	No treatment
Testicular Cancer	186.9	Painless mass	More commonly adolescent or young adult	Secondary hydrocele may be present. Abdominal mass, prominent inguinal lymph nodes	N/A	Referral to urology and oncology

OTHER
DIAGNOSES
TO CONSIDER

- Henoch-Schönlein purpura

- Leukemic infiltration

- Intraperitoneal hemorrhage

- Inguinal lymphadenopathy

- Generalized edema

WHEN TO
CONSIDER
FURTHER
EVALUATION
OR TREATMENT

- Acute scrotal swelling that suggests the possibility of testicular torsion requires emergent evaluation by a urologist or general surgeon.

- Newborns with a noncommunicating hydrocele can be observed for resolution.

- During the examination of a suspected hydrocele, fluctuation of the volume of fluid suggests a communicating hydrocele or hernia. Communicating hydroceles and hernias should be referred for surgical evaluation and treatment.

- If a hernia is incarcerated or strangulated, the patient should be referred for emergent surgical evaluation.

- Treatment of varicoceles in adolescents is controversial. Patients should be referred to a urologist or pediatric surgeon to discuss treatment options.

- A suspected tumor of the testis requires further evaluation and referral to a urologist. Ultrasound will localize the tumor and may be helpful in differentiating benign tumors from malignant tumors.

SUGGESTED READINGS

Fleisher GR, Ludwig S, Baskin MN. *Atlas of pediatric emergency medicine*. Philadelphia, PA: Lippincott Williams & Wilkins; 2004:304.
Kass EJ. Adolescent varicocele. *Pediatr Clin North Am*. 2001;48:1559–1569.
Katz DA. Evaluation and management of inguinal and umbilical hernias. *Pediatr Ann*. 2001;30:729–735.
Leslie JA, Cain MP. Pediatric urologic emergencies and urgencies. *Pediatr Clin North Am*. 2006;53:513–527.
Sheldon CA. The pediatric genitourinary examination. *Pediatr Clin North Am*. 2001;48:1339–1380.
Wan J, Bloom DA. Genitourinary problems in adolescent males. *Adolesc Med*. 2003;14:717–731.

FOURTEEN

Perianal Area and Buttocks

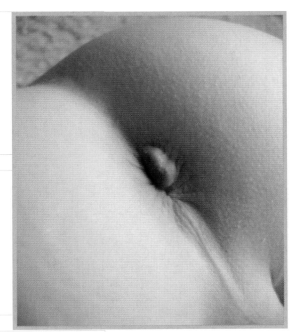

(Courtesy of Michael J. Wilsey, Jr, MD, FAAP.)

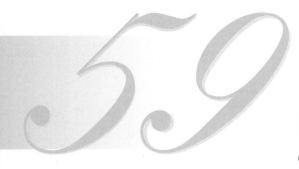

MICHAEL J. WILSEY, JR.
AND KARINA IRIZARRY

Perianal and Buttock Swelling

| APPROACH TO THE PROBLEM | Pediatricians will often encounter concerns about symptoms related to the anorectal region. Most of these conditions in children are benign and seldom require surgical interventions. They present with similar symptoms, such as perianal masses, rectal pain, bleeding, and pruritus, which makes diagnosis a challenging task. A careful review of the history, paying attention to bowel movements pattern and associated symptoms, can guide the physical examination and facilitate diagnosis. |

| KEY POINTS IN THE HISTORY | • Perirectal abscesses are more common in infants and children who are less than 1 year of age. |

- Inflammatory bowel disease, HIV, diabetes mellitus, and neutrophil dysfunction may predispose children to develop perirectal abscesses.

- Perirectal abscesses present with perianal pruritus, redness, swelling, or a lump near the anus. They are very painful, and the pain worsens with movement, sitting, defecation, and diaper changing in infants.

- Multiple, draining, midline sinus tracts that often soil underclothes with cloudy or blood-stained discharge may accompany pilonidal abscesses.

- Skin tags, rectal prolapse, and hemorrhoids in children usually result from functional constipation. Look for a history of large, hard, and/or painful bowel movements and encopresis.

- A history of bright-red-blood-streaked stools, blood dripping into the toilet, or blood seen on toilet paper after wiping is suggestive of a perianal fissure.

- A fibrotic "sentinel" skin tag may be present over a chronic fissure.

- Large, edematous, shiny, perianal skin tags should raise concern about the presence of Crohn disease.

- External hemorrhoids are varicose veins involving the skin of the anoderm and rarely cause symptoms.

- Acutely thrombosed external hemorrhoids present as a sudden onset of throbbing, burning pain at the end of defection associated with a new bulge in the anal region.

- Internal hemorrhoids, which arise from the rectal submucosa, are uncommon in children and should raise concern about underlying portal hypertension.

- Anogenital warts are often asymptomatic and found incidentally by parents or physicians.

- Anogenital warts in children may be acquired vertically during birth or by autoinoculation from common hand warts.

KEY POINTS IN THE PHYSICAL EXAMINATION

- A localized, tender, well-defined, fluctuant mass may be palpated on the anal verge or on digital examination if there is a perirectal abscess.

- Ischiorectal abscesses are often large and visible on the surface of the buttock, although occasionally an examination may be completely normal.

- A pilonidal abscess may occur at the site of an ingrown hair follicle and often presents as a midline sacral boil approximately 1 to 2 cm above the anus. If the boil spontaneously drains, it can be associated with a fistulous tract.

- A hard, painful, bluish lump may be seen in the anal opening if there is an external thrombosed hemorrhoid.

- Ninety percent of anal fissures are located at the 6 o'clock position (midposterior region), with the 12 o'clock position (midanterior region) being the next most common. Anal fissures in unusual locations should raise concern about inflammatory bowel disease, occult abscesses, and infections, such as herpes simplex virus infection or syphilis.

- Anogenital warts will turn white when soaked in 3% to 5% acetic acid (vinegar).

- Rectal prolapse may involve only the mucosa or all layers of the rectum (most commonly). In complete prolapse, concentric rings of rectal mucosa are seen herniating through the anus on examination.

- After reduction of rectal prolapse, the anal tone may be absent or decreased during rectal examination. The normal tone will generally return after several hours.

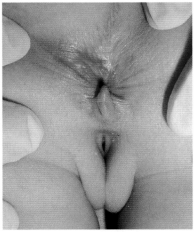

Figure 59-1 Perianal skin tag.
A "sentinel" perianal skin tag seen in a female infant.
(Courtesy of Mary L. Brandt, MD.)

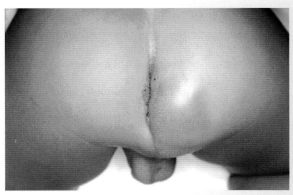

Figure 59-2 Perirectal abscess. A 12-month-old male presenting with a perirectal mass.
(Courtesy of Mark A. Ward, MD.)

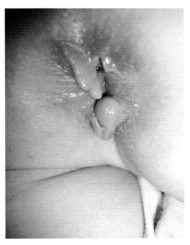

Figure 59-3 Perianal Crohn disease in a child with multiple large, edematous skin tags and a perianal fissure at the 7 o'clock position.
(Courtesy of Martin Fried, MD.)

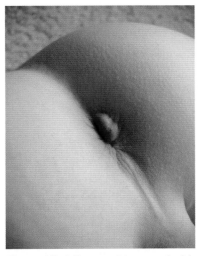

Figure 59-4 External hemorrhoid in a 2-yr-old male with recurrent straining because of chronic constipation.
(Courtesy of Michael J. Wilsey, Jr, MD, FAAP.)

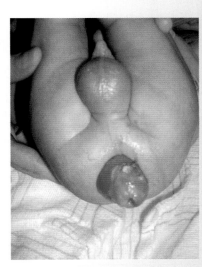

Figure 59-5 Rectal prolapse seen in a male infant.
(Courtesy of Mary L. Brandt, MD.)

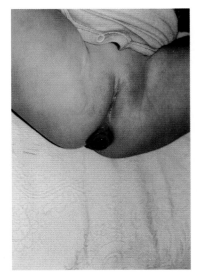

Figure 59-6 Rectal prolapse. Concentric rings of rectal mucosa (all the layers of the rectum) are seen herniating through the anus, indicating a complete prolapse.
(Courtesy of Fernando L. Heinen, MD.)

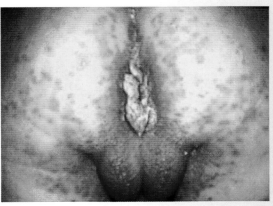

Figure 59-7 Perianal condylomata seen following sexual abuse.
(Courtesy of Fernando L. Heinen, MD.)

DIFFERENTIAL DIAGNOSIS

DIAGNOSIS	ICD-9	DISTINGUISHING CHARACTERISTICS	DISTRIBUTION	DURATION CHRONICITY	
Perirectal Skin Tag	455.9	Painless, shapeless lumps or flaps of skin or flesh Painful defecation when associated with anal fissure	Anal verge Sentinel tags form above Chronic anal fissures	Chronic	
Perirectal Abscess	566	Tender, fluctuant mass near anus or on digital exam Pilonidal abscess; mid-line boil and/or fistula	Perianal—60% Ischiorectal Intersphincteric Supralevator	Present until it drains spontaneously or is surgically drained	
Hemorrhoids	455.6	Firm bulge at anal verge, may have bluish discoloration Usually asymptomatic External hemorrhoids may be acutely painful when thrombosed	External (below dentate line)—most common Internal (above dentate line)—rare in pediatrics	Acute pain lasts hours to 1–2 wks (until spontaneously or surgically drained)	
Rectal Prolapse	569.1	Painless, bright red tissue protruding from anus In mucosal prolapse, radial folds are seen at junction with anal skin. In complete rectal prolapse, circular folds are seen at junction with anal skin. Highest incidence in the first year of life	Anal herniation of rectal mucosa	May become chronic, occurring with most bowel movements (weeks to months)	
Anogenital Warts	078.19	Four types: 1. Condyloma acuminatum-cauliflower-like lesions 2. Flat-macular 3. Papular 4. Keratotic-thick, crusty; usually multiple	May be found as discrete lesions or may coalesce to form plaques	N/A	

ASSOCIATED FINDINGS	COMPLICATIONS	PREDISPOSING FACTORS	TREATMENT GUIDELINES
Anal pruritus Rectal bleeding	Hygienic problems—may impair cleaning of perineum when wiping	Constipation Fissures Fistulae Injury from rectal surgery Hemorrhoids	Treatment of underlying constipation with stool softeners and high-fiber diet
Fever Perianal pruritus Pain worse with defecation	Fistula Recurrence Stricture Incontinence	Infancy More common in immunosupressed patients and those with diabetes mellitus	Pediatric surgery referral for incision, drainage, and debridement
Painless rectal bleeding Occasional discomfort with defecation Anal pruritus	Thrombosis Prolapse Strangulation	Constipation often precedes external hemorrhoids Portal hypertension may precede internal hemorrhoids	Treatment with stool softeners, high-fiber diet, Sitz baths, and topical and systemic analgesics Pediatric surgery referral for acutely thrombosed external hemorrhoids
Pruritus Bleeding Urgency	Edema and necrosis of prolapsed tissue Fecal incontinence	Constipation Acute or chronic diarrhea Chronic lung disease Cystic fibrosis Pelvic floor weakness due to myelomeningocele, post anal surgery or Ehlers-Danlos Parasitic infestations, especially with trichuriasis (whipworm) Hirschsprung disease Malnutrition Congenital hypothyroidism	Often can be reduced at home with a warm washcloth and gentle manual pressure Emergency center evaluation and surgical consultation for irreducible rectal prolapse
May be friable, pruritic and painful	Cancer (very rarely)	HPV infection (low risk types: 6,11) Child sexual abuse Autoinoculation from hand wart	Evaluate for child sexual abuse Dermatology referral for close observation or ablative therapy with cryotherapy or surgical excision

OTHER
DIAGNOSES
TO CONSIDER

- Inflammatory bowel disease (Crohn disease)

- Protruding colonic polyp

- Protruding ileocecal intussusception

- Chronic solitary ulcer

WHEN TO
CONSIDER
FURTHER
EVALUATION
OR TREATMENT

- Presence of skin tags, fissures, abscesses, and fistulae associated with abdominal pain, diarrhea, and weight loss warrants evaluation for inflammatory bowel disease.

- An acutely thrombosed external hemorrhoid, which presents as a painful firm bluish mass, should be evaluated by a pediatric surgeon.

- Obtain a sweat test for cystic fibrosis and infectious stool studies for parasitic infestations, especially trichuriasis or whipworm, in patients with rectal prolapse.

- Consider evaluation for child sexual abuse for a child that presents with anogenital warts.

SUGGESTED READINGS

Blumberg D, Wald A. Other diseases of the colon and rectum. In: Feldman, ed. *Sleisenger & Fordtran's gastrointestinal and liver disease.* 7th ed. Philadelphia, PA: W.B. Saunders, 2002:2294–2296.

Budayr M, Ankney RN, Moore RA. Condyloma acuminata in infants and children. *Dis Colon Rectum.* 1996;39(10):1112–1115.

Johnson S, Jaksic T. Benign perianal lesions. In: Walker WA, Goulet O, Kleinman RE, et al., eds. *Pediatric gastrointestinal disease: pathophysiology, diagnosis, management.* 4th ed. Vol. 1. Hamilton, Ontario: B.C. Decker Inc., 2004:598–601.

Pfenninger JL, Zainea GG. Common anorectal conditions: part II. lesions. *Am Fam Physician.* 2001;64(1):77–88.

Raimer SS. Family violence, child abuse and anogenital warts. *Arch Dermatol.* 1992;128:842–844.

Siafakas C, Vottler TP, Andersen, JM. Rectal prolapse in pediatrics. *Clin Pediatr (Phila).* 1999;38(2):63–72.

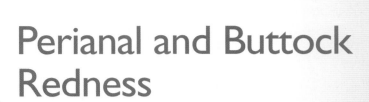

JAN EDWIN DRUTZ

Perianal and Buttock Redness

APPROACH TO THE PROBLEM

The leading cause for erythema involving the buttock and/or perianal skin surfaces of infants and younger children is diaper dermatitis. This term is used to describe many skin conditions that happen to be confined to the area covered by the diaper. Because of variability in the presentation and distribution of the erythema, confusion and controversy often arise as to the correct etiology, treatment, and prognosis. Of the various forms, contact diaper dermatitis is the most common. Urine and feces in combination have a tendency to increase skin pH making skin more susceptible to irritants. The normal skin pH is 4.0 to 5.5. As skin wetness increases, so do frictional resistance, abrasive damage, and skin permeability. Pancreatic enzymes, including protease and lipase, irritate skin directly, especially as the pH increases. Bile salts act as skin irritants, potentiating the activity of lipases.

KEY POINTS IN THE HISTORY

- As increased and prolonged moisture in the diaper area may be a significant contributing factor to skin irritation, it is important to determine whether the patient has had increased stooling and/or frank diarrhea and how often diapers have been changed.

- Contact with chemical agents should be considered as a possible explanation for an erythematous rash in the diaper area.

- Children wearing highly absorbent diapers as opposed to cloth diapers have lower tendencies to develop diaper dermatitis.

- *Candida albicans* infection, the most common complication of contact diaper dermatitis, may produce diffuse erosions, particularly in deep flexural areas.

- Perianal erythema, pain/tenderness, and pruritus are the most common presenting signs and symptoms for group A beta-hemolytic streptococci (*Streptococcus pyogenes*).

- Nighttime and early morning perianal itching, insomnia, and abdominal cramping are manifestations of pinworm infestation.

KEY POINTS IN THE PHYSICAL EXAMINATION

- The earliest manifestation of contact diaper dermatitis is mild perianal redness, particularly among infants less than 4 months old.

- The most common sites for contact diaper dermatitis in older infants are the lower abdomen, anterior-medial thighs, scrotum, and labia, where chafing due to friction is common.

- Contact diaper dermatitis causes papules and mild erythema with a shiny, glazed surface, and the depths of skin folds generally are spared. In some areas, the skin appears dry and somewhat wrinkled with mild-to-moderate, ill-defined, erythematous borders.

- A common variant of contact diaper dermatitis, the "tidemark" rash, involves areas bordered by the constriction bands of the diaper, including the waist and proximal thighs.

- With *Candida albicans* infections, individual pustular lesions generally erode and spread to develop satellite lesions, which generally are concentrated within the warm, moist confines of the diaper area.

- Bright-red, erythematous lesions in the perianal area with well-defined borders, accompanied by a mucopurulent discharge, are consistent with a *S. pyogenes* infection.

- Perianal desquamation and erythema may be seen with staphylococcal and streptococcal infections, and Kawasaki disease.

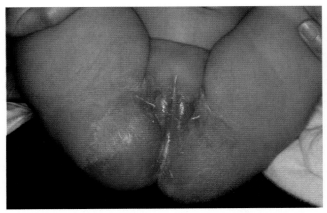

Figure 60-1 Primary irritant diaper dermatitis. Confluent areas of shiny erythema over labia majora and buttocks. (Courtesy of Jan Edwin Drutz, MD.)

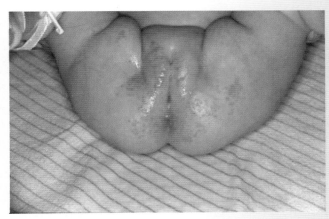

Figure 60-2 Candidal diaper dermatitis. Infant with erythematous rash with satellite lesions in the groin. (Courtesy of Jan Edwin Drutz, MD.)

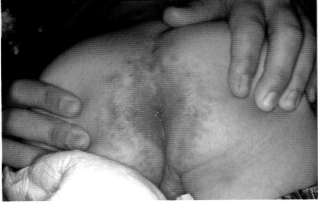

Figure 60-3 Perianal group A beta-hemolytic streptococcus (GABHS). Intense erythema is noted in the immediate perianal area of this toddler. (Courtesy of Jan Edwin Drutz, MD.)

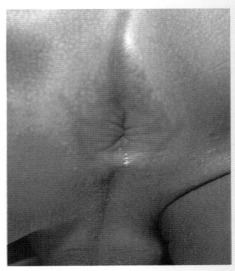

Figure 60-4 Perianal group A beta-hemolytic streptoccal infection (GABHS). Perianal streptococcal disease in an African-American child. (Courtesy of George A. Datto, III, MD.)

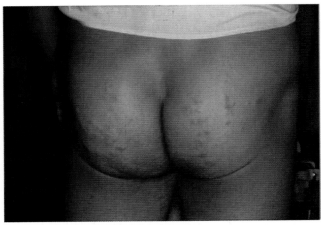

Figure 60-5 Buttock folliculitis. A child with erythematous papules over the posterior buttocks consistent with folliculitis. (Courtesy of Jan Edwin Drutz, MD.)

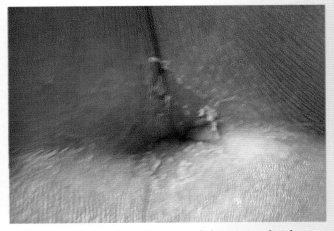

Figure 60-6 Perianal erythema and desquamation in a patient with Kawasaki disease. (Courtesy of Esther K. Chung, MD, MPH.)

DIFFERENTIAL DIAGNOSIS

DIAGNOSIS	ICD-9	DISTINGUISHING CHARACTERISTICS	DISTRIBUTION	ASSOCIATED FINDINGS
Contact Diaper Dermatitis	691.0	Mild erythema with papules Shiny glazed surface Sparing of skin fold depths	Lower abdomen, anteromedial thighs, and genitalia	Some dry/wrinkled areas evident Erythematous borders clearly defined by diaper constriction bands "Tidewater rash"
Candidiasis	112.2	Individual lesions have raised, white-scaly margins. Distinctive vesiculopustular satellite lesions	Diffuse erythematous rash involving lower abdomen, medial thighs, and buttocks	Frequently, concomitant oral moniliasis (thrush)
Perianal Streptococcal Infection	041.0	Bright-red, perianal erythema Perianal tenderness, pain, and pruritus Mucopurulent secretion	Immediate perianal area	Pharyngitis
Jacquet Erosive Dermatitis	691.0	Small, distinct papules and nodules approximately 5 mm in diameter Central umbilication and superficial ulcerations	Localized to occluded skin of perianal and/or genital areas	Mucosa frequently spared Lesions are typically painless.
Seborrheic Dermatitis	690.1	Salmon-colored, greasy lesions May be accompanied by erythematous, well-demarcated rash and peripheral satellite lesions, but generally no pustules or erosions Patient generally asymptomatic	Initially may be confined to diaper area After few days, rash extends to involve other body parts with predilection for flexural creases	Usually begins in the scalp during infancy Scalp lesions may be somewhat red with yellow, flaky scale.
Allergic Contact Dermatitis	692.9	Erythematous lesions; spares skin folds	Convex surfaces of diaper area	Erythematous papules and some skin flaking
Intertrigo	695.89	Moderately erythematous superficial rash with ill-defined borders, generally accompanied by a white-yellow exudate	Deep folds of thighs and lower abdomen	Mild to moderate tenderness

COMPLICATIONS	PRECIPITATING FACTORS	TREATMENT GUIDELINES
Secondary candidal and/or bacterial infection	Increased and prolonged moisture in the diaper area Type of diaper being used	Encourage frequent diaper changes. Use mild cleansing agents. Avoid harsh soaps. Maintain clean dry skin. Use barrier agents, for example, zinc oxide, sucralfate, or petroleum jelly. Use highly absorbent diapers.
N/A, unless patient immunosuppressed	Preceding/concomitant generic or other form of diaper dermatitis Recent history of systemic antibiotic therapy	Topical application of antifungal preparations
Acute glomerulonephritis	Self inoculation of the perianal area from organisms in the pharynx	Oral antibiotics for coverage of group A beta-hemolytic streptococcus
Secondary candidal and/or bacterial infection	Prolonged skin contact with urine/feces under occlusion Resultant friction and maceration render skin permeable to proteases/lipases. Fecal urea-splitting bacteria raise ammonia level with subsequent elevated pH and further fecal enzyme involvement.	Encourage frequent diaper changes. Use mild cleansing agents. Maintain clean dry skin Use barrier agents, for example, zinc oxide, sucralfate, or petroleum jelly
Secondary candidal and/or bacterial infection	Specific etiology unknown Appears to be related to inflammatory reaction of the skin	Clearing of scalp lesions (when present) using anti-seborrheic shampoo is generally beneficial. Low-potency topical corticosteroid application for short period of time helps clear remaining lesions.
Vesicles and eruptions occasionally	Any number of topical substances/agents (e.g., ethylenediamine or rubber) to which patient is highly sensitized	Avoid known sensitizing agents; use mildly potent topical steroids; and consider oral antihistamine
Secondary bacterial or fungal infection	Chafing secondary to friction and heat in areas of diaper moisture leading to skin maceration	Moist compresses and gentle debridement Low-potency topical corticosteroids Antimicrobial agents when indicated

OTHER
DIAGNOSES
TO CONSIDER

- Acrodermatitis enteropathica

- Psoriasis

- Granuloma gluteale infantum

- Histiocytosis X

- Scabies

- Congenital syphilis

- Child sexual abuse

- Folliculitis

- Infections with microbial organisms other than group A beta-hemolytic streptococcus or *Staphylococcus aureus*

- Irritation from laxative use

WHEN TO
CONSIDER
FURTHER
EVALUATION
OR TREATMENT

- Contact diaper dermatitis should be treated with mild cleaning agents, frequent diaper changes, and barrier creams.

- Candidal diaper rash should be treated with a topical antifungal agent.

- If the diaper dermatitis fails to respond to the appropriate topical agents, evaluation for less common etiologies such as psoriasis should be considered.

SUGGESTED READINGS
Arnsmeier SL, Paller AS. Getting to the bottom of diaper dermatitis. *Contemp Pediatr.* 1997;14(11):115–129.
Berg RW, Milligan MC, Sarbaugh FC. Association of skin wetness and pH with diaper dermatitis. *Pediatr Dermatol.* 1994;11(1):18–20.
Lane AT. Resolving controversies in diaper dermatitis. *Contemp Pediatr.* 1986;3(4):45–54.
Leventhal JM, Griffin D, Duncan KO, et al. Laxative-induced dermatitis of the buttocks incorrectly suspected to be abusive burns. *Pediatrics.* 2001;107(1):178–180.
Mogielnicki NP, Schwartzman JD, Elliott JA. Perineal group A streptococcal disease in a pediatric practice. *Pediatrics.* 2000;106(2)(part 1):276–281.
Zimmerer RE, Lawson KD, Calvert CJ. The effects of wearing diapers on skin. *Pediatr Dermatol.* 1986;3(2):95–101.

FIFTEEN

Skin

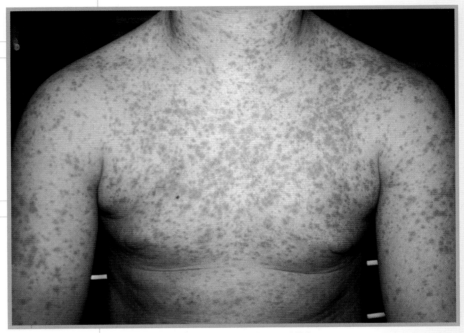

(Courtesy of Kathleen Cronan, MD.)

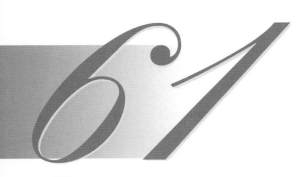

GARY A. EMMETT

Facial Rashes

APPROACH TO THE PROBLEM

Facial rashes may be local processes or signs of systemic illness. The distribution (dermatomal, asymmetric or symmetric, or well-defined shape), the anatomical location of the rash within the skin (superficial or subcutaneous), the classification of the rash (vesicle, papule, or plaque), and the color of the rash are all potential clues to their etiology. Acne is the most common chronic facial rash seen among adolescents. The psychological consequences of all facial rashes must be considered when addressing their treatment and when counseling families.

KEY POINTS IN THE HISTORY

- Acne is often the first sign of adrenal gland activation associated with the onset of puberty.

- The facial lesions of tuberous sclerosis often are misdiagnosed as acne.

- With impetigo, the gradual spread of golden-crusted, inflamed sores from the nares across the face is caused by bacterial spread from scratching.

- A family history of eczema, allergies, or asthma is frequently found in children with significant eczema.

- Facial rashes associated with skin dryness, including eczema, pityriasis alba, and lip-licking dermatitis, are often worse in the winter when there is relatively low humidity.

KEY POINTS IN THE PHYSICAL EXAMINATION

- Impetigo or tinea corporis usually presents with focal facial rashes.

- Skin lesions resulting from acute infectious systemic illnesses, such as erythema infectiosum or scarlet fever, usually are symmetric.

- Acne can present with the following types of lesions: open and closed comedones, papules, pustules, and nodulocystic lesions.

- Contact dermatitis occurs in areas exposed to the offending agent, such as under nickel-containing jewelry.

- Vesicles are seen with herpes virus infections, contact dermatitis (including poison ivy), and eczema.

- Vesicular lesions that are grouped or that follow a dermatome are classic for herpes virus (simplex and zoster) infections.

- Many forms of papules are associated with specific diseases such as the very hard, subcutaneous papules seen in tuberous sclerosis; comedones seen in acne; the small, rough papules of scarlet fever; and the polished, pearl-like lesions of molluscum contagiosum.

- Eczema, seborrhea, psoriasis, and pityriasis alba are scaly facial rashes that can be found elsewhere on the body.

- Pityriasis alba can be differentiated from fungal infections by performing a KOH examination of the scale.

- Seborrhea has a predilection for areas in which there is hair, including the scalp, eyebrows, eyelashes, and beard, but it is also found just under and behind the earlobes.

- Chronic facial rashes associated with signs of inflammation, including fever and arthritis, raise concerns for and should prompt further evaluation for autoimmune diseases.

- Rashes that disappear temporarily on compression are intravascular and can result from either hemangiomata or vascular inflammation.

- Scarlet fever in the absence of an infected throat may be seen with perianal streptococcal infection.

PHOTOGRAPHS OF SELECTED DIAGNOSES

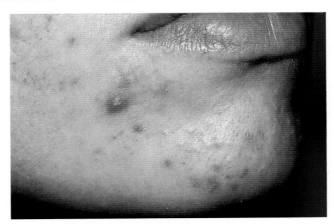

Figure 61-1 Inflammatory acne. Erythematous papules and
pustules on chin.
(Used with permission from Goodheart HP. *Goodheart's photoguide to
common skin disorders.* 2nd ed. Philadelphia, PA: Lippincott Williams &
Wilkins; 2003:14.)

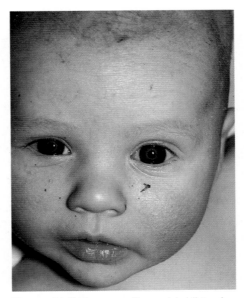

Figure 61-2 Eczema. Symmetric bilateral
scaly rash on cheeks.
(Used with permission from Goodheart HP.
Goodheart's photoguide to common skin disorders.
2nd ed. Philadelphia, PA: Lippincott Williams &
Wilkins; 2003:46.)

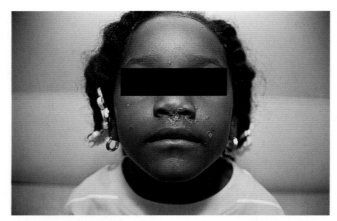

Figure 61-3 Impetigo. Honey-crusted lesions at base of nares that are self-inoculated onto other parts of the face.
(Courtesy of George A. Datto, III, MD.)

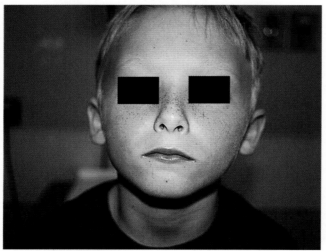

Figure 61-4 Erythema infectiosum. Bilateral erythematous macular rash on cheeks—"slapped cheeks."
(Courtesy of George A. Datto, III, MD.)

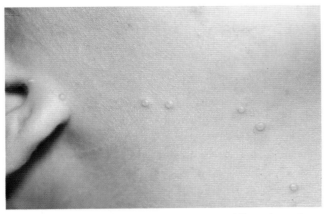

Figure 61-5 Molluscum contagiosum. Umbilicated papules on face of child.
(Used with permission from Goodheart HP. *Goodheart's photoguide to common skin disorders*. 2nd ed. Philadelphia, PA: Lippincott Williams & Wilkins; 2003:138.)

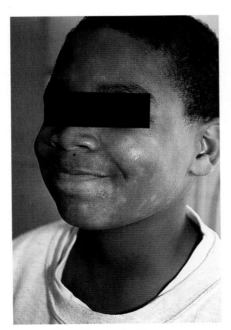

Figure 61-6 Pityriasis alba.
Hypopigmented scaly macules on cheeks.
(Courtesy of George A. Datto, III, MD.)

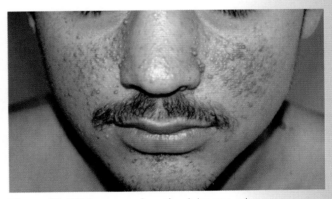

Figure 61-7 Tuberous sclerosis. Adenoma sebaceum (angiofibroma).
(Used with permission from Goodheart HP. *Goodheart's photoguide to common skin disorders*. 2nd ed. Philadelphia, PA: Lippincott Williams & Wilkins; 2003:388.)

DIFFERENTIAL DIAGNOSIS

DIAGNOSIS	ICD-9	DISTINGUISHING CHARACTERISTICS	DISTRIBUTION	ASSOCIATED FINDINGS
Acne	706.1	Open comedones—blackhead Closed comedones—whitehead Papules Nodules in dermis	Forehead Chest and back in males	Other signs of puberty (i.e., adrenarche, pubic hair)
Eczema	691.8	Scaly Erythema Exudate Microvesicles (acute) Lichenification (chronic)	Symmetric Cheeks, chin, forehead	Extremity lesions Pruritus Asthma Allergic symptoms
Impetigo	684.0	Golden-crusted lesions	Nares	May spread to other parts of body by self-inoculation
Seborrhea	706.3	Greasy, scaly, papules	Scalp Retroauricular Eyebrows Blepharitis External ear canal	Pruritus
Scarlet Fever	034.1	Small "sandpaper" papules	Diffuse	Pharyngitis Strawberry tongue Fever Circumoral pallor Evidence of streptococcal infection Perianal streptococcal infection
Erythema Infectiosum	057.0	Erythematous "slapped cheeks"	Cheeks Trunk Proximal extremities	Prodrome of fever, headache, symptoms of upper respiratory tract infection (URI)
Molluscum Contagiosum	078.0	Firm, pearly papules Central umbilication	Eyelids Cheeks	N/A
Pityriasis Alba	696.5	Hypopigmented Oval shaped Fine scale	Cheeks	Lesions may also be on trunk and upper arms.
Adenoma Sebaceum (seen with Tuberous Sclerosis)	759.5 (tuberous sclerosis)	Pink firm papules	Nasolabial folds Cheeks	Ash leaf spots Shagreen patch
Herpes Simplex Virus Infection	054	Vesicular lesions	Often perioral, but can be seen around the eye from contact spread	With primary infection, there may be fever and other systemic signs.

COMPLICATIONS	PREDISPOSING FACTORS	TREATMENT
Scarring Emotional impact	Adolescent Increased sebum production *Propionibacterium acnes*	Start with topical agents such as benzoyl peroxide, benzoyl peroxide-clindamycin and a topical retinoid. Systemic antibiotics, including doxycycline, are often useful (although there is increasing antibiotic resistance of *P. acnes*). In females, consider systemic estrogens in the form of oral contraceptive pills. If severe, consider an oral retinoid and referral to dermatology.
Superinfection	Family history of atopic disease	Moisturize skin immediately following a shower or bath. Minimize use of drying agents such as soaps. Use cutaneous steroids for acute flares, short course oral steroids for severe outbreaks, oral antibiotics against *S. aureus* for bacterial superinfection, and immunomodulators such as tacrolimus or pimecrolimus in severe chronic disease.
Cellulitis Post-streptococcal glomerulonephritis	Skin trauma *Staphylococcus aureus* Group A beta-hemolytic streptococci (GABHS)	If well localized, use mupirocin, soap and water. If generalized, use trimethoprim-sulfamethoxizole or clindamycin orally.
Loss of hair	Infants Adolescents	Use selenium sulfide shampoo every 2–3 days along with mechanical removal of scales with a soft brush or fine-toothed comb.
Glomerulonephritis Rheumatic fever	Pyrogenic exotoxins GABHS	Penicillin or amoxicillin If allergic to penicillins, use azithromycin
Arthritis Arthralgias Aplastic crisis	Parvovirus B19	Follow serial CBCs and intervene if bone marrow suppression is excessive.
Conjunctivitis	Poxvirus	Self-limited Will resolve with time (months to years) Surgical removal may be followed by recurrence; cantharidin, potassium hydroxide, or podophyllum may also be used.
N/A	Skin dryness	Self-limited Moisturizers may alleviate itching.
Seizure Cardiac rhabdomyoma CNS tubers	Chromosome 9q34 and 16q13.3 mutations Autosomal dominant 50% new mutations	Surgical removal of tumors, if necessary
Herpes keratoconjunctivitis	Known contact with herpes simplex virus	Self-limited Treat pain with acetaminophen or ibuprofen. Acyclovir is helpful if started within the first 48–72 hr of outbreak. For frequent recurrent outbreaks, consider prophylaxis with acyclovir.

OTHER
DIAGNOSES
TO CONSIDER

- Hemangiomas

- Lipomas

- Purpura

- Dermatomyositis

WHEN TO
CONSIDER
FURTHER
EVALUATION
OR TREATMENT

- Scarring acne that does not respond quickly to topical medication should be referred to a skin specialist.

- Suspect secondary infection with *Staphylococcus aureus* in eczema that does not respond to steroid creams.

- Widely separated or numerous skin lesions of impetigo need systemic antibiotics.

- Treating seborrhea capitis (with selenium based shampoos) usually clears up seborrhea in other areas including the eyebrows.

- A pregnant mother's obstetrician should be informed of a diagnosis of erythema infectiosum (fifth disease).

SUGGESTED READINGS
Barron RP, Kainulainen VT, Forrest CR. Tuberous sclerosis: clinicopathologic features and review of the literature. *J Craniomaxillofac Surg.* 2002;30:361–366.
Goodheart HP. *Goodheart's photoguide to common skin disorders.* 2nd ed. Philadelphia, PA: Lippincott Williams & Wilkins; 2003:14, 46, 138, 388.
Gupta AK, Bluhm R, Cooper EA, et al. Seborrheic dermatitis. *Dermatol Clin.* 2003;21(3):401–412.
Hurwitz S. *Clinical pediatric dermatology.* 2nd ed. Philadelphia, PA: WB Saunders; 1993:45–59, 62, 66, 136–149, 279–281, 319–321, 338–339, 357, 379–381, 629–632.
Illi S, von Mutius E, Lau S, et al. The natural course of atopic dermatitis from birth to age 7 years and the association with asthma. *J Allergy Clin Immunol.* 2004;113(5):925–931.
Krowchuk DP. Managing acne in adolescents. *Pediatr Clin North Am.* 2000;47:841–857.
Silverberg N. Pediatric molluscum contagiosum: optimal treatment strategies. *Paediatr Drugs.* 2003;5:505–512.
Smolinski KN, Yan AC. Acne update: 2004. *Curr Opin Pediatr.* 2004;16:385–391.

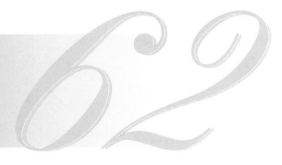

BETHLEHEM L. ABEBE

Diffuse Red Rashes

APPROACH TO THE PROBLEM

The evaluation of a diffuse red rash can be challenging. This type of rash has a vast differential diagnosis ranging from minor and self-resolving illnesses to life-threatening illnesses that require prompt management decisions. Etiologies of diffuse erythematous rashes include exposure to sunlight, a variety of infections, and medications.

KEY POINTS IN THE HISTORY

- Drug-related eruptions usually occur within 5 to 14 days after starting medications, such as antibiotics, nonsteroidal anti-inflammatory drugs (NSAIDs), or anticonvulsants. Pruritus is often an associated symptom.

- Erythema, flushing, and pruritus of the face and upper body are typical of Red Man syndrome, a common adverse reaction to the rapid infusion of vancomycin.

- The typical prodrome of measles (rubeola) includes fever, malaise, dry cough, coryza, conjunctivitis, and Koplik spots (small red lesions on mucous membranes with a white central spot) followed on day 3 by the rash that spreads in a cephalocaudal fashion.

- The diffuse painless or painful erythema of sunburn occurs 3 to 5 hours, usually peaking at 12 to 24 hours, after ultraviolet (UV) radiation of as little as 30-minutes duration.

- Exaggerated and accelerated sunburn reactions may result from the combination of UV light exposure and the use of photosensitizing medications such as NSAIDs, quinolones, tetracyclines, furosemide, thiazides, amiodarone, and phenothiazines. Erythema that occurs in sun-exposed areas can occur minutes after sun exposure.

- Polymorphous light eruption is a light-induced, pruritic eruption that usually occurs with the first sun exposure of the year.

- Initial symptoms of staphylococcal scalded skin syndrome (SSSS) include fever, irritability, conjunctivitis, pharyngitis, and impetigo prior to the onset of the rash.

- Toxic shock syndrome (TSS) is characterized by fevers, hypotension, and diffuse erythroderma with subsequent desquamation. Three or more of the following organ systems need to be involved to make the diagnosis: gastrointestinal (vomiting, diarrhea), musculoskeletal (myalgias), mucous membranes (hyperemia), renal, hepatic, hematologic, and/or central nervous system.

- In TSS, there is a focus of infection such as a tampon, skin lesion, or abscess.

KEY POINTS IN THE PHYSICAL EXAMINATION

- The rash of measles is a blotchy, erythematous, blanching, maculopapular rash that spreads in a cephalocaudal manner.

- The appearance of erythema on sun-exposed areas with sparing of covered skin aids with diagnosing sunburn.

- Drug-related eruptions are usually morbilliform in nature and start on the face and trunk, and then spread distally.

- Polymorphous light eruption can present on the extremities with slight involvement of the face.

- Parvovirus B19 infection, or erythema infectiosum, causes an intense erythema specifically on the face and a reticulated erythematous rash on the rest of the body.

- Flushed face, pharyngitis, and fever in association with a diffuse, blanching, erythematous rash with a sandpaper quality are consistent with scarlet fever.

- The diffuse erythroderma of SSSS is tender to touch and appears similar to a sunburn, and then progresses to bullous lesions that easily rupture.

- The diffuse erythroderma of TSS, which can resemble sunburn, also involves mucous membranes.

- The typical petechial rash of Rocky Mountain Spotted Fever may start as a maculopapular eruption peripherally, which then spreads centrally before becoming petechial.

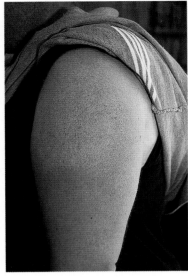

Figure 62-1 Sunburn. Diffuse erythema on lateral aspect of arm.
(Courtesy of George A. Datto, III, MD.)

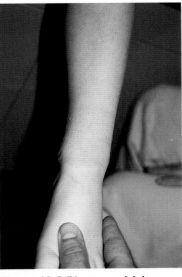

Figure 62-2 Photosensitivity. Edematous and erythematous sharp-bordered lesion that developed on ankle after sun exposure.
(Courtesy of George A. Datto, III, MD.)

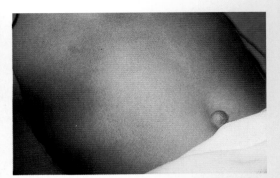

Figure 62-3 Drug rash. Erythroderma with fine morbilliform rash that developed after antibiotic exposure.
(Courtesy of George A. Datto, III, MD.)

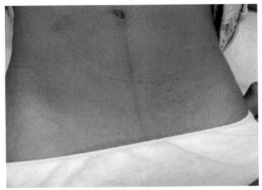

Figure 62-4 Rash seen with scarlet fever. Note the diffuse distribution of this rash that is more intense in the lower abdomen and groin.
(Courtesy of Esther K. Chung, MD, MPH.)

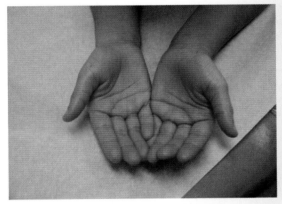

Figure 62-5 Palmar erythema. Note the intense palmar redness seen in a child with scarlet fever.
(Courtesy of Esther K. Chung, MD, MPH.)

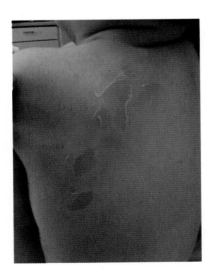

Figure 62-6 Staphylococcal scalded skin syndrome. A 4-year-old boy with the characteristic skin sloughing seen with SSSS.
(Courtesy of Bethlehem L. Abebe, MD.)

DIAGNOSIS	ICD-9	DISTINGUISHING CHARACTERISTICS	DISTRIBUTION	DURATION, CHRONICITY
Sunburn	692.71	Diffuse painless or painful erythema to sun-exposed areas	Sun-exposed skin	Peaks at 12–24 hrs after exposure, resolves several days later but may take longer if the sunburn is severe
Photosensitivity	692.72	Accelerated and/or exaggerated sunburn	Sun-exposed skin	Improves after discontinuation of drug
Drug Rash	693.0	Rapid onset erythema (vancomycin and Red Man syndrome) or gradual development of a morbilliform rash	Generalized; may start on upper body then spread distally	Resolves over 1–2 wks following discontinuation of drug
Scarlet Fever	034.1	Blanching, erythematous rash with a sandpapery quality Rash is prominent in skin folds forming Pastia lines (petechiae along the skin creases).	May be diffuse or limited to the upper body	
Staphylococcal Scalded Skin Syndrome (SSSS)	695.1	Diffuse erythroderma is tender to touch, appears similar to a sunburn, then progresses to bullous lesions that easily rupture with epidermal separation (Nikolsky sign). Majority of cases seen in patients <6 years of age	May be patchy or generalized	Resolution of rash in 1–2 wks
Parvovirus B19 (Erythema Infectiosum)	057.0	Intense, nontender erythema specifically on the face Reticulated erythematous rash on the rest of the body	Face with intense erythema, often spares the nasolabial folds Body with diffusely lacy erythema	Resolves 3–7 days after onset
Toxic Shock Syndrome (TSS)	040.82	Diffuse erythroderma resembling a sunburn with mucous membrane involvement as well as involvement of palms and soles May have nonpitting edema	Generalized	Can be fatal

ASSOCIATED FINDINGS	COMPLICATIONS	PRECIPITATING FACTORS	TREATMENT GUIDELINES
Blisters Edema Skin peeling	Systemic symptoms if burn is severe Secondary infections Increased risk of skin cancer	Lack of sunscreen use Lack of protective clothing Sun exposure during the hottest part of the day	Avoid sun exposure until symptoms resolve. Symptomatic relief from aloe, moisturizing lotions, NSAIDs, acetaminophen, antihistamines, cool compresses, topical steroids
Blisters Edema Skin peeling	Same as for sunburn above	Drug-induced Baseline sensitivity to sun	Avoid causative drug. Symptomatic relief agents similar to those used with sunburn Liberal use of sunscreen
Pruritus	Secondary infection	Rash occurs within 5–14 days after starting a medication such as antibiotics, NSAIDs, or anticonvulsants	Discontinuing the drug leads to resolution of the rash. Symptomatic treatment with antihistamines, topical steroids/antipruritic agents
Fever, pharyngitis, headache, desquamation, occasionally pruritus	Rheumatic fever, peritonsillar/retropharyngeal abscess, post-streptococcal glomerulonephritis	Group A streptococcal infection	Penicillin, amoxicillin, macrolides if penicillin-allergic, antihistamines for pruritus
Fever, irritability, conjunctivitis, pharyngitis, and impetigo prior to the onset of the rash	Fluid losses Bacteremia Sepsis	Staphylococcal infection	Topical wound care, antibiotics to cover staphylococcus
Occasionally arthralgias	Aplastic crisis in patients with hemoglobinopathies	Nonspecific prodrome of fever, headache, nausea	Usually none needed Symptomatic treatment of arthralgias and pruritus with NSAIDs and antihistamines, respectively
Fever, hypotension, desquamation, multiorgan involvement	Shock, 3–5% mortality	Tampon use, abscess, skin lesions, sinusitis	Fluid resuscitation, vasopressors, antibiotics

OTHER
DIAGNOSES
TO CONSIDER

- Systemic lupus erythematosus

- Dermatomyositis

- Kawasaki disease

- Infectious mononucleosis

- Porphyria cutanea tarda

- Toxic epidermal necrolysis

WHEN TO
CONSIDER
FURTHER
EVALUATION
OR TREATMENT

- Avoid sun exposure until the resolution of sunburn or photosensitivity rash. Liberal use of sunscreen is encouraged.

- Discontinuation of the causative agent in drug-related rashes is imperative for resolution of symptoms.

- In patients with strep throat and/or scarlet fever, treat with penicillin to prevent rheumatic fever.

- SSSS requires topical wound care similar to that for thermal burns as well as careful and repeated fluid status assessments because of increased fluid losses seen in this syndrome.

- Watch for aplastic crisis in patients with hemoglobinopathies who present with parvovirus B19 infection.

- Prompt recognition of TSS is essential to enable treatment with fluid resuscitation, antibiotics, and vasopressors.

SUGGESTED READINGS

Byer RL, Bachur RG. Clinical deterioration among patients with fever and erythroderma. *Pediatrics.* 2006;118:2450–2460.

Hensley DR, Hebert AA. Pediatric photosensitivity disorders. *Dermatol Clin.* 1998;16:571–578.

Patel GK, Finlay AY. Staphylococcal scalded skin syndrome: diagnosis and management. *Am J Clin Dermatol.* 2003;4:165–175.

Roelandts R. The diagnosis of photosensitivity. *Arch Dermatol.* 2000;1136:1152–1157.

Stevens, DL. The toxic shock syndromes. *Infect Dis Clin North Am.* 1996;10:727–746.

Segal AR, Doherty KM, Leggott J, et al. Cutaneous reactions to drugs in children. *Pediatrics.* 2007;120:e1082–e1096.

Todd JK. Staphylococcal infections. *Pediatr Rev.* 2005;26:444–450.

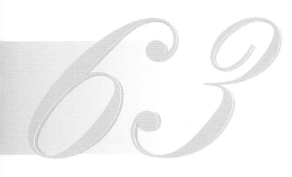

GARY A. EMMETT

Red Patches and Swellings

APPROACH TO THE PROBLEM

Red patches and swellings are common, presenting complaints in the pediatric office. These lesions may be caused by immune-mediated reactions, by infections (or the toxins from infections), and by vascular overgrowth or malformation. Immune-mediated lesions tend to be pruritic. Infections may have associated systemic symptoms, such as fever and malaise. Vascular lesions blanch when pressure is applied to them. This chapter will divide common red patches and swellings into three groups—immune-mediated lesions, lesions from infection, and vascular lesions—to enable the reader to improve their differential diagnosis and quality of care.

KEY POINTS IN THE HISTORY

- Immune-mediated lesions

  - Urticaria (hives) tend to change location, shape, and size over minutes to hours.

  - Allergic reactions often manifest as urticaria, erythema, and pruritus.

  - Insect bites may result in large welt-like areas around them as the body reacts to the insect saliva that is deposited at the time of the bite.

- Lesions from infection

  - Systemic symptoms such as chills, fever, and malaise are commonly found in association with rashes of infectious origin, or just before the rash appears.

  - Erythematous lesions from infection are often swollen and tender.

  - A break in the skin associated with surrounding erythema strongly suggests infection, such as cellulitis.

  - An expanding macular red "bull's eye" rash around an insect bite with a central area of clearing, called erythema chronicum migrans, is strongly associated with Lyme disease. Erythema chronicum migrans occurs in over half of those with Lyme disease and occurs 1 to 2 weeks after the deer tick bite.

  - The majority (75%) of persons infected with Lyme disease do not recall having a tick bite. Other Lyme disease manifestations, and there are many, are may be. The sudden onset of an isolated arthritis in a large joint, such as the knee, in a Lyme endemic area should raise suspicion for Lyme disease.

- Erythema nodosum is often of infectious origin. It is commonly found in association with the following infections: cat scratch fever, Epstein-Barr virus infection or mononucleosis, fungal infections, group A streptococcal infections, tuberculosis, and tularemia.

- Vascular lesions

  - Hemangiomas may start off as flat areas of telangiectasia and tend to increase in size over the first year of life prior to involuting.

  - Nevus simplex (Stork's bite or Angel's kiss) is frequently found on the occiput or nape of the neck, and on the eyelids, glabella, and/or philtrum.

KEY POINTS IN THE PHYSICAL EXAMINATION

- Immune-mediated lesions

  - Insect bites that are within 40 cms (about 15 in.) from the ground (remember children are often on the ground) suggest flea bites, and pets should be examined.

  - Mosquito bites may also be in the lower extremities near the ankles, and in other exposed areas.

  - Urticarial lesions have a classic wheal and flare appearance, and can evolve during the course of examination.

- Lesions from infection

  - Erysipelas is raised with well-defined edges.

  - The bull's eye lesion of erythema migrans may occur as a solitary lesion or there may be multiple lesions.

  - Cellulitis typically has rubor (a reddish appearance), tumor (a raised lesion), calor (warmth), and dolor (tenderness).

  - Pretibial, tender, raised, reddish blue nodules found deep in the dermis are characteristic of erythema nodosum.

- Vascular lesions

  - Vascular lesions may be either superficial or deep.

  - A superficial lesion such as nevus simplex typically blanches completely with pressure, and may be more prominent with crying and increased warmth.

  - A deep lesion such as a cavernous hemangioma or a port-wine stain (nevus flammeus) may feel elevated, and blanch incompletely on pressure.

  - Hemangiomata generally become flesh colored or grey as they involute from the center outward between 9 months and 5 years. Suspect deeper hemangioma when there is a bluish discoloration noted as more superficial lesions tend to be intensely red.

PHOTOGRAPHS OF SELECTED DIAGNOSES

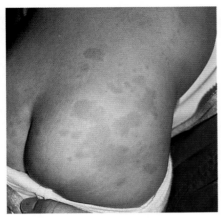

Figure 63-1 Urticaria. Erythematous wheals on buttocks of child.
(Courtesy of George A. Datto, III, MD.)

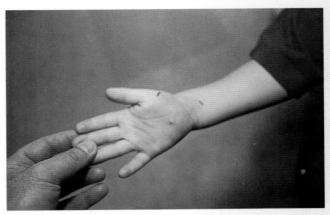

Figure 63-2 Cellulitis. Poorly defined erythematous lesion on hand that developed after skin abrasion.
(Courtesy of George A. Datto, III, MD.)

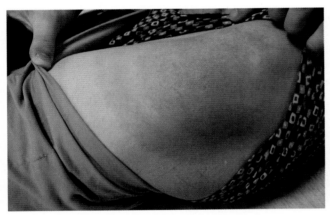

Figure 63-3 Erythema (chronicum) migrans. Note the central punctum following a tick bite and the ring-like appearance.
(Courtesy of Paul S. Matz, MD.)

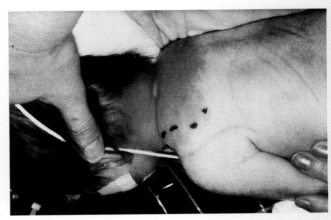

Figure 63-4 Erysipelas. Very erythematous rash on neck with sharply demarcated borders.
(Courtesy of George A. Datto, III, MD.)

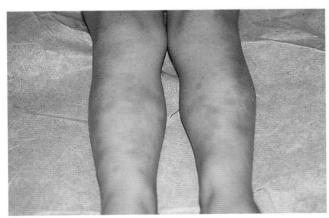

Figure 63-5 Erythema nodosum. Tender erythematous nodules on extensor aspects of lower legs.
(Courtesy of George A. Datto, III, MD.)

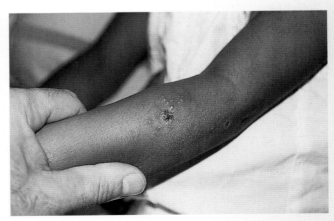

Figure 63-6 Spider bite. Erythematous lesion with central eschar following a spider bite.
(Courtesy of George A. Datto, III, MD.)

DIFFERENTIAL DIAGNOSIS

DIAGNOSIS	ICD-9	DISTINGUISHING CHARACTERISTICS	DISTRIBUTION	ASSOCIATED FINDINGS
Urticaria	708.9	Evanescent, erythematous wheals	Localized or diffuse	Angioedema Pruritus
Cellulitis	528.3	Warm, tender, raised erythematous lesion	Typically surrounding a break in the skin May occur anywhere on the body	Fever Pain Chills
Erythema Chronicum Migrans	088.81	Bull's eye lesion with central clearing and erythematous borders May see expanding ring lesion	Solitary Multiple lesions with disseminated Lyme disease	Fever Myalgias Arthralgias Arthritis Pain Pruritus
Erysipelas	035	Well-circumscribed, warm, erythematous, raised lesion	May occur anywhere on the body	Fever Pain Chills Malaise
Erythema Nodosum	695.2	Reddish blue, tender, raised nodules	Face Arms Pretibial area	Fever Arthralgias Aches Adenopathy
Insect Bite	919.4	Pruritic, raised, warm lesion with central punctum	Anywhere, but typically exposed areas including head and neck, arms, lower legs	Pruritus
Spider Bites	E905.1	Painful, erythematous lesions with central hemorrhage and/or necrosis	Most commonly on extremities	Fever Myalgias Headache Vomiting Pain Severe abdominal pain
Hemangioma	228.0	Raised, nontender, erythematous or bluish lesions	Head and neck Trunk Extremities Internally, affecting spleen, liver, and other organs	Multiple superficial lesions may be associated with internal hemangioma.

COMPLICATIONS	PREDISPOSING FACTORS	TREATMENT GUIDELINES
If severe allergic reaction, may see hypotension, respiratory distress, and other symptoms of anaphylaxis	Food Drugs Infections including group A streptococcus Physical factors	Antihistamines, such as diphenhydramine, and systemic steroids have been used but they are not consistently effective.
Abscess Lymphangitis Sepsis Osteomyelitis	Skin trauma, including lacerations, abrasions, insect bites and other puncture wounds Immunocompromise	In some areas of United States, the rate of methicillin-resistant Staphylococcus aureus is so high that cephalexin is no longer effective for community-acquired staphylococcus and trimethoprim-sulfamethoxazole or clindamycin is recommended as first-line therapy.
Arrhythmias Meningitis Cranial neuropathies Carditis	Ixodes (deer) tick bite and infection with the spirochete, Borrelia burgdorferi	Antibiotic therapy Appropriate antibiotic therapy should be initiated.
Abscess Sepsis Streptococcal toxic shock syndrome Osteitis Arthritis	Diabetes mellitus Immunocompromise Nephrotic syndrome Streptococcal infection	Penicillin is first-line therapy.
Arthritis	Streptococcal, mycobacterial, mycoplasmal, or fungal infections Yersinia, salmonella, or campylobacter Inflammatory bowel disease Sarcoidosis Hodgkin lymphoma Behçet disease Sulfonamides Oral contraceptive pills	Depends on underlying condition
Cellulitis	Preceding insect bite Mosquito bites tend to occur at dusk and dawn, but may occur at other times	Oral antihistamines Topical corticosteroids
Tachycardia Hypertension Thrombocytopenia Disseminated intravascular coagulopathy (DIC)	Black widow spider bite Recluse spider bite	Wash wound with soap and water. Apply antibiotic ointment if wound infected. If muscle spasms or other systemic sequelae, admit to hospital for supportive care and further evaluation
Visual problems Airway compromise Rarely bleeding Consumptive coagulopathy Kasabach-Merritt syndrome	Generally nonhereditary but 10% of patients have a positive family history of such lesions	Lesions typically involute. Unless lesion is causing sequelae (obstructing vision or breathing or chronically bleeding), do not treat. Treatment may include corticosteroid injection, excision, or laser therapy performed by a trained dermatologist.

- Pityriasis rosea

- Measles (rubeola)

- German measles (rubella)

- Dermatographia

- Superficial trauma, including abrasions and petechial lesions

- Cutaneous anthrax

WHEN TO
CONSIDER
FURTHER
EVALUATION
OR TREATMENT

- An insect bite that lasts more than 7 days should be evaluated.

- An insect bite that is associated with a fever greater than 38°C suggests bacterial superinfection and warrants treatment with oral or parenteral antibiotics.

- Urticaria has been described with group A beta-hemolytic streptococcal pharyngitis; therefore, it is important to send a throat culture if urticaria is accompanied by a red or sore throat.

- Cellulitis that does not improve within 72 hours of starting systemic antibiotics may need either incision and drainage or broader antibiotic coverage. If there is drainage initially, a culture with sensitivity can help to guide therapy.

- Hemangiomas near the eye should be evaluated and treated by a dermatologist to prevent obstruction of vision and amblyopia. Similarly, hemangiomas near the airway should be evaluated and treated by a dermatologist to prevent airway compromise.

- Multiple hemangiomas on the skin may be associated with internal hemangiomas and should be evaluated by a dermatologist. Further radiographic imaging may be indicated.

SUGGESTED READINGS

Bisno A. Current concepts: streptococcal infections of the skin and soft tissues. *N Engl J Med.* 1996;334(4):240–245.

Diekema DS, Reuter DG. Environmental emergencies. *Clin Pediatr Emerg Med.* 2001;2(3):155–167.

Edlow JA. Tick-borne diseases. *Med Clin North Am.* 2002;86(2):239–260.

Kakourou T, Drosatou P, Psychou F, Aroni K, Nicolaidou P. Erythema nodosum in children: a prospective study. *J Am Acad Dermatol.* Jan 2001;44(1):17–21.

Khangura S, Wallace J, Kissoon N, et al. Management of cellulitis in a pediatric emergency department. *Pediatr Emerg Care.* 2007;23:805–811.

Sadick N. Current aspects of bacterial infections in the skin. *Dermatol Clin.* 1997;15(2):341–349.

Sicherer S, Leung D. Advances in allergic skin disease, anaphylaxis, and hypersensitivity reactions to foods, drugs and insects in 2007. *J Allergy Clin Immunol.* 2008;121:1351–1358.

Wenner KA, Kenner JR. Anthrax. *Dermatol Clin.* 2004;22(3):247–256.

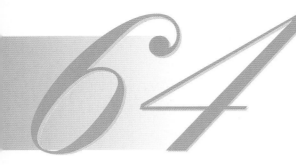

LIANA K. McCABE

Linear Red Rashes

APPROACH TO THE PROBLEM

The pattern of a rash can be quite helpful in identifying its etiology. Linear patterns of rashes may be seen in many conditions. In particular, linear red rashes are commonly seen in infectious and inflammatory conditions. In addition, they may be the result of other systemic processes.

KEY POINTS IN THE HISTORY

- A linear red rash that develops after outdoor activity should raise the suspicion of rhus dermatitis due to exposure to poison ivy, oak, or sumac.

- Rhus dermatitis, scabies and cutaneous larva migrans are intensely pruritic lesions.

- Children with scabies may have a close contact who also has an itchy rash. It is helpful to inquire if the parent has a rash as well.

- Lichen striatus is twice as common in girls than in boys.

- Lichen striatus may start as a small area of papules that then spreads into a linear distribution.

- Outdoor exposure to soil that is shared with dogs or cats, particularly sandboxes, is often found with cutaneous larva migrans.

- Linear epidermal nevus, which is not typically pruritic, appears at birth or shortly afterward.

KEY POINTS IN THE PHYSICAL EXAMINATION

- Rhus dermatitis is seen on exposed skin, particularly the areas that were exposed while outdoors.

- Excoriation surrounding a linear rash suggests pruritus and scratching, which may lead to bacterial superinfection.

- Red rashes may not be as apparent in individuals with darker skin.

- Lichen striatus may appear mildly hypopigmented or flesh colored.

- Infants with scabies often have a generalized rash that includes the soles of their feet. In young children, the rash of scabies is typically seen in the axilla and groin. Older children will often have lesions in the web spaces of their fingers and toes.

- An advancing serpiginous tunnel in the skin that is intensely pruritic is virtually pathognomonic for cutaneous larva migrans.

- Koebner phenomenon is seen commonly in linear rashes such as rhus dermatitis, linear psoriasis, and lichen planus.

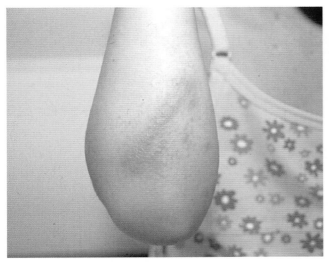

Figure 64-1 Rhus dermatitis. Linear papules and vesicles following exposure to poison ivy.
(Courtesy of George A. Datto, III, MD.)

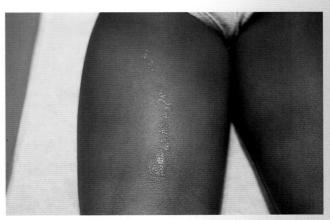

Figure 64-2 Lichen striatus. Small, shiny, hypopigmented papules in a linear distribution on the posterior thigh.
(Courtesy of George A. Datto, III, MD.)

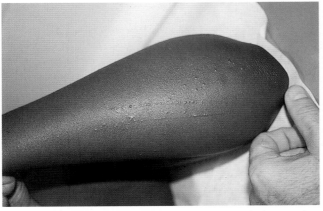

Figure 64-3 Koebner phenomenon. Papulovesicular eruption in a linear distribution on the forearm of a child with an id reaction (autosensitization dermatitis) associated with tinea capitis.
(Courtesy of George A. Datto, III, MD.)

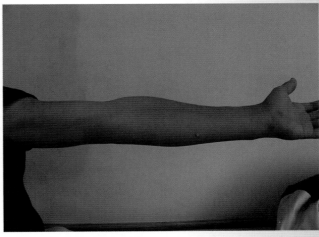

Figure 64-4 Lymphangitis. Linear red streak proximal to skin infection.
(Courtesy of Paul S. Matz, MD.)

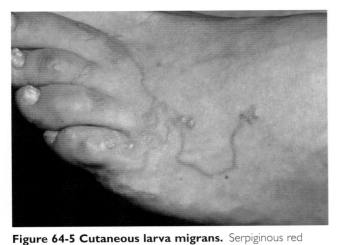

Figure 64-5 Cutaneous larva migrans. Serpiginous red streaks on sole of foot.
(Used with permission from Goodheart HP. *Goodheart's photoguide of common skin disorders.* 2nd ed. Philadelphia, PA: Lippincott Williams & Wilkins; 2003:315.)

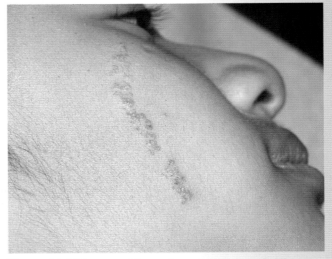

Figure 64-6 Linear epidermal nevus. Warty, linear lesions on face.
(Used with permission from Goodheart HP. *Goodheart's photoguide of common skin disorders.* 2nd ed. Philadelphia, PA: Lippincott Williams & Wilkins; 2003:9.)

DIFFERENTIAL DIAGNOSIS

DIAGNOSIS	ICD-9	DISTINGUISHING CHARACTERISTICS	DISTRIBUTION
Rhus Dermatitis	692.6	Multiple types of lesions including papules, vesicles, or bullae with straw-colored fluid inside that are pruritic	Often on arms and legs or other exposed surfaces of the skin. May be transmitted to other sites by scratching
Lichen Striatus	697.8	Flat-topped papules in unilateral streaks and swirls Overlying dusky scale with mild erythema	Along lines of Blaschko Usually on extremities, upper back, or neck
Scabies	133.0	Linear burrows with adjacent papules Often seen are areas of excoriation due to the intense pruritus.	Infant—lesions are often generalized to the entire body. Toddler—lesions may be pronounced in the axilla and groin. Children—lesions often seen specifically within the webs of fingers and toes
Lymphangitis	682.3	Warm, painful, erythematous streak(s) that extends proximal to an injury or infection	Usually proximal to site of infection along the lymphatic drainage lines
Cutaneous Larva Migrans	126.8	Erythematous, tortuous or serpent-like lesions that may progress Larvae migrate at about 1–2 cm per day Occasional bullae	Often found on the lower extremities or hands
Linear Epidermal Nevus	216.9	Linear papules that appear smooth and then may become wart-like or scaly.	May occur on any part of the body, but commonly found on the face, trunk, or extremities

ASSOCIATED FINDINGS	COMPLICATIONS	PREDISPOSING FACTORS	TREATMENT GUIDELINES
Pruritus Koebner phenomenon (new lesions develop after trauma) Edema	Bacterial superinfection secondary to pruritus	Contact with poison oak, ivy, or sumac Indirect contact with clothing, pets that brushed against plant, or smoke from burning plant	Antihistamine for itch Topical or systemic corticosteroids
Hypopigmentation may be associated Asymptomatic	None	Unclear cause May be triggered by viral infection	Fades without treatment in 1–2 yrs Lubricants and topical steroids may decrease scale and inflammation.
Intense pruritus Other family members with similar symptoms	Bacterial superinfection	*Sarcoptes scabiei*	5% permethrin cream for patients >2 months Oral antihistamines and topical steroids may be used to treat symptoms.

Local lymphadenopathy
Fever
	Bacteremia
	Sepsis
		Infection due to:
		  Staphylococcus aureus
		  Group A streptococci
			Culture
			Antibiotic active against gram-positive organisms

Local lymph nodes are enlarged and tender. Pruritus	N/A	Most commonly caused by dog/cat hookworm: *A. brazilienes*	If untreated, larvae will die in a few months. Topical antifungals will hasten treatment.
Most lesions appear at birth, and 95% present by 7 yr of age.	Cosmetic concern	N/A	Topical retinoids or keratolytics May be excised or ablated with laser therapy

OTHER DIAGNOSES TO CONSIDER

- Striae

- Linear morphea (localized scleroderma)

- Linear psoriasis

- Contact dermatitis

WHEN TO CONSIDER FURTHER EVALUATION OR TREATMENT

- Rhus dermatitis may be treated with systemic corticosteroids when severe or extensive in distribution. If systemic steroids are used, start with a 48-hour course of steroids, followed by a 2- to 3-week taper.

- Scabies should be treated with 5% permethrin if the patient is older than 2 months. The lotion should be applied from head to toe, and then washed off 8 to 14 hours later. Treatment may need to be repeated 1 week later if symptoms worsen. Treatment is recommended for all household contacts when possible.

- For scabies, all bedding and clothing worn next to the skin during the 3 days before the initiation of therapy should be laundered in a washer with HOT water. Mites do not survive more than 3 days in the absence of skin contact.

- If desired by the patient for cosmetic reasons, linear epidermal nevus may be treated with topical retinoids or keratolytics. If these agents are unsuccessful, the lesion can be excised or ablated by laser therapy.

SUGGESTED READINGS

American Academy of Pediatrics. *Red Book, 2006 Report of the Committee on Infectious Diseases.* 27th ed. Elk Grove Village, IL: AAP; 2006: 272, 584–587.

Cohen BA. *Pediatric dermatology.* 3rd ed. Baltimore, MD: Elsevier Mosby; 2005.

Goodheart HP. *Goodheart's photoguide of common skin disorders.* 2nd ed. Philadelphia, PA: Lippincott Williams & Wilkins; 2003:9, 315.

Paller AS, Mancini AJ. *Hurwitz clinical pediatric dermatology: A textbook of skin disorders of childhood and adolescence.* 3rd ed. Philadelphia, PA: Elsevier Saunders; 2005.

Weston WL, Lane AT, Morelli JG. eds. *Color textbook of pediatric dermatology.* 4th ed. St. Louis, MO: Mosby; 2007.

Zitelli B, Davis H. *Atlas of pediatric physical diagnosis.* 4th ed. Philadelphia, PA: Mosby; 2002.

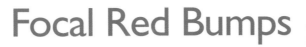
Focal Red Bumps

APPROACH TO THE PROBLEM

Focal red bumps are commonly seen in pediatric patients. The most common bumps are insect bites, which affect nearly 100% of the pediatric population. Also common are hemangiomas—superficial, known as "strawberry" or capillary hemangiomas, and deep, or cavernous hemangiomas—cherry angiomas, and pyogenic granulomas, although these are likely to be more chronic in nature than insect bites. Most newborns develop erythema toxicum neonatorum, and many toddlers will have panniculitis. Infectious etiologies at any age include abscesses, furuncles, carbuncles, or lesions such as with cat scratch disease.

KEY POINTS IN THE HISTORY

- Acute versus chronic onset of the rash may differentiate insect bites or infectious causes from growths or tumors. Sometimes an unrelated incident may draw attention to a pre-existing bump.

- Insect bites often do not have a known contact. There are differences among the symptoms and appearance of spider, mosquito, ant, bee, flea, and fly bites.

- Insect bites often present with pruritus and even pain.

- Superficial hemangiomas may not be present at birth, but will be seen within the first few weeks, grow rapidly over the first 6 months, and slowly involute over years.

- Pyogenic granulomas regularly have bleeding associated with minor or incidental trauma.

- Abscesses may develop after a preceding break in the skin and are often exquisitely tender.

- Fevers may be associated with some spider bites, but are more commonly associated with abscesses or furuncles.

- The time of day or activity the child was undertaking at the time of onset can help differentiate the etiology. For example, onset while asleep may be associated with bed bug bites, while on a hike with insect bites, and while playing with cats with cat scratch disease. If the lesion develops in a spot where the child had been scratching, consider the diagnosis of an abscess from open skin.

- Panniculitis can develop after a precipitating trauma. The classic popsicle panniculitis with fat necrosis occurs from contact of a cold object with the patient's cheek.

- Ecthyma, also known as "deep impetigo" can occur with a history of immunocompromise or after prior skin damage via a bite, eczema, or a wound.

- Insect bites may be seen on other family members. They may be very specific to the individual's care and interaction with family members.

- Insect bites may have swelling and warmth, but should not be particularly tender.

- Hemangiomas may be more erythematous or violaceous depending on the child's overall body temperature and baseline skin color, and on the depth of the lesion. Cavernous hemangiomas are more bluish with less-defined borders and strawberry/ capillary hemangiomas are more erythematous with clearly defined edges.

- Pyogenic granulomas may develop a collarette at the base, but hemangiomas do not.

- A perifollicular abscess with one opening is a furuncle, whereas a carbuncle has multiple openings or is associated with multiple hair follicles.

- Classic impetigo has honey-crusted lesions.

- Impetigo may be differentiated from an inflicted cigarette burn, in that a lesion of impetigo may have a bullous rim. Cigarette burns affect a deeper skin thickness than lesions of impetigo.

- Allergic contact dermatitis, such as from a nickel allergy, will have a characteristic distributions that is associated with contact with an object or substance. For example, a rash along the waistband or the sock line may be due to an allergy to elastic.

PHOTOGRAPHS OF SELECTED DIAGNOSES

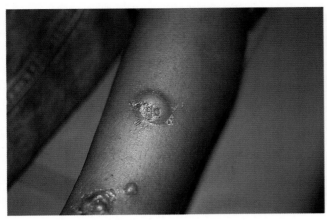

Figure 65-1 Insect bite. Located on the extensor surface of lower leg, this insect bite occurred during the summer. (Courtesy of George A. Datto, III, MD.)

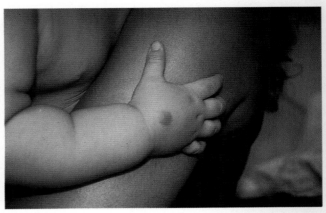

Figure 65-2 Insect bite. Erythematous wheal on dorsum of hand. (Courtesy of George A. Datto, III, MD.)

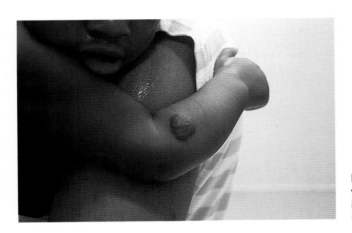

Figure 65-3 Hemangioma on the forearm of an infant with darkly pigmented skin. The lesion appears more purple in color than red. (Courtesy of George A. Datto, III, MD.)

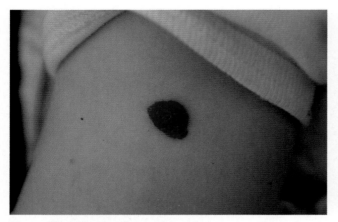

Figure 65-4 Hemangioma. Note the uneven surface.
(Courtesy of Susan A. Fisher-Owens, MD, MPH.)

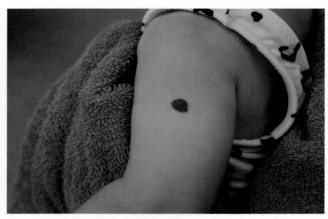

Figure 65-5 Involuting hemangioma. Note the central grey
discoloration as the hemangioma begins to involute.
(Courtesy of Susan A. Fisher-Owens, MD, MPH.)

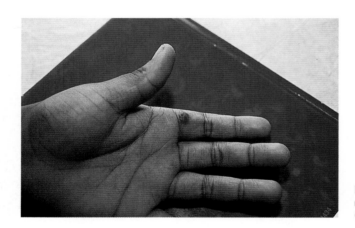

Figure 65-6 Pyogenic granuloma. A lobulated vascular
nodule on the finger.
(Courtesy of George A. Datto, III, MD.)

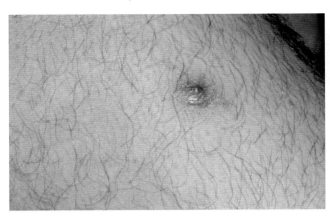

Figure 65-7 Furuncle. Painful, red, tender nodule on thigh.
(Used with permission from Goodheart HP. *Goodheart's photoguide of common skin disorders.* 2nd ed. Philadelphia, PA: Lippincott Williams & Wilkins; 2003:126.)

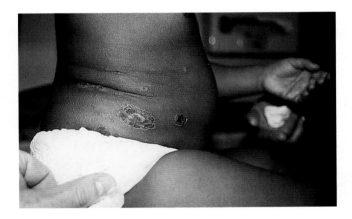

Figure 65-8 Ecthyma. Erythematous papules that develop an adherent central crust.
(Courtesy of George A. Datto, III, MD.)

DIAGNOSIS	ICD-9 (if followed by .X, it needs a location modifier)	DISTINGUISHING CHARACTERISTICS	DISTRIBUTION
Insect Bites	910.4–919.4 (not infected) 910.5–919.5 (infected)	May be warm and swollen May have central punctum or mark May be pruritic Generally not tender Bee/wasp stings, fire ant bites—painful Mosquito, flea, mite bites—pruritic	Anywhere, but most commonly on exposed skin
Erythema Toxicum Neonatorum	778.8	Neonates (0–1 month) Erythematous macules with white pustules or papules superimposed Child asymptomatic May be a handful or extensive Common among term infants (20%–60% of term infants >2,500 g)	May be anywhere; generally spares palms/soles, but may be present there
Superficial Hemangioma	228.X	Clearly defined borders with erythematous to violaceous color	Anywhere, but more likely on face
Deep Hemanioma	228.X	Less defined borders with bluish hue Palpable softness under skin	Anywhere
Pyogenic Granuloma	686.1	Small, red, glistening papule; can be pedunculated Bleeds easily	Most often on face or extremity
Abscess	681.X–682.X	Warm, swollen, tender	Anywhere
Carbuncle, Furuncle	680.X	Warm, swollen, tender, central necrosis with purulent discharge	Perifollicular, particularly hairy areas
Spitz Nevus (Spindle Cell Nevus)	190.0	Benign neoplasm; smooth-surface pinkish red nodule	Usually on face
Impetigo	684	Can be honey crusted or bullous	Bullous impetigo caused by staphylococcus most often on trunk Lesions due to staphylococcus on the face Lesions due to streptococcus on the lower extremities
Cat Scratch Disease	078.3	Raised nodules at site of scratch	Exposed skin most commonly
Allergic/Irritant Contact Dermatitis	692.X	Pruritic eczematous eruption, or erythematous papules, bullae, or vesicles	Location specific to irritant exposure, although in cases such as the oil of poison ivy, can be spread by scratching

ASSOCIATED FINDINGS	PREDISPOSING FACTORS	TREATMENT GUIDELINES
None	Exposure to outdoors, particularly at dusk or dawn	Supportive Consider topical low potency steroid or topical antihistamine if very pruritic
Smear shows the presence of eosinophils	Normal newborn finding	N/A Self-limited
None	Very low birth weight (VLBW) babies Male:female ratio is 1:3	Observe and follow Refer if midline on head, elbows, perineum, around eyes or beard distribution, or over spine
None	VLBW babies Male:female ratio is 1:3	Observe and follow Refer if midline on head, elbows, perineum, around eyes or beard distribution, or over spine
None	Can arise at site of trauma	Cauterization, excision, or laser therapy
None	Skin trauma; more common in families with MRSA	Incision and drainage ± antibiotics
None	Use of occlusive oils or other agents, folliculitis, or skin trauma	Incision and drainage ± antibiotics
Can have overlying telangiectasia	None	Conservative management or complete excision
Less surrounding erythema with staphylococcal than with streptococcal impetigo	More common in warm, humid areas; poor hygiene and crowded living conditions; more common with disorders of skin integrity, such as eczema	Appropriate bacterial coverage Know local MRSA rates and antibiotic resistance
Painful regional lymphadenopathy with erythema—often more striking than the primary site Constitutional symptoms such as malaise, fever	Exposure to cats, but may come from dogs or other points (splinters, needles, thorns) Male:female ratio is 3:2	Supportive care except in most severe cases
Id reaction	Metal (especially nickel, in belts, snaps, or earrings) Plants (poison ivy, oak, sumac) Fragrance/dyes (including cosmetics, henna tattoos, deodorant) Rubber	Topical steroids Oral steroids, if severe Irritant avoidance

- Kasabach-Merritt syndrome

- Maffucci syndrome (multiple angiomas with enchondromas—benign cartilaginous tumors)

- Port-wine stain (nevus flammeus)

- Traumatic hematoma

- Nonaccidental trauma

- PHACES syndrome (posterior fossa abnormalities, hemangioma, arterial anomalies, cardiac abnormalities, eye anomalies, sternal defects or supraumbilical raphe)

- Spitz nevus

- Erythema nodosum (in setting of Crohn disease)

- Vascular malformations

- Mastocytoma

WHEN TO
CONSIDER
FURTHER
EVALUATION
OR TREATMENT
- Hemangiomas that are midline on the head, near the eye area, in the beard distribution, or in the mouth, diaper area, or elbows should be further evaluated by a dermatologist because of concerns for underlying compression of structures with growth or increased risk for ulceration and bleeding.

- Fully formed vascular lesions at birth, particularly over the spine, warrant further evaluation.

- Rapidly changing vascular lesions should be evaluated by a dermatologist.

- A nevus arising on top of a congenital nevus should be evaluated by a dermatologist.

- Recurrent abscesses should prompt an evaluation for an underlying immunodeficiency.

SUGGESTED READINGS

American Academy of Pediatrics. Committee on infectious diseases. *AAP red book*. Elk Grove Village, IL: American Academy of Pediatrics; 2006.

Cohen BA, Davis HW. Dermatology. In: Zitelli BJ, Davis HW, eds. *Atlas of pediatric physical diagnosis*. 4th ed. St. Louis, MO: Mosby; 2002:257–314.

Johr RH, Schachner LA. Neonatal dermatologic challenges. *Pediatr Rev.* 1997;18(3):86–94.

Militello G, Jacob SE, Crawford GH. Allergic contact dermatitis in children. *Curr Opin Pediatr.* 2006;18:385–390.

Morelli JG. Vascular disorders. In: Kliegman RM, ed. *Nelson textbook of pediatrics*. 18th ed. Philadelphia, PA: Saunders; 2007.

Wahrman JE, Honig PJ. Hemangiomas. *Pediatr Rev.* 1994;15(7):266–271.

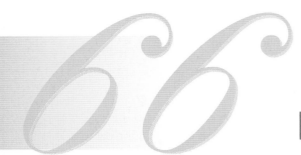

LEE R. ATKINSON-McEVOY
AND KATHLEEN CRONAN

Raised Red Rashes

APPROACH TO THE PROBLEM

Raised red rashes, common in pediatrics, often present cause for concern among parents and practitioners. The majority of raised red rashes are not indicative of serious illness. Many red rashes have associated symptoms that may be helpful in making a final diagnosis. For example, symptoms of fatigue, fever, and lymphadenopathy suggest infectious mononucleosis. Complications occur in some individuals with certain red rashes. For example, exposure of a pregnant woman to parvovirus may place her fetus at risk. At times, typical eruptions may not follow a predicted pattern—the distribution may be atypical, the season may not fit, or the age may be unusual. These diagnostic challenges emphasize the importance of a detailed history and astute observation.

KEY POINTS IN THE HISTORY

- High fever for 3 to 5 days followed by acute defervescence that precedes the rash eruption is characteristic of roseola.

- Classic characteristics in the history aid in the diagnosis. For example, a history of "slapped cheeks" indicates Fifth disease; the presence of Koplik spots denotes measles.

- Individuals acutely affected by infectious mononucleosis are at risk for rash development following exposure to penicillin.

- Antibiotic exposure is associated with a drug rash and erythema multiforme.

- Pruritus is typical in erythema multiforme, hot tub folliculitis, and scabies.

- Seasonal occurrence can provide clues to the diagnosis: late summer and fall, (coxsackie virus); spring and fall, (erythema multiforme).

- Family members with a similar rash may suggest scabies.

- The location of rash origin is important. For example, a red rash that begins on the scalp and travels downward is characteristic of measles.

KEY POINTS IN THE PHYSICAL EXAMINATION

- Erythema may be more apparent in light-skinned children.

- The size and types of papules may support specific diagnoses: fine micropapules indicate scarlet fever; target lesions denote erythema multiforme.

- The color of the lesions aids in the diagnosis of the rash: rose pink lesions are seen in roseola; red maculopapular lesions, in measles; and brownish lesions on the palms and soles, in syphilis.

- Red lesions on the palms and soles are present in syphilis, measles, erythema multiforme, scabies, and Gianotti-Crosti syndrome.

- Symmetric lesions may be noted in erythema multiforme, syphilis, and Gianotti-Crosti syndrome.

- Diffuse mucosal inflammation (urethritis, conjunctivitis, pharyngitis) is seen in Kawasaki disease.

- There are often oral mucous membrane findings in infectious mononucleosis, erythema multiforme, Kawasaki disease, and measles.

- Conjunctivitis is seen in Kawasaki disease and measles.

- In syphilis, the rash follows lines of cleavage.

- Periorbital edema is associated with roseola and infectious mononucleosis.

- Measles presents with Koplik spots (grey-white papules) on the buccal mucosa and dark red macules and papules that start on the head and spread caudally.

PHOTOGRAPHS OF SELECTED DIAGNOSES

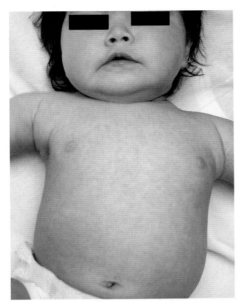

Figure 66-1 Roseola. Rose pink–colored rash on the trunk of an infant. (Courtesy of John Loiselle, MD.)

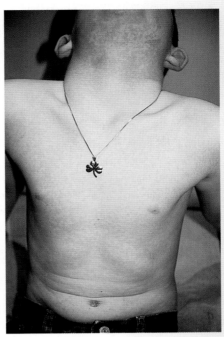

Figure 66-2 Scarlet fever. Fine, sandpapery rash on the trunk and neck. (Courtesy of George A. Datto, III, MD.)

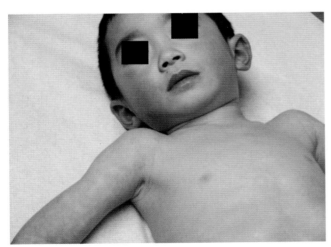

Figure 66-3 Erythema infectiosum. Erythematous "slapped" cheeks along with erythematous rash on extensor surfaces of arms. (Courtesy of Philip Siu, MD.)

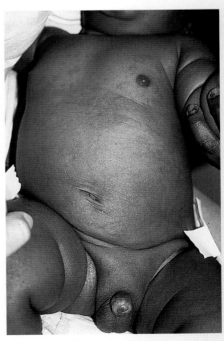

Figure 66-4 Kawasaki disease. Erythematous maculopapular rash that started in the groin and spread onto the trunk. (Courtesy of George A. Datto, III, MD.)

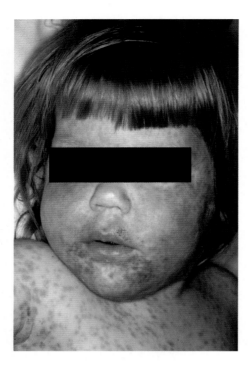

Figure 66-5 Infectious mononucleosis.
(Courtesy of Kathleen Cronan, MD.)

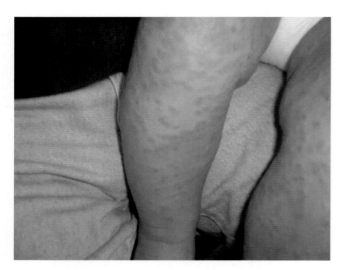

Figure 66-6 Gianotti-Crosti syndrome. Note the reddish-brown papular lesions on the extremities.
(Courtesy of John Loiselle, MD.)

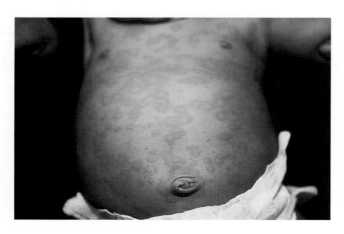

Figure 66-7 Erythema multiforme. Target-shaped lesions in an infant.
(Courtesy of George A. Datto, III, MD.)

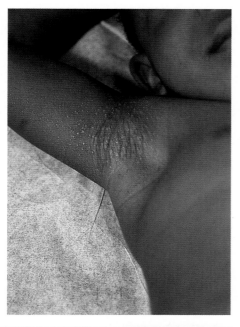

Figure 66-8 Scabies. Note the lesions in the axilla of a child.
(Courtesy of George A. Datto, III, MD.)

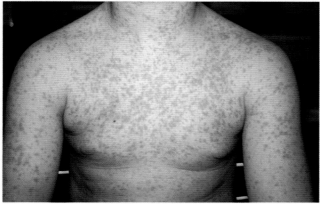

Figure 66-9 Measles. Lesions typically start on the head and travel downward.
(Courtesy of Kathleen Cronan, MD.)

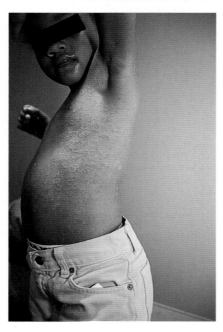

Figure 66-10 Unilateral laterothoracic exanthem. Pink, scaly rash involving the axilla and trunk on the right side of this child.
(Courtesy of George A. Datto, III, MD.)

DIAGNOSIS	ICD-9	DISTINGUISHING CHARACTERISTICS	DISTRIBUTION	DURATION/ CHRONICITY
Roseola	057.8	Rose-pink lesions that blanch with pressure Rarely coalesce <2 yr of age	Trunk Extremities Neck	Brief Self-limited
Scarlet Fever	034.1	Erythematous punctate rash that blanches with pressure Generalized sandpaper rash School age	Begins in axillae and groin, then generalizes Often seen on the face and neck areas	Brief Self-limited
Erythema Infectiosum (Fifth Disease)	079.99	Three stages: • Erythematous malar blush "slapped cheeks" • Erythematous maculopapular eruption on extensor surfaces of the extremities • Lacy reticulated pattern	Face Extremities Trunk Proximal extremities	Brief Self-limited
Kawasaki Disease	446.1	Maculopapular to morbilliform rash <5 yrs of age	Often starts in groin	Can last from days to weeks
Infectious Mononucleosis	075	Macular or maculopapular, morbilliform eruption Exanthem occurs in 10%–15% of patients Adolescents	Trunk Upper arms Face Forearms Thighs	Brief Self-limited
Gianotti-Crosti Syndrome	782.1	Monomorphous red to red-brown papules 1–6 yrs of age	Begins on extensor surfaces of legs and arms Buttocks Cheeks Symmetric distribution	Lasts 2–8 wks
Erythema Multiforme (Minor)	695.1	Papules that develop into erythematous ring with dusky center (target lesion)	Trunk, face, neck, palms, soles, dorsal hands, and feet; extensor surfaces of arms and legs Oral lesions—buccal mucosa	Usually lasts 3–4 wks
Scabies	133	Papules, pustules, vesicles Linear burrows	Infants—trunk, palms, soles, neck, face Older children—flexural areas, interdigital spaces, wrists, axillae	Can last several weeks
Measles	055	Erythematous maculopapular lesions followed by brawny desquamation Enanthem—Koplik spots	Progresses from scalp to hairline to face to neck to upper extremities to trunk to upper and lower extremities to feet	Lasts 1–2 wks
Asymmetric Lateral Exanthem of Childhood (Asymmetric Periflexural Exanthem OR Unilateral Laterothoracic Exanthem)	05.78	Pink-red, scaly papules Initial eruption—unilateral palms, soles, and face spared	Lesions initially start around the axilla. Also frequently involves the trunk, arms, and thigh Becomes bilateral within 2 wks	Lasts 3–6 wks (occasionally up to 4 months)
Hot Tub Folliculitis	704.8	Pruritic papules may change to pustules or nodules. Occurs 1–2 days after exposure	Torso Hot tub exposed areas	Brief Self-limited

ASSOCIATED FINDINGS	COMPLICATIONS	PRECIPITATING FACTORS	TREATMENT GUIDELINES
Rash preceded by high fever Periorbital edema Leukopenia	Febrile seizures	Human herpes virus 6	None needed
Fever, malaise, sore throat, palatal petechiae, abdominal pain, tonsillopharyngitis, strawberry tongue Pastia lines	Glomerulonephritis Rheumatic fever	Group A beta-hemolytic streptococcus (GABHS)	Treat with penicillin for 10 days (consider clindamycin or erythromycin in penicillin allergic patient)
Low-grade fever Aches and pains Mild arthritis Arthralgia Cold symptoms	Red-cell aplasia Nonimmune fetal hydrops	Parvovirus B19	None needed
High fever for 5 days Lymphadenopathy Swelling of hands and feet Mucositis	Coronary artery aneurysms	Unknown	IVIG and aspirin
Fever Headache Malaise Pharyngitis Lymphadenopathy Periorbital swelling Splenomegaly Hepatomegaly	Splenic rupture Neurological symptoms Hemolytic anemia	Epstein-Barr virus	Treat symptoms (fever, pharyngitis) as needed
Fever Cough Lymphadenopathy Hepatomegaly in hepatitis B–associated cases	None	Viral infections Hepatitis B virus infection	None needed
Low-grade fever Arthralgias Malaise	None	Viral infections Recurrent herpes infections Drugs	Removal of inciting antigen if possible Oral antihistamines If recurrent, consider acyclovir prophylaxis
Intense pruritus	Secondary infection Id reaction Eczematous changes	*Sarcoptes scabiei*	Permethrin 5% cream is the treatment of choice, may need to be repeated in 1 wk
Cough Coryza Fever Conjunctivitis Ill appearance	Pneumonia Encephalitis	Paramyxovirus	No specific treatment Single oral dose of 200,000 IU of vitamin A recommended in children older than 1 yr
Pruritus Localized lymphadenopathy Usually follows low-grade fever, sore throat, rhinorrhea, or diarrhea	None	Unknown	None supportive
Occasional fever Malaise Headache	Cellulitis	*Pseudomonas aeruginosa*	Topical antipruritic agents can help relieve symptoms. When severe, consider antibiotics with antipseudomonal coverage.

OTHER DIAGNOSES TO CONSIDER	• Drug eruptions
	• Urticaria
	• Contact dermatitis
	• Henoch-Schönlein purpura
	• Meningococcal disease
	• Varicella (particularly in children who have received varicella vaccine for whom the rash appears atypically)

WHEN TO CONSIDER FURTHER EVALUATION OR TREATMENT

• A second course of permethrin 5% cream is often necessary 1 week later in the treatment of scabies. Family members should also be treated, and bedding and clothing should be washed in the hottest water possible or dry-cleaned.

• In patients with diagnosed measles and poor nutrition or vitamin A deficiency, vitamin A supplementation is recommended. Measles is associated with significant complications including pneumonia, encephalitis, myocarditis, and the late-occurring (years) subacute sclerosing panencephalitis. If these are suspected, appropriate referrals and inpatient management should be sought.

• Fever and petechiae or purpura should always be considered as high risk for meningococcemia, and appropriate testing and treatment should be instituted.

• Patients with Kawasaki disease should be evaluated for aneurysm formation in the coronary arteries.

• Acute abdominal pain in a child with infectious mononucleosis should warrant an evaluation of the spleen for possible rupture.

• Patients with roseola should be instructed to avoid contact with pregnant women until the infection subsides due to the risk of nonimmune hydrops in the fetus.

SUGGESTED READINGS
Carder KR, Weston WL. Atypical viral exanthems: new rashes and variations on old themes. *Contemp Pediatr.* 2003;12:111–127.
Cohen BA. A baby, a cutaneous lesion—and an efficient approach to recognition and management. *Contemp Pediatr.* 2004;July:28–50.
Dyer JA. Childhood viral exanthems. *Pediatr Ann.* 2007;36(1):21–29.
Mancini AJ. Exanthems in childhood: an update. *Pediatr Ann.* 1998;27:163–170.
Paller AS, Mancini AJ. *Hurwitz clinical pediatric dermatology: a textbook of skin disorders of childhood and adolescence.* 3rd ed. Philadelphia, PA: Elsevier Saunders; 2005.
Shwayder T. Five common skin problems—and a string of pearls for managing them. *Contemp Pediatr.* 2003;34–54.

DARREN M. FIORE

Vesicular Rashes

APPROACH TO THE PROBLEM

A vesicle is a raised skin lesion filled with clear fluid that is less than 1 cm in diameter. A raised, clear-fluid-filled lesion larger than 1 cm is referred to as a bulla. In childhood, there are many diseases that manifest as vesicular rashes, the most familiar of which is the rash seen with herpes simplex virus (HSV) infection. Other viral and bacterial infections also may present with vesiculobullous lesions as may many noninfectious processes, including allergic and immune-mediated diseases, mechanical disorders of the skin, burns, and insect bites.

Vesicular eruptions may be benign and self-limited or may be progressive and life threatening. Early identification of potentially serious disease and prompt attention to complications are critical, particularly in infants and immunocompromised hosts.

KEY POINTS IN THE HISTORY

- Recurrent herpetic skin outbreaks in the same location almost always represent the reactivation of a latent infection rather than a new primary infection.

- Immunocompromised hosts may have disseminated disease due to HSV, varicella zoster virus (VZV), and coxsackie virus infections.

- Primary HSV lesions are often associated with fever and systemic symptoms, whereas, secondary lesions or reactivation of HSV lesions are usually not.

- The reactivation of HSV or VZV, known as "shingles", is typically preceded by a prodrome of pain, tingling, itching, or burning at the site.

- In assessing vesicular rashes in the neonate, a detailed maternal history is necessary to elicit possible HSV exposure.

- Lethargy, poor feeding, temperature instability, jaundice, irritability, or seizures in an infant with vesicular lesions should raise suspicion for neonatal HSV infection.

- Frequently accompanying genital HSV is painful inguinal adenopathy, dysuria, urinary retention, and vaginal discharge. However, most primary genital HSV infections are asymptomatic.

- Primary VZV infection or chickenpox is very contagious; therefore, a history of household or school exposure in a child with characteristic lesions is highly suggestive.

- Children vaccinated against VZV may still develop chickenpox, though the disease course is milder.

- When contact dermatitis is suspected, a detailed environmental exposure history is warranted.

- Symptoms of allergic contact dermatitis may not manifest for 6 to 24 hours after the exposure. Symptoms are often worse with second or subsequent exposures.

- A history of outdoor exposure can indicate rhus dermatitis—poison oak, poison ivy, or poison sumac.

KEY POINTS IN THE PHYSICAL EXAMINATION

- Grouped vesicles on an erythematous base are the hallmark of HSV infection; however, in immunocompromised patients, the erythematous base is not always apparent.

- HSV lesions on skin or mucous membranes may appear vesicular or, if they have ruptured, the lesions may appear eroded or ulcerated.

- Lesions of neonatal herpes often appear at 5 to 14 days of life; lesions appearing in the first 2 days of life suggest intrauterine exposure. Intrauterine-acquired HSV may not present with vesicles but rather scarring.

- The oral vesicles and ulcers of HSV tend to form more anteriorly on the gingivae, tongue, and hard palate, whereas, the lesions of hand-foot-and-mouth disease are typically more posterior on the soft palate, tonsillar pillars, and posterior oropharynx.

- Primary HSV infection of the eye may appear as blepharitis or keratoconjunctivitis. Signs include corneal or conjunctival erythema, watery discharge, lid swelling, and preauricular adenopathy.

- Lesions of primary VZV infection or chickenpox progress from papules to vesicles to erosions with crust. They occur in successive crops over 2 to 5 days and are predominant on the trunk, face, and scalp and progress in a centripetal distribution.

- Smallpox lesions spread centrifugally, with lesions concentrated on the extremities and spreading inward. A distinguishing feature of smallpox is the central umbilication of the lesions. Children with this disease are typically very ill.

- The presence of a dermatomal vesicular eruption is consistent with the diagnosis of shingles or reactivation of VZV infection.

- Extensive herpes zoster skin lesions may indicate an underlying immunodeficiency and an increased risk of visceral involvement.

- Lesions of contact dermatitis are typically limited to the area of exposure. The skin is often erythematous and edematous with vesiculation and weeping.

- Papular urticaria is characterized by recurrent crops of pruritic papulovesicles on skin areas exposed to insect bites.

PHOTOGRAPHS OF SELECTED DIAGNOSES

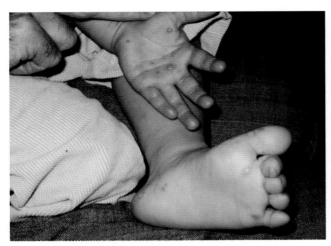

Figure 67-1 Hand-foot-and-mouth disease. Vesicles on palms and soles.
(Courtesy of Philip Siu, MD.)

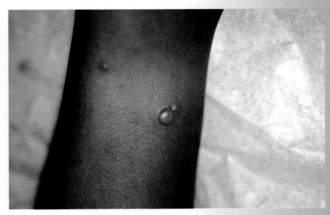

Figure 67-2 Papular urticaria. Vesicular lesion following an insect bite on the lower leg of a child.
(Courtesy of Shirley P. Klein, MD, FAAP.)

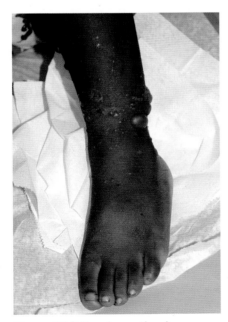

Figure 67-3 Papular urticaria. Vesiculobullous eruption secondary to insect bites on exposed area.
(Courtesy of Ilona J. Frieden, MD.)

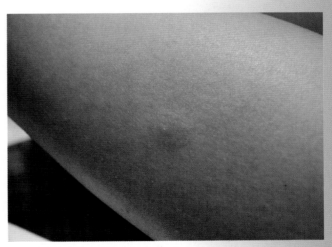

Figure 67-4 Breakthrough varicella. Note the "dewdrop-on-a-rose-petal" appearance of this lesion in a child previously immunized against varicella.
(Courtesy of Esther K. Chung, MD, MPH.)

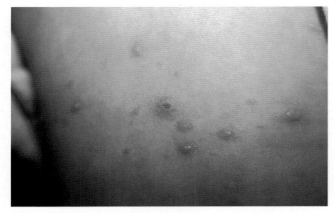

Figure 67-5 Varicella. Note the various stages of the lesions: papular, vesicular, and crusted.
(Courtesy of Shirley P. Klein, MD, FAAP.)

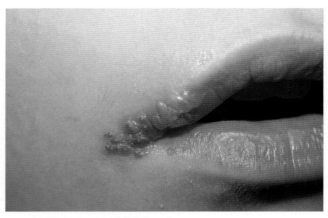

Figure 67-6 Herpes labialis. Grouped vesicles predominantly on one portion of the lip.
(Courtesy of Ilona J. Frieden, MD.)

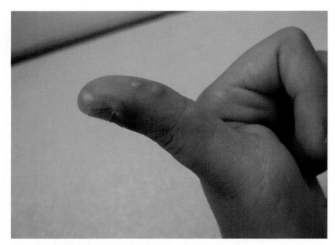

Figure 67-7 Herpetic whitlow. A group of vesicular lesions on the distal phalanx.
(Courtesy of Paul S. Matz, MD.)

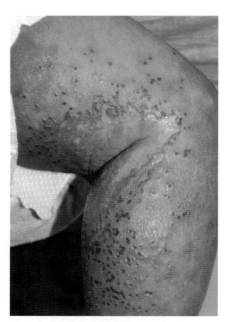

Figure 67-8 Eczema herpeticum. Multiple eroded vesicles with umbilication and crusting overlying a patch of eczematous skin.
(Courtesy of Ilona J. Frieden, MD.)

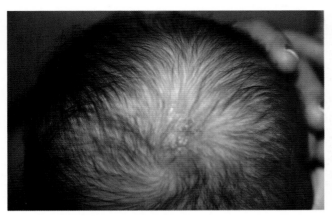

Figure 67-9 Neonatal herpes. Scalp erythema and vesicle at site of scalp electrode.
(Courtesy of Shirley P. Klein, MD, FAAP.)

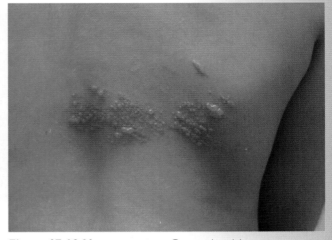

Figure 67-10 Herpes zoster. Grouped vesicles on an erythematous base in a dermatomal distribution.
(Courtesy of Hans B. Kersten, MD.)

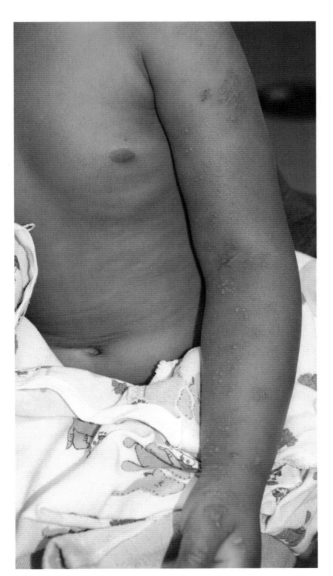

Figure 67-11 Herpes zoster. Grouped vesicles and erosions on an erythematous base in a C6 dermatomal distribution.
(Courtesy of Ilona J. Frieden, MD.)

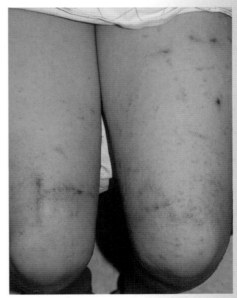

Figure 67-12 Contact dermatitis. Erythema and vesicle formation in a linear pattern characteristic of poison ivy. Also seen is the "black lacquer sign," a grey/black discoloration caused by plant resin deposition in the stratum corneum.
(Courtesy of Ilona J. Frieden, MD.)

DIAGNOSIS	ICD-9	DISTINGUISHING CHARACTERISTICS	DISTRIBUTION	DURATION/ CHRONICITY
Hand-Foot-and-Mouth-Disease	074.3	Elongated, thin-walled vesicles that may ulcerate	Palms, soles, palate, and posterior pharynx Characteristic lack of truncal involvement	5–7 days
Papular Urticaria	698.2	Erythematous papules with urticarial flare in clusters, may progress to vesicles or bullae	Clustered lesions on shoulders, arms, legs, buttocks	Recurrent crops last 2–10 days The illness may persist for months.
Primary Herpes Simplex Virus Infections (see below)				
• **Gingivostomatitis**	054.2	Perioral and intraoral vesicles and crusting	Perioral skin, gingivae, buccal mucosa, palate, tongue	7–10 days
• **Herpes Labialis**	054.9	Grouped vesicles on one portion of the lip; often recurrent	Most common location is lower lip.	7–10 days
• **Keratoconjunctivitis**	054.43	Red, irritated eye with concomitant periocular vesicles	Vesicles on eyelid or face Conjunctivitis (often bilateral) Corneal ulcerations	14–21 days
• **Herpetic Whitlow**	054.6	Grouped vesicles on fingers	One or more fingers; often on terminal phalanx (thumb is most common)	7–10 days
• **Genital Herpes**	054.1	May range from asymptomatic infection to painful, grouped vesicles in genital area	External genitalia, labia, vaginal mucosa, cervix, penis, scrotum, thighs	5–15 days
• **Eczema Herpeticum**	054.0	Generalized HSV infection in patients with atopic dermatitis, characterized by wide spread vesicles and crusting associated with fever and malaise	Seen in skin areas affected by atopic dermatitis, with predilection for upper body and head	2–6 wks
Neonatal HSV	054.9	Three disease patterns: mucocutaneous, CNS, and disseminated—all may have vesicular and/or eroded lesions Onset in first 4 wks of life	Lesions can appear anywhere on skin (or at site of fetal scalp electrode) and commonly on oral mucosa	14–21 days
Secondary (Recurrent) HSV	054.9	Grouped vesicles at or near site of primary eruption	At or near site of initial lesion, often less severe	5–7 days
Varicella (Chickenpox)	052.9	Crops of lesions in different stages (papules, vesicles on erythematous base, crusted erosions)	Entire body and oral mucous membranes	10 days
Herpes Zoster (Shingles)	053.9	Clustered vesicles on erythematous base	Dermatomal distribution Unilateral thoracic dermatomal eruption is most common, but head, neck, buttocks eruptions do occur.	10 days
Variola (Smallpox)	050.9	Papular and vesicular rash; often papules have central umbilication	Face, arms, and legs > trunk Lesions may be seen in mouth and throat.	10–14 days
Contact Dermatitis	692.9	Erythema, vesiculation, and oozing	Limited to area of contact with offending substance Often linear pattern in rhus dermatitis	2–3 wks

ASSOCIATED FINDINGS	COMPLICATIONS	PRECIPITATING FACTORS	TREATMENT GUIDELINES
Fever Sore throat Painful oral lesions Anorexia	Mouth pain Dehydration	Exposure to coxsackievirus, most commonly A16, and other enteroviruses	Supportive care Analgesia Hydration
Pruritus	Bacterial superinfection Recurrent lesions if exposure continues	Delayed hypersensitivity reaction to fleas, mosquitoes, lice, scabies, or other mites	Remove offending insect or minimize child's exposure. DEET-containing insect repellants may help. Treat urticaria and pruritus with antihistamines.
Fever, cervical adenopathy, irritability, mouth pain	Pain Dehydration	HSV-1 (or less commonly HSV-2) exposure via infected saliva	Analgesics, antipyretics, and hydration Consider systemic antiviral therapy.
Usually after febrile illness or URI (hence, colloquial term "cold sore")	Pain	HSV-1 (or less commonly HSV-2) exposure via infected saliva	OTC topical anesthetics may temporarily reduce pain associated with eroded lesions
Eye pain, photophobia, blurred vision	Corneal scarring Visual impairment	Typically HSV-1 exposure (HSV-2 conjunctivitis more often seen in neonates)	Topical or systemic antiviral therapy is required. Referral to an ophthalmologist is typically recommended.
Often a concomitant oral HSV infection (fingers are auto-inoculated via saliva) Pain and tingling of finger	Pain Recurrences are common.	Skin breakdown (e.g., torn cuticle or thumb-sucking)	Analgesics Topical antiviral therapy may shorten duration of symptoms and viral shedding. Systemic therapy generally not recommended
Fever, lymphadenopathy, malaise, dysuria	Vesicle rupture leading to painful ulcers Cervicitis Urethritis	Predominantly caused by HSV-2 transmitted via sexual contact	Analgesia and systemic antiviral therapy are required for primary genital herpes. Chronic suppressive therapy is required for recurrent disease.
Atopic dermatitis, fever, fatigue, keratoconjunctivitis	Pain Secondary bacterial infection Systemic viremia	Atopic dermatitis and HSV exposure	Parenteral acyclovir therapy
Temperature instability, poor feeding, lethargy, jaundice	Sepsis, DIC, shock, meningitis, seizures, death	Maternal HSV at time of delivery (increased with primary infection)	Parenteral acyclovir therapy
Prodrome of pain, burning, or tingling Lymphadenopathy Usually no fever or systemic symptoms (as in primary infection)	Pain Recurrence	Physical or emotional stress (e.g., bacterial infection, URI, surgery, sunburn) or immunocompromise	Analgesics Treatment of recurrent HSV with systemic antiviral therapy early during prodromal phase may abort or shorten the duration of the eruption. Chronic suppressive therapy may benefit children with frequent recurrences.
Prodrome of fever, malaise, sore throat, anorexia Lesions are pruritic.	Secondary bacterial infection of skin lesions Scarring Pneumonia Reye's syndrome and encephalitis are rare.	Exposure to varicella zoster virus, particularly day care or household exposure.	Self-limited disease (in immunocompetent patients) requiring no systemic treatment Pruritus can be managed with cool compresses, calamine lotion, and antihistamines. Vaccination universally recommended to children ≥12 months of age VZIG postexposure prophylaxis exists for certain high-risk populations.
Outbreak is often preceded by dermatomal pain. Lesions can be pruritic.	Pain Recurrent outbreaks	Represents reactivation of a prior varicella infection	Supportive care and analgesics
Prodrome of fever, malaise, myalgia	Disseminated infection (sepsis, osteomyelitis, pneumonia, encephalitis)	Exposure to variola virus Considered a possible agent of bioterrorism	Supportive care Vaccine exists for exposed individuals. Confirmed or suspected cases should be isolated.
Pruritus Pain	Repeated exposure may cause more widespread eruption of an Id reaction	Delayed hypersensitivity reaction Common sources of contact allergens include poison ivy and oak, nickel, shoes, perfumes, soaps, cosmetics, topical medications, and alcohol.	Topical corticosteroids for localized lesions Systemic corticosteroids for more widespread (>10% skin surface) involvement Avoidance of offending contact allergen is critical.

OTHER DIAGNOSES TO CONSIDER

- Incontinentia pigmenti
- Photosensitivity reactions
- Bullous impetigo
- Eczema herpeticum
- Staphylococcal scalded skin syndrome
- Langerhans cell histiocytosis
- Pemphigus
- Rhus dermatitis

WHEN TO CONSIDER FURTHER EVALUATION OR TREATMENT

- HSV infections are often diagnosed clinically; however, diagnostic testing should be performed in uncertain or complex cases. A Tzank smear is a rapid, but nonsensitive and nonspecific test. For more definitive results, consider viral culture, DNA detection, or direct fluorescent antibody testing.

- The use of systemic antiviral therapy in uncomplicated cutaneous HSV infections is not always warranted; treatment *may* shorten the duration of illness if initiated early in the first 72 hours of symptoms or in cases of severe disease.

- HSV and VZV infections in immunocompromised hosts or neonates may disseminate rapidly, and consultation with an infectious disease specialist and/or a neonatologist is recommended.

- The presence of HSV-2 in young children should raise concerns for child sexual abuse.

- Vesicular lesions may become bacterially superinfected, typically by staphylococci, and may require systemic antibiotics.

- HSV or VZV keratoconjunctivitis should be referred to an ophthalmologist for evaluation and treatment.

- Recurrent episodes of genital herpes may be treated with episodic or chronic suppressive antiviral medication.

- The last documented case of smallpox in the United States was in 1949, and the last case in the world was in 1977. Any confirmed or suspected case of smallpox must be reported to public health officials.

- Immunocompromised patients exposed to VZV are candidates for varicella zoster immune globulin (VZIG) and should be referred to an infectious disease specialist.

- Atypical, recurrent or poorly healing, contact dermatitis should be referred to a dermatologist for further evaluation.

SUGGESTED READINGS

Cohen, B. *Pediatric dermatology*. 3rd ed. London: Mosby; 2005:101–120.
Eichenfield LF, Frieden IJ, Esterly NB, eds. *Neonatal dermatology*. 2nd ed. Philadelphia, PA: Elsevier, 2008:131–158.
Gnann JW Jr, Whitley RJ. Clinical practice: herpes zoster. *N Engl J Med*. 2002;347:340–346.
Waggoner-Fountain LA, Grossman LB. Herpes simplex virus. *Pediatr Rev*. 2004;25:86–93.
Weston WL, Lane AT, Morelli JG. *Color textbook of pediatric dermatology*. 4th ed. Philadelphia, PA: Mosby; 2007:127–138, 195–212.

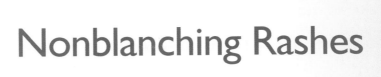

WILLIAM R. GRAESSLE

Nonblanching Rashes

APPROACH TO THE PROBLEM

The child who presents with a nonblanching rash requires careful evaluation. Purpuric lesions, including petechiae and ecchymoses, usually result from vascular injury or disorders of hemostasis. The underlying etiology may be trauma, a simple viral infection, or a more serious condition such as leukemia or a bleeding disorder. When a nonblanching rash is seen in association with fever, serious bacterial infection, including meningococcemia, must be considered.

KEY POINTS IN THE HISTORY

- A history of fever makes an infectious etiology more likely.

- Acute presentation of a nonblanching rash is more concerning than a rash that has been present for more than a couple of weeks.

- The location and pattern of spread may give a clue to the diagnosis: Rocky Mountain spotted fever (RMSF) tends to begin peripherally; Henoch-Schönlein purpura (HSP) tends to primarily involve the lower extremities and buttocks.

- The presence of photophobia, headache, or both, in association with a nonblanching rash raises the suspicion for meningococcal or other bacterial meningitis.

- A history of trauma may be the cause of the nonblanching lesions: localized bruising may follow blunt trauma, and petechiae may be seen in areas of friction or scratching.

- Significant ecchymotic lesions in the absence of a history of trauma should raise the suspicion for child physical abuse or a bleeding disorder.

- Forceful coughing or vomiting may cause petechiae, particularly on the face and upper chest.

- Accompanying fatigue may be caused by anemia because of bone marrow suppression or infiltration as seen with leukemia.

- A history of tick bites or opportunity for exposure to ticks by geography or activities should raise suspicion for RMSF or ehrlichiosis.

- Mongolian spots are present at birth and, though they may fade, they generally do not undergo color changes over time. In contrast, ecchymoses change color over time and eventually resolve.

- A history of easy bruising or excessive bleeding in the patient or a family history of a bleeding disorder should raise the suspicion for hemophilia or von Willebrand disease.

- Familiarity with home remedies found in certain Asian cultures, such as coining and cupping, is essential.

KEY POINTS IN THE PHYSICAL EXAMINATION

- Petechiae are nonblanching macules up to 2 mm in diameter caused by the extravasation of blood from capillaries. Mucosal bleeding sometimes is referred to as "wet purpura."

- Forceful coughing or vomiting may cause petechiae on the face and chest, above the nipple line.

- Purpura, seen with inflammatory injury to the smaller blood vessels, are elevated, firm, hemorrhagic plaques located predominantly on dependent surfaces.

- Ecchymoses are larger areas of bleeding into the skin. There is a characteristic change in color as they age, changing from red to purple to green to yellow-brown as the heme is degraded.

- Deep bleeding and hemarthroses are seen with clotting factor deficiencies, whereas petechiae are more commonly seen with thrombocytopenia.

- Ecchymoses that are not explained easily by accidental trauma should raise the suspicion of child abuse. Ecchymoses, uncommonly caused by infection, usually are indicative of trauma—accidental and nonaccidental—or a bleeding disorder. Bruising in normally active children is predominately on the pretibial surfaces.

- Cupping and coining are practices used by some Asian cultures to treat acute illnesses. Each has a characteristic appearance, and petechiae and ecchymoses may be seen in both.

PHOTOGRAPHS OF SELECTED DIAGNOSES

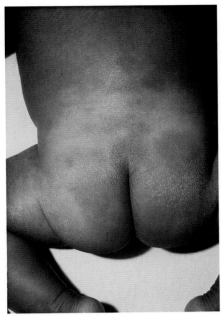

Figure 68-1 Mongolian spots. Blue nevi in the typical sacral area.
(Courtesy of Sidney Sussman, MD.)

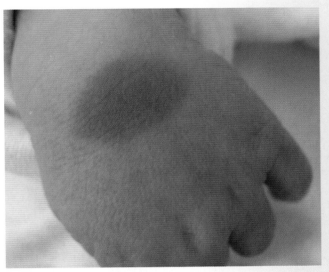

Figure 68-2 Mongolian spot on the hand.
(Courtesy of Esther K. Chung, MD, MPH.)

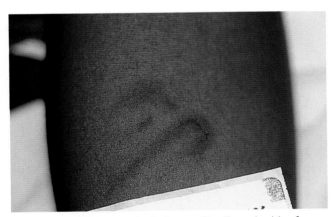

Figure 68-3 Child physical abuse. Curvilinear bruising from a looped cord.
(Used with permission from Fleisher GR, Ludwig S, Baskin MN. *Atlas of pediatric emergency medicine.* Philadelphia, PA: Lippincott Williams & Wilkins; 2004:425.)

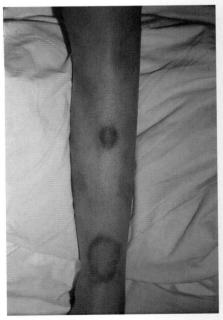

Figure 68-4 Ecchymoses in a patient with hemophilia.
(Courtesy of Sidney Sussman, MD.)

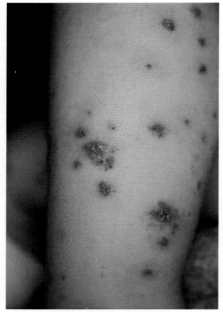

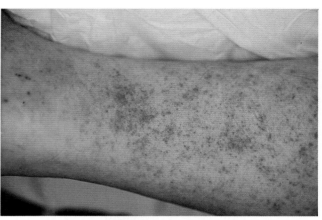

Figure 68-6 Rocky mountain spotted fever. Note the multiple petechial lesions on the forearm. (Courtesy of Steven Manders, MD.)

Figure 68-5 Henoch-Schönlein purpura. Note the palpable purpura on the posterior aspects of this child's leg. (Courtesy of Steven Manders, MD.)

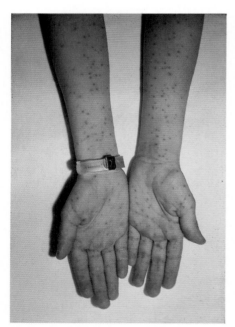

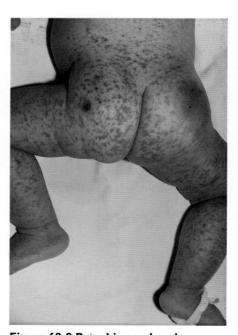

Figure 68-7 Rocky mountain spotted fever.

(Courtesy of Sidney Sussman, MD.)

Figure 68-8 Petechiae and ecchymoses in a patient with idiopathic thrombocytopenic purpura.

(Courtesy of Sidney Sussman, MD.)

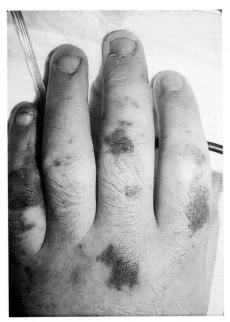

Figure 68-9 Purpura fulminans in a patient with meningococcemia.
(Courtesy of Steven Manders, MD.)

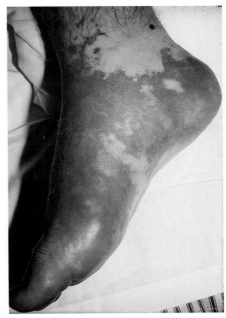

Figure 68-10 Purpura fulminans.
Purpura on the foot of the same patient in Figure 68.9.
(Courtesy of Steven Manders, MD.)

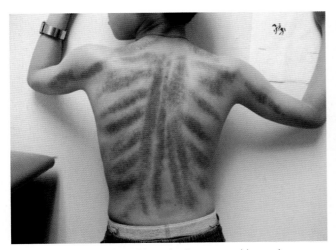

Figure 68-11 Coining. Note the linear petechiae and ecchymoses over the back that are characteristic for this healing practice used by some Asian cultures.
(Courtesy of Philip Siu, MD.)

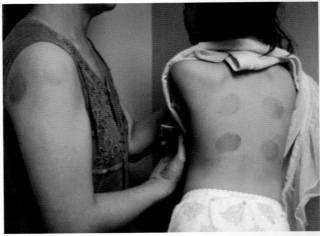

Figure 68-12 Cupping. Note the circular bruises on the mother's arm and the child's back that are the result of cupping, a healing practice used by some Asian cultures.
(Courtesy of Philip Siu, MD.)

DIFFERENTIAL DIAGNOSIS

DIAGNOSIS	ICD-9	DISTINGUISHING CHARACTERISTICS	DISTRIBUTION
Mongolian Spots	757.33	Blue-gray lesions with indistinct borders present at birth No color or size changes with time as one would see with ecchymoses	Most commonly in lumbosacral area, but upper back, shoulders, and extremities also commonly affected
Child Physical Abuse	995.54	Ecchymoses in unusual locations or unusual patterns	Anywhere on the body
Henoch-Schönlein Purpura	287.0	Initially urticarial, progresses to palpable purpura	Typically, buttocks and extensor surfaces of extremities, but any area of body may be involved
Rocky Mountain Spotted Fever	082.0	Initially macular, gradually develops petechial, purpuric, and ecchymotic features	Begins around ankles and wrists; progresses to involve the entire body, including palms and soles
Idiopathic Thrombocytopenic Purpura	287.3	Petechiae, ecchymoses, and mucosal bleeding	Generalized petechiae
Purpura Fulminans	286.6	Palpable purpura, undergoes necrosis	Symmetrical distribution Often begins on dependent surfaces
Coining	782.7	Linear ecchymotic lesions	Usually back or chest
Cupping	782.7	Petechiae, ecchymoses, and occasionally first-degree and second-degree burns	Cups placed in area of discomfort—back, abdomen

ASSOCIATED FINDINGS	PREDISPOSING FACTORS	COMPLICATIONS	TREATMENT GUIDELINES
No reddened appearance	Congenital Ethnicities with darker skin, including Asians, Hispanics, and those of African descent	N/A	No treatment required
Retinal hemorrhages, swelling of extremities, unusual skin marks, bucket-handle fractures, spiral fractures, multiple rib fractures, subdural hematomas	Teens and single parents, poverty, substance abuse, domestic violence, and parents who were physically abused as children Young and mentally retarded children are at greater risk	Head injury Internal injury (liver and spleen laceration, intestinal rupture)	Remove from situation where injury occurred Refer to child protective services Consult ophthalmology in young children to rule out retinal hemorrhages
Abdominal pain, vomiting, periarticular and joint swelling, scrotal edema Elevated ESR (erythrocyte sedimentation rate) and thrombocytosis	Preceding upper respiratory tract infection (URI) or other viral syndrome	Gastrointestinal (GI) bleeding Intussusception Renal disease	Consider steroid treatment
Fever, chills, severe headache, myalgias, and GI symptoms (nausea, vomiting, and diarrhea)	Tick bite Most commonly eastern and southern United States 90% occur between April and September	Hyponatremia DIC Shock	Doxycycline
Child otherwise well appearing	Preceding viral illness in 50–65% of cases Most commonly 1 to 4 yr of age	Intracranial hemorrhage	Steroids and IVIG are used Treatment is controversial
Ill-appearing child with features of septic shock—hypotension, poor perfusion	Commonly caused by meningococcemia, but may be seen with other bacterial causes of sepsis	Septic shock	Fluids Broad-spectrum antibiotics Admit with close monitoring
Usually performed on an individual with an acute illness	Vigorous rubbing with coin or spoon sometimes after application of a medicated ointment	N/A	Lesions self-resolve
Usually performed on an individual with an acute illness	Cup applied to skin after igniting alcohol to create a vacuum	N/A	Lesions self-resolve

OTHER
DIAGNOSES
TO CONSIDER

- Leukemia

- Aplastic anemia

- Hemolytic-uremic syndrome

- Systemic lupus erythematosus

- Liver disease

- Coagulation disorders

- Drug-induced thrombocytopenia

- Wiskott-Aldrich syndrome

WHEN TO
CONSIDER
FURTHER
EVALUATION
OR TREATMENT

- Patients with generalized petechiae or petechiae that are not easily explained by trauma should have a complete blood count. If the diagnosis of thrombocytopenia is established, further evaluation for a specific etiology should occur.

- An ill-appearing child with petechiae or purpura requires urgent evaluation and may need empiric treatment for an infectious etiology, such as bacterial sepsis or RMSF.

- Patients with ecchymoses suspicious for nonaccidental trauma should be evaluated further with coagulation studies and radiographic studies. Referral to child protective services should also be made.

- Patients with significant thrombocytopenia or involvement of other cell lines (anemia and/or white cell abnormalities) should be evaluated by a hematologist.

SUGGESTED READINGS

Browning J, Levy M. Purpura. In: Long SS, ed. *Principles and practice of pediatric infectious diseases.* 3rd ed. New York, NY: Elsevier; 2008:446–448.

Fleisher GR, Ludwig S, Baskin MN. *Atlas of pediatric emergency medicine.* Philadelphia, PA: Lippincott Williams & Wilkins; 2004:425.

Leung AKC, Chan KW. Evaluating the child with purpura. *Am Fam Physician.* 2001;64(3):419–428.

Mudd SS, Findlay JS. The cutaneous manifestations and common mimickers of physical child abuse. *J Pediatr Health Care.* 2004;18(3):123–129.

Singh-Behl D, LaRosa SP, Tomecki KJ. Tick-borne infections. *Dermatol Clin.* 2003;21(2):237–244.

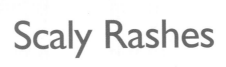

ESTHER K. CHUNG

Scaly Rashes

APPROACH TO THE PROBLEM

The most common scaly rash in pediatrics is atopic dermatitis (eczema), which affects 15% to 20% of the pediatric population. While eczema tends to be chronic in nature, some patients have symptoms primarily during cold and dry weather. Other common causes of scaly rash include pityriasis rosea, tinea corporis, and seborrhea. Psoriasis and ichthyosis are less common. Initial lesions of pityriasis may at times be mistaken for tinea corporis, and ichthyosis may at times be mislabeled as severely dry skin. In general, most dry and scaly rashes tend to be pruritic in nature.

KEY POINTS IN THE HISTORY

- The duration of symptoms will help to distinguish acute and subacute rashes, such as tinea corporis, from more chronic conditions, such as eczema.

- A family history of atopy should raise suspicion for eczema.

- Eczema generally spares the groin and diaper areas, whereas seborrhea does not.

- A solitary lesion may suggest tinea corporis or may be the herald patch seen in pityriasis rosea.

- Tinea corporis worsens with topical steroids, whereas eczema generally improves.

- Eczema on the face of young infants may have a circular area of erythema and may be mistaken by less experienced providers for tinea corporis.

- Cold weather generally exacerbates eczema.

- In pityriasis rosea, the rash often starts as a single isolated lesion followed by a more generalized rash occurring 5 to 10 days later.

- In the event a child shares a bed with another individual who denies pruritus or rash, a diagnosis of scabies is unlikely.

- Psoriasis affects 1% to 3% of the population, but it is uncommon in African-American populations.

KEY POINTS IN THE PHYSICAL EXAMINATION

- Patients with eczema often have dry skin, keratosis pilaris, or both.

- Lichenification is pathognomic of chronic atopic dermatitis when it appears in the expected distribution.

- Often, allergic shiners and Dennie-Morgan lines are seen in individuals with atopic dermatitis.

- Seborrhea generally stays within the hairline, whereas psoriasis extends beyond the hairline.

- In ectopic allergic contact dermatitis, the rash may not be in the expected location as can be seen with nail polish (tosylamide/formaldehyde) allergy.

- Lesions associated with tinea corporis tend to be round, whereas the herald patch in pityriasis rosea is oval.

- The generalized rash of pityriasis rosea classically runs parallel to the lines of skin cleavage, in a "Christmas-tree" distribution.

- Postinflammatory hypopigmentation commonly occurs following eczema, pityriasis, and tinea. Hypopigmentation can be distressing to families; therefore, discussing this early in the course of the disease may be helpful.

PHOTOGRAPHS OF SELECTED DIAGNOSES

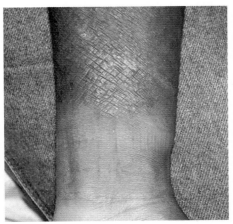

Figure 69-1 Atopic dermatitis. This lesion shows no evidence of active inflammation. Lichenification and postinflammatory hyperpigmentation are apparent.
(Used with permission from Goodheart HP. *Goodheart's photoguide to common skin disorders.* 2nd ed. Philadelphia, PA: Lippincott Williams & Wilkins; 2003:44.)

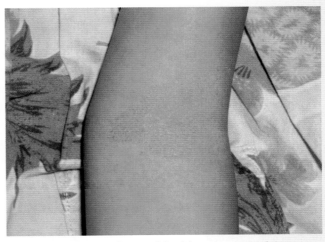

Figure 69-2 Atopic dermatitis. Note the areas of dryness, hypopigmentation and hyperpigmentation and lichenification in the antecubital fossa of this 5-year-old.
(Courtesy of Esther K. Chung, MD, MPH.)

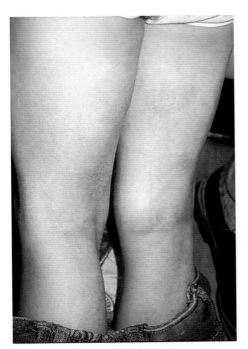

Figure 69-3 Nummular eczema. "Coin-shaped" patches and plaques are located on the legs.
(Used with permission from Goodheart HP. *Goodheart's photoguide to common skin disorders.* 2nd ed. Philadelphia, PA: Lippincott Williams & Wilkins; 2003:87.)

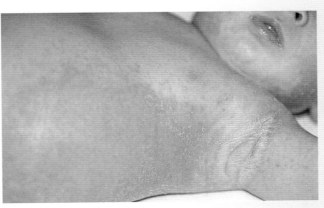

Figure 69-4 Seborrhea.
(Used with permission from Fleisher GR, Ludwig S, Baskin MN. *Atlas of pediatric emergency medicine.* Philadelphia, PA: Lippincott Williams & Wilkins; 2004:85.)

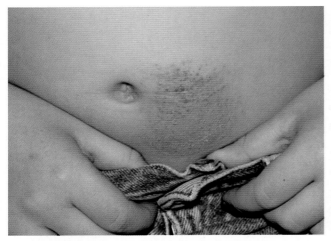

Figure 69-5 Allergic contact dermatitis. This boy developed an eczematous eruption at the site where the nickel snap on his blue jeans contacted his skin.
(Used with permission from Goodheart HP. *Goodheart's photoguide to common skin disorders*. 2nd ed. Philadelphia, PA: Lippincott Williams & Wilkins; 2003:67.)

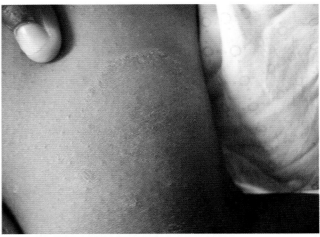

Figure 69-6 Herald patch of pityriasis rosea.
(Courtesy of Paul S. Matz, MD.)

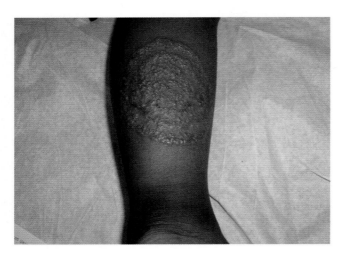

Figure 69-7 Tinea corporis. Note the large size of this lesion that was made worse by the use of topical steroids.
(Courtesy of Esther K. Chung, MD, MPH.)

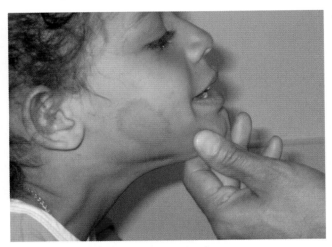

Figure 69-8 Tinea corporis on the face.
(Courtesy of George A. Datto, III, MD.)

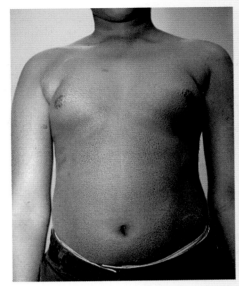

Figure 69-9 Ichthyosis vulgaris.
(Courtesy of George A. Datto, III, MD.)

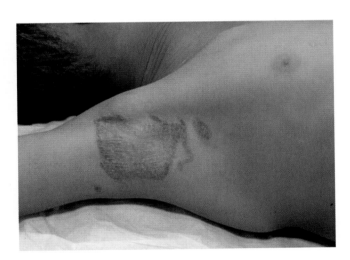

Figure 69-10 Psoriasis.
(Courtesy of George A. Datto, III, MD.)

DIFFERENTIAL DIAGNOSIS

DIAGNOSIS	ICD-9	DISTINGUISHING CHARACTERISTICS	DISTRIBUTION
Atopic Dermatitis	691.8	Erythema, papules, vesicles in early infancy Dry, pruritic, scaly patches in young children May present after the newborn period Many individuals only have the condition as young children; some adults are affected	Often begins on the face in young infants Often begins on extensor surfaces and trunk in older infants Antecubital and popliteal fossae, face, and neck in older children and adults Frequently spares the groin
Nummular Eczema	692.9	Starts as vesicles, papules Erythematous, coin-shaped lesions May or may not see pruritus May only occur in the winter months	Extensor surfaces of the extremities
Seborrhea	690.12 (infantile) 690.10 (dermatitis)	Greasy, yellow, or salmon-colored Nonpruritic or very mildly pruritic Appears at 1 month of age and disappears between 8 and 12 months of age. Reappears in adolescence	Scalp (as cradle cap), nasolabial folds, postauricular areas, cheeks, trunk, extremities, diaper area, intertriginous areas
Irritant Contact Dermatitis	692.9	Focal, mild erythema Resolves shortly after the irritant is removed	Chin, cheeks, extensor surfaces, diaper area
Allergic Contact Dermatitis	692.9	May occur in children as young as 6 months Increased risk in females Pruritic, eczematous dermatitis appears 24–48 hrs after exposure	Geometric or linear configuration "Jean snap dermatitis"—periumbilical area Midline chest with nickel snaps on infant clothing
Pityriasis Rosea	696.3	70%–80% begin with a single patch followed by a general eruption 5–10 days later of smaller, more ovoid lesions Oval shape with flat, pink, brown center with an elevated border that is erythematous with a collarette of fine scales The rash may be more common in young children and in African Americans Peak incidence in adolescence	Trunk, upper arms, neck, and thighs but may occur anywhere on the body
Tinea Corporis	110.5	Round, scaly patches with a papular, vesicular, or pustular border with clear center Most commonly in children, but may be seen at any age	Predilection for nonhairy areas of the face, trunk, and extremities Asymmetric distribution
Ichthyosis Vulgaris	757.1	Scales on the tibia may be thick and plate-like Hyperkeratosis Rarely occurs before 3 months of life Scaling on the face is generally limited to childhood and decreases with age.	Extensor surfaces Flexural surfaces generally spared May see chapping and accentuation of palmar markings
Psoriasis	696.1	Round, sharply demarcated, deep-red lesion with a silvery scale attached at the center of the lesion Droplike lesions are seen in guttate psoriasis. Unpredictable exacerbations and remissions Prolonged course	Extensor surfaces, scalp, genital regions, and lumbosacral areas Typically, a bilateral, symmetric pattern of lesions

ASSOCIATED FINDINGS	PREDISPOSING FACTORS	TREATMENT GUIDELINES
Keratosis pilaris Ichthyosis vulgaris 4%–12% of patients develop cataracts Cutaneous infection resulting from *S. aureus,* strep Eczema herpeticum (herpes simplex) Eczema vaccinatum (vaccinia) Id reaction Irritability Daytime tiredness	Worse during the winter months Worsened by frequent bathing Allergenic foods Inhalant allergens Dust mites	Topical steroids Calcineurin inhibitors (second line) Antibiotics for skin infections (e.g., staphylococcal infections) Antihistamines to reduce itching and to possibly improve overall sleeping Moisturizers Humidified air Avoidance of irritant and allergic triggers
N/A	Worse during winter months Manifestation of dry skin (xerosis), ichthyosis (but not necessarily atopy)	Lukewarm, cool baths Emollients Topical steroids Tar preparations Oral antihistamines
N/A	Puberty	Antiseborrheic shampoos containing selenium sulfide, salicylic acid, or zinc pyrithione Topical steroids in some instances
N/A	Soaps, detergents Salivary secretions Urine and feces	Irritant avoidance/removal
Id reaction	Nickel-containing snaps, piercings, belts Cosmetic products Fragrant and deodorant products Leather materials (potassium dichromate) Rubber materials (carba mix, thiuram) Poison ivy (urushiol) Para-phenylenediamine (PPD) found in hair dye, henna tattoos	Allergen avoidance Epicutaneous patch testing can help in some instances to identify allergens. Short courses of topical or oral steroids
Prodrome of headache, malaise, pharyngitis may be reported. The rash, seen in secondary syphilis, may be similar and should not be overlooked.	Associated with preceding viral illness	Self-limited Topical antipruritics, sparingly Oral antihistamines Exposure to UV light hastens resolution
N/A	Warm, humid climates Contact with an infected individual Systemic disease such as diabetes mellitus, immunodeficiency	Topical antifungal creams
Keratosis pilaris	Worse in cold and dry weather Atopy	Emollients Topical retinoids Antihistamines for itching Topical steroids for itching Alpha-hydroxy acids (including lactic and glycolic acids)
25–50% with nail pits Geographic tongue Psoriatic arthritis Psoriatic uveitis	Stress, trauma, strep infection (such as guttate psoriasis), climate, and certain medications may be precipitating factors in fewer than half of patients.	Emollients Topical steroids Avoid irritants Tar preparations

OTHER
DIAGNOSES
TO CONSIDER

- Scabies

- Letterer-Siwe disease (a form of histiocytosis consisting of lymphadenopathy, hepatosplenomegaly, and a seborrhea-like rash)

- Leiner disease (seborrhea-like dermatitis, diarrhea, wasting and dystrophy, recurrent Gram-negative infection)

- Netherton syndrome ("bamboo hair," congenital ichthyosiform erythroderma, and atopic diathesis)

- Acrodermatitis enteropathica (listlessness, diarrhea, failure to thrive, and low-serum zinc)

- Wiskott-Aldrich syndrome (diarrhea, purpura, and susceptibility to infection)

- Phenylketonuria (mental retardation, seizures, blond hair, and eczema)

- Hyper IgE syndrome (recurrent sinopulmonary and cutaneous infections, markedly elevated IgE levels, chronic dermatitis)

- Lichen striatus

WHEN TO
CONSIDER
FURTHER
EVALUATION
OR TREATMENT

- Further evaluation and treatment should be considered for dry scaly rashes that fail to improve in spite of frequent moisturizing.

- Most dry, scaly rashes are due to atopic dermatitis and will respond to emollients and the use of mild topical steroids.

- Severe and complicated cases of eczema warrant consultation with a dermatologist.

- Because tinea corporis worsens with the use of topical steroids, only use these agents when there is a low suspicion for tinea corporis.

- Pityriasis rosea is generally self-limited and resolves by 6 weeks generally; however, it may last as long as 5 months.

- With pityriasis rosea, exposure to UV light hastens resolution.

- Keep in mind that allergic contact dermatitis may last for weeks to months after the removal of the allergen, even with the use of topical steroids.

SUGGESTED READINGS

Fleisher GR, Ludwig S, Baskin MN. *Atlas of pediatric emergency medicine*. Philadelphia, PA: Lippincott Williams & Wilkins; 2004:85.

Goodheart HP. *Goodheart's photoguide to common skin disorders*. 2nd ed. Philadelphia, PA: Lippincott Williams & Wilkins; 2003:44, 67, 87.

Krol A, Krafchik B. The differential diagnosis of atopic dermatitis in childhood. *Dermatol Ther*. 2006(19);73–82.

Larsen S, Hanifin JM. Epidemiology of atopic dermatitis. *Immunol Clin North Am*. 2002;22:1–24.

Militello G, Jacob SE, Crawford GH. Allergic contact dermatitis in children. *Curr Opin Pediatr*. 2006;18:385–390.

Paller AS, Mancini AJ. *Hurwitz clinical pediatric dermatology: a textbook of skin disorders of childhood and adolescence*. 3rd ed. Philadelphia, PA: Elsevier Saunders; 2006:49–64, 67–69, 85–94, 99–101, 451–458.

Schon MP, Boehncke WH. Psoriasis. *N Engl J Med*. 2005;352:1899–1912.

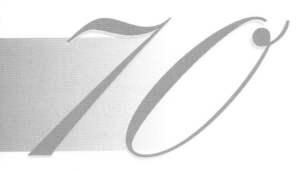

Fine, Bumpy Rashes

APPROACH TO THE PROBLEM

Fine, bumpy rashes are a common complaint seen in the pediatric outpatient setting. They may be acute or chronic, and may be so subtle and asymptomatic that they are not noted for a period of time. The most classic example of a fine, bumpy rash is the sandpaper rash of scarlet fever, but this category of rashes also includes nonspecific rashes such as viral exanthems, heat rashes, drug reactions, and rarer lichenoid eruptions. Most of these conditions are benign and self-limited, and at times it may not be possible to make the exact diagnosis. It is important to note, however, that there are serious conditions such as toxic shock syndrome that may initially present as a mild rash. It is important to have a high clinical suspicion for these serious disorders, particularly when systemic symptoms accompany the rash.

KEY POINTS IN THE HISTORY

- Scarlet fever is generally seen with the accompanying symptoms of fever, headache, sore throat, and abdominal pain; the rash usually appears 24 to 48 hours after the onset of symptoms.

- Folliculitis, which occurs in all skin types, is not always infectious but may also be caused by chemical irritation or physical injury from shaving.

- Keratosis pilaris is often prominent in patients with underlying atopic dermatitis or obesity. Many patients with keratosis pilaris have a family member with this condition.

- Lichen nitidus is usually a chronic, nonpruritic, asymptomatic condition.

- Though usually precipitated by heat, miliaria can occur in the winter in association with fever, overbundling, or the use of certain ointments.

- Fine papular eruptions are the most frequent of all cutaneous drug reactions, classically due to ampicillin or amoxicillin, and are often identical to viral exanthems.

- Penicillin therapy in patients with Epstein-Barr virus infection may result in a morbilliform (measles-like) exanthem, which is considered to be a drug reaction.

KEY POINTS IN THE PHYSICAL EXAMINATION

- Scarlet fever often produces Pastia lines, linear rows of petechiae, in the skin folds, particularly the antecubital and popliteal fossae and the inguinal area.

- Scarlet fever is most often associated with pharyngitis, but may also be seen with other group A streptococcal skin infections such as cellulitis.

- In patients with more skin pigmentation, the rash of scarlet fever may not readily appear erythematous; therefore, it is important to examine patients in bright lighting.

- The Koebner phenomenon, linear papules along the lines of skin trauma, is a hallmark of lichen nitidus and presents in almost all cases.

- Keratosis pilaris, which is rough in texture, occurs along the extensor surfaces of extremities.

- Folliculitis, which may consist of pustules of varying size, is usually confined to hair-bearing areas such as the scalp, forearms, groin, and legs. Often the hair follicle cannot be seen in folliculitis.

- Miliaria is often found on the face and upper trunk.

PHOTOGRAPHS OF SELECTED DIAGNOSES

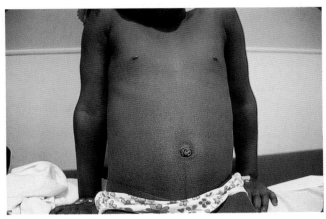

Figure 70-1 Scarlet fever. Fine papules, "sandpaperlike" rash on trunk of child with scarlet fever.
(Courtesy of George A. Datto, III, MD.)

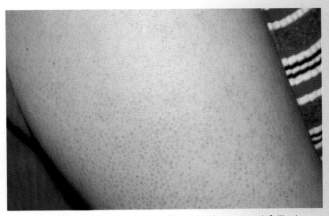

Figure 70-2 Keratosis pilaris. Tiny, rough-textured, follicular papules on lateral upper arms.
(Used with permission from Goodheart HP. *Goodheart's photoguide to common skin disorders.* 2nd ed. Philadelphia, PA: Lippincott Williams & Wilkins; 2003:49.)

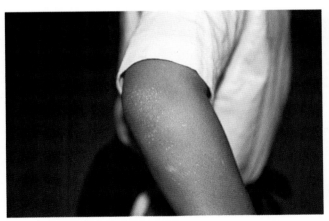

Figure 70-3 Lichen nitidus. Shiny small papules on elbow.
(Courtesy of George A. Datto, III, MD.)

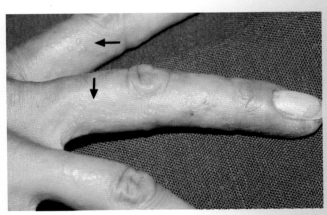

Figure 70-4 Dyshidrotic eczema. Note the fine, fluid-filled bumps on the fingers as depicted by the *arrows.*
(Used with permission from Goodheart HP. *Goodheart's photoguide to common skin disorders.* 2nd ed. Philadelphia, PA: Lippincott Williams & Wilkins; 2003:60.)

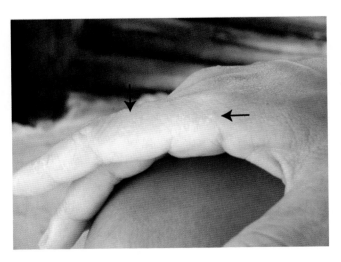

Figure 70-5 Dyshidrotic eczema. Note the fine, fluid-filled bumps on the finger (as depicted by the *arrows*) and the distal area of peeling.
(Courtesy of Esther K. Chung, MD, MPH.)

DIFFERENTIAL DIAGNOSIS

DIAGNOSIS	ICD-9	DISTINGUISHING CHARACTERISTICS	DISTRIBUTION	DURATION/ CHRONICITY
Scarlet Fever	034.1	Erythematous "sandpaperlike" pinpoint papules Desquamation of tips of fingers and toes	Generalized Concentrates on trunk and skin folds Palms and soles are often erythematous	Rash appears 2–4 days after onset of other symptoms
Keratosis Pilaris	701.1	Perifollicular Rough 1–2 mm papules	Posterolateral upper arms Anterior thighs	Chronic
Folliculitis	704.8	Perifollicular inflammation May be painless or tender	Any hair-bearing area—most commonly affecting the face, arms, legs, and axillae	Acute onset
Lichen Nitidus	697.1	Flesh-colored, monomorphous papules Sharply demarcated	Cluster in groups Trunk Upper extremities Glans penis	Slowly progressive May remain for years Spontaneously resolves
Miliaria Rubra (Heat Rash)	705.1	Erythematous, fine papules	Face Neck Upper trunk	Spontaneous resolution in 2–3 days
Drug Allergy	995.27	Erythematous maculopapular rash May be confluent	Generalized Mucous membranes Often spares palms and soles	Begins 7–10 days after starting drug Resolves 1–2 wks after discontinuation

ASSOCIATED FINDINGS	COMPLICATIONS	PRECIPITATING FACTORS	TREATMENT GUIDELINES
Fever Exudative pharyngitis Strawberry tongue Pastia lines	Suppurative complications Rheumatic fever Glomerulonephritis	Group A streptococcus	Antimicrobial therapy—penicillin, macrolides, cephalosporins
Dry skin	None	Obesity Family history of keratosis pilaris Atopic dermatitis Insulin resistance	Keratolytics Retinoids Mild topical corticosteroids
Hair shaft Pustules present when infected	Cellulitis	Shaving Curly hair Chemical irritants Staphylococcal infection	Modified shaving techniques Laser hair removal Antibiotics, only if infected
Not pruritic Koebner phenomenon	None	Unknown	If persistent, trial of topical corticosteroids
"Prickly" or itchy sensation	None	Heat Tight-fitting clothes Emollients	Cool baths Loose-fitting clothes Avoid oil-based lubricants
Itching Fever Exfoliation	Generally does not progress to anaphylaxis if not urticarial	Ampicillin Amoxicillin Sulfonamides Any medication	Stop offending drug Cool compresses Topical corticosteroids for symptom relief

OTHER
DIAGNOSES
TO CONSIDER

- Nonspecific viral exanthem

- Toxic shock syndrome (TSS) (early phase)

- Kawasaki disease

- "Id" reaction (autoeczematization to various stimuli, particularly fungi, that results in a symmetrical eczematous, maculopapular, or papulovesicular rash)

- Lichen spinulosus (papular rash with a spine or horn at each hair follicle)

- Keratosis follicularis or Darier disease (hereditary skin disorder where keratotic papules coalesce to form crusty warty plaques)

- Dyshidrotic eczema

WHEN TO
CONSIDER
FURTHER
EVALUATION
OR TREATMENT

- Most fine, bumpy rashes are benign and self-limited. Any persistent rash or a rash associated with systemic symptoms such as fever or altered mental status warrants further evaluation.

- If a rash is bothersome and does not respond to initial therapy, further management should be determined after consultation with a pediatric dermatologist.

- The initial rash of TSS may mimic scarlet fever. The presence of high fever, mental status changes, headache, or early shocklike symptoms should raise suspicion for TSS and warrants immediate evaluation and management.

SUGGESTED READINGS

Bisno AL. Practice guidelines for the diagnosis and management of Group A streptococcal pharyngitis. *Clin Infect Dis.* 2002:35:113–125.
Goodheart HP. *Goodheart's photoguide to common skin disorders.* 2nd ed. Philadelphia, PA: Lippincott Williams & Wilkins; 2003:60.
Habif T. *Clinical dermatology.* 4th ed. St. Louis, MO: Mosby; 2004:116–117, 279–283, 464–466, 486–488.
Hurwitz S. *Clinical pediatric dermatology.* 3rd ed. Philadelphia, PA: WB Saunders; 2006:106–107.
Tilly JT, Drolet BA. Lichenoid eruptions in children. *J Am Acad Dermatol.* 2004;51:606–624.

LEE R. ATKINSON-McEVOY

Hypopigmented Rashes

APPROACH TO THE PROBLEM

Disorders of pigment are often an important concern to parents. Even for benign conditions, the cosmetic impact is of importance to patients and families. Hypopigmented lesions may be congenital or acquired, with the latter often occurring in association with inflammation or infection. Congenital lesions appear within the first year of life; as the skin is exposed to sunlight, the normal skin acquires more color and the lesions remain light relative to the normal skin.

KEY POINTS IN THE HISTORY

- A history of rash or other lesion prior to the development of a hypopigmented area suggests postinflammatory hypopigmentation. This condition resolves with time.

- There is a positive family history of vitiligo in 30% of cases.

- Half of the cases of vitiligo present in childhood (usually adolescence).

- Pityriasis alba is common in children with atopy.

- Ash leaf spots may occur in isolation or in association with tuberous sclerosis.

- Piebaldism is an autosomal dominant condition.

KEY POINTS IN THE PHYSICAL EXAMINATION

- Nevoid hypopigmentation (formerly known as Hypomelanosis of Ito) follows the lines of Blaschko in a linear pattern on the extremities and in whorls on the trunk.

- Vitiligo, which may be irregularly shaped, displays hypopigmented and depigmented macules of varying sizes. Vitiligo may involve mucous membranes and hair.

- Patients with piebaldism have a white forelock with hypopigmentation of the adjacent scalp and forehead. The pattern is triangular and enhances with a Wood lamp.

- Ash leaf macules enhance under a Wood lamp.

- Scale frequently accompanies tinea versicolor and may be seen with pityriasis alba. Tinea versicolor infections by *Microsporum* sp. and *Malassezia furfur* tend to fluoresce with Wood lamp examination.

PHOTOGRAPHS OF SELECTED DIAGNOSES

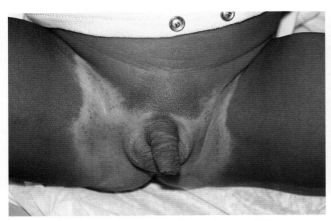

Figure 71-1 Postinflammatory hypopigmentation following a diaper dermatitis.
(Courtesy of Ilona J. Frieden, MD.)

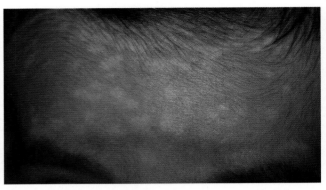

Figure 71-2 Tinea versicolor. Hypopigmented scaly lesions on the forehead of a 22-month-old boy.
(Courtesy of Ilona J. Frieden, MD.)

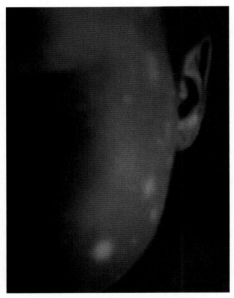

Figure 71-3 Tinea versicolor under Wood lamp. Note the blue-whitish fluorescence.
(Courtesy of Paul S. Matz, MD.)

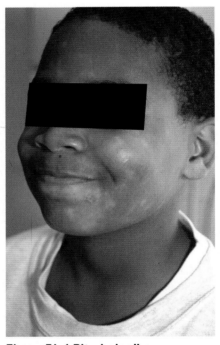

Figure 71-4 Pityriasis alba.
(Courtesy of George A. Datto, III, MD.)

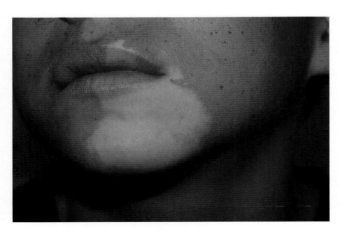

Figure 71-5 Vitiligo. Segmental vitiligo in an 11-year-old child.
(Courtesy of Ilona J. Frieden, MD.)

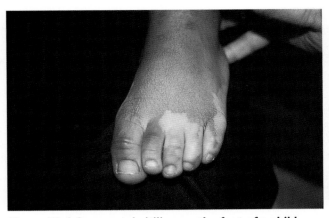

Figure 71-6 Segmental vitiligo on the foot of a child.
(Courtesy of George A. Datto, III, MD.)

Figure 71-7 Ash leaf macule. Hypopigmented macules on the torso of a child with tuberous sclerosis.
(Courtesy of Ilona J. Frieden, MD.)

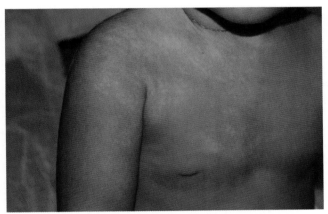

Figure 71-8 Nevoid hypopigmentation (formerly referred to as hypomelanosis of Ito). Linear swirl pattern of hypopigmentation on shoulder.
(Courtesy of Ilona J. Frieden, MD.)

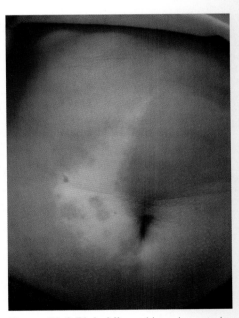

Figure 71-9 Piebaldism. Hypopigmented lesion on a child associated with a white forelock.
(Courtesy of Amy Gilliam, MD.)

DIFFERENTIAL DIAGNOSIS

DIAGNOSIS	ICD-9	DISTINGUISHING CHARACTERISTICS	DISTRIBUTION	DURATION/ CHRONICITY
Postinflammatory Hypopigmentation	709.00 (dyschromia)	Area of hypopigmentation	Diffuse	Subacute to chronic
Tinea Versicolor	111.0	Scaly annular confluent hypopig-mented lesions on the chest, shoulder, and/or back	Upper chest, shoulder, and/or back	Subacute to chronic
Pityriasis Alba	696.5	Hypopigmented macules on the face, moving from place to place	Usually in sun-exposed areas Most often on the face	Chronic, waxing and waning
Vitiligo	709.01	Hypopigmented macules involving mucous membranes	Extensor surfaces of the extremi-ties, face, and neck, but can be diffuse	Chronic
Ash Leaf Macule	759.5 (tuberous sclerosis) 709.00 (isolated Ash leaf macule)	Discrete hypopigmented macule that enhances with Wood's lamp	Diffuse	Chronic
Nevoid Hypopigmentation (Hypomelanosis of Ito)	709.00	Linear or whorled hypopigmented macule	Follows Blaschko lines on trunk or extremities	Chronic
Piebaldism	709.09	Rare condition Segmented white patch of scalp involving hair and skin Enhances with a Wood lamp	Often on scalp, usually frontal	Chronic
Nevus Depigmentosus	709.00	Hypopigmented macule present at or shortly after birth	May occur anywhere	Chronic

ASSOCIATED FINDINGS	COMPLICATIONS	PRECIPITATING FACTORS	TREATMENT GUIDELINES
Areas of inflammation	None	Previous area of inflammation or infection	Sunscreen to protect the area from UV rays Treat inflammation or infection appropriately to minimize development.
Rare complaints of pruritus	May be difficult to treat	Fungal infection with *M. furfur* or *Microsporum* sp. Thrives in hot, humid climates	Ketoconazole shampoo or selenium sulfide 2.5% applied daily for 1 wk then monthly for 3 months
Other signs of atopy such as atopic dermatitis, allergic rhinitis, or asthma	None	Sun exposure Dry skin	Sunscreen to prevent inflammation from sun exposure Emollients/moisturizers to face
None	Cosmetic concerns	Often genetic/familial	Sunscreen to protect the area from UV rays Cosmetic cover up if considered disfiguring Psoralen with UVA radiation in children over 12 yrs has been successful. Refer to dermatologist for treatment
When associated with tuberous sclerosis: angiofibromas on face and nose, seizures, renal tumors, periungual fibromas, Shagreen patch (connective tissue nevus)	Lesions themselves do not cause complications, but many with associated findings in tuberous sclerosis	Autosomal dominant, 100% penetrance 60% spontaneous mutation rate	None for macules If associated with tuberous sclerosis, should see appropriate specialists for associated symptoms
None	None	None	Sunscreen to protect the area from UV rays
None	None	Autosomal dominant inheritance	Sunscreen to protect the area from UV rays
None	None	None	Sunscreen to protect the area from UV rays

OTHER
DIAGNOSES
TO CONSIDER

- Idiopathic guttate hypomelanosis

- Chemical-induced hypopigmentation

- Albinism partial

- Nevus anemicus

- Waardenburg syndrome (autosomal dominant condition with white forelock, white patches on skin, heterochromia of irises, sensorineural deafness, and other defects)

WHEN TO
CONSIDER
FURTHER
EVALUATION
OR TREATMENT

- When tuberous sclerosis is suspected in a child with an Ash leaf macule, referrals for the management of associated conditions should be made to genetics, pediatric neurology, and pediatric dermatology. Imaging should be done to identify tubers, which can occur in any organ and lead to sequelae.

- Patients with vitiligo should be seen by pediatric dermatologists for potential treatment to minimize the cosmetic disfigurement.

SUGGESTED READINGS

Chan Y, Tay Y. Hypopigmentation disorders. In: Eichenfield, LF, Frieden IJ, Esterly NB, eds. Neonatal dermatology. 2nd ed. Philadelphia, PA: Saunders Elsevier; 2008:375–396.

Lio PA. Little white spots: an approach to hypopigmented macules. Arch Dis Child Educ Pract Ed. 2008;93:98–102.

Taïeb A, Picardo M. Vitiligo. N Eng J Med. 2009;360:2:160–169.

Weinberg S, Prose NS, Kristal L, eds. Color atlas of pediatric dermatology. 4th ed. New York, NY: McGraw Hill; 2007:267–284.

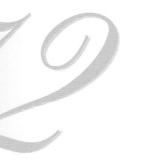

LEE R. ATKINSON-McEVOY

Hyperpigmented Rashes

APPROACH TO THE PROBLEM

Hyperpigmented lesions are caused by an increased melanin deposition in the skin. Congenital lesions may occur over time as sun exposure increases the amount of melanin contained within these lesions. Patients and their families frequently have concerns about the cosmetic effects of these lesions and the malignant potential of certain lesions. A careful history and examination, following the lesions closely over time, and referring to appropriate specialists when needed, can reassure patients and families and often result in the correct diagnosis and management.

KEY POINTS IN THE HISTORY

- A history of pustules present at birth that evolve into hyperpigmented macules is characteristic of neonatal pustular melanosis.

- Café au lait spots grow proportionally to overall body growth in the first few years of life and then stabilize.

- Café au lait spots may be a benign familial trait. A family history of neurofibromatosis and the presence of more than six lesions should raise suspicion for café au lait spots in association with neurofibromatosis.

- Only 1% of pigmented lesions at birth are congenital melanocytic nevi.

- Freckles are common in light-skinned, red-haired individuals, and are an autosomal dominant, inherited trait.

- Freckles are induced by sunlight and are more prominent in the summer and fade in the winter.

- Acanthosis nigricans is associated with overweight/obesity, polycystic ovary syndrome, and the metabolic syndrome—particularly in association with diabetes mellitus with insulin resistance.

- Congenital Dermal Melanocytosis (previously called Mongolian spots), fade after the first 5 to 10 years of life.

KEY POINTS IN THE PHYSICAL EXAMINATION

- A combination of small 1 to 3 mm hyperpigmented macules and pustules is seen in neonatal pustular melanosis.

- A complaint of a "dirty neck" is frequently associated with the physical finding of acanthosis nigricans, which is commonly seen in association with an elevated body mass index.

- Acanthosis nigricans has a velvety quality and may have papillomatous growths within the area of hyperpigmentation.

- Weight loss can result in improvement or resolution of acanthosis nigricans.

- Congenital dermal melanocytosis is often seen in the sacral or gluteal areas, but may also be present elsewhere on the body, including the dorsum of the hand, the upper back, and the shoulders.

- Congenital melanocytic nevi vary in size and may be associated with hair often darker and longer than in surrounding areas.

- Tinea versicolor may be hyperpigmented or hypopigmented and often has scale.

- Blue nevi get their bluish color from the location of the melanocytes deep in the dermis.

- Nevoid hypermelanosis follows Blaschko's lines on the extremities and appears linear; on the trunk, it can have a whorled pattern.

- In neurofibromatosis type 1, there are greater than six café au lait macules at least 0.5 cm in size in prepubertal children, and there are associated findings of axillary or inguinal freckling, Lisch nodules (iris hamartomas), and neurofibromas.

PHOTOGRAPHS OF SELECTED DIAGNOSES

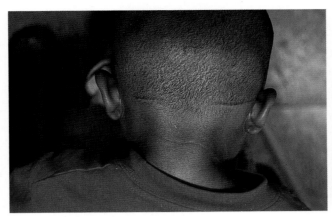

Figure 72-1 Postinflammatory hyperpigmentation. Hyperpigmented linear lesions following skin trauma from a razor.
(Courtesy of George A. Datto, III, MD.)

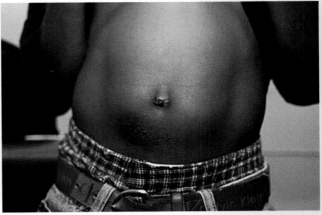

Figure 72-2 Hyperpigmentation resulting from nickel dermatitis.
(Courtesy of George A. Datto, III, MD.)

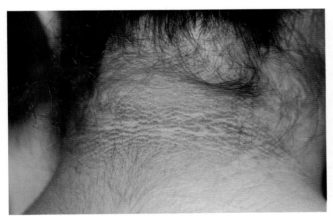

Figure 72-3 Acanthosis nigricans. Thickened velvety, hyperpigmented epidermis in the neck of obese child.
(Courtesy of Ilona J. Frieden, MD.)

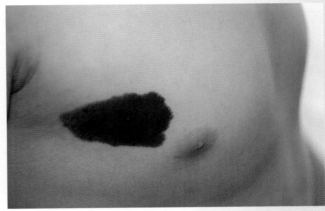

Figure 72-4 Congenital melanocytic nevus. A medium-sized, congenital, pigmented nevus on the trunk of an infant.
(Courtesy of Ilona J. Frieden, MD.)

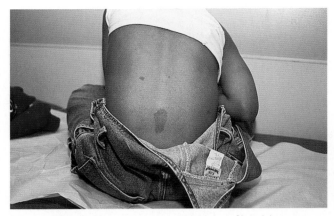

Figure 72-5 Café au lait spots. Multiple café au lait spots on the back of a child.
(Courtesy of George A. Datto, III, MD.)

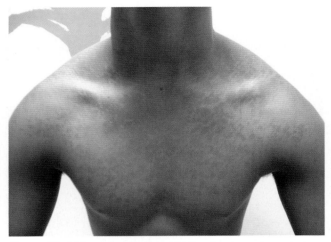

Figure 72-6 Tinea versicolor. While often hypopigmented, this rash may be hyperpigmented as in this individual.
(Courtesy of Paul S. Matz, MD.)

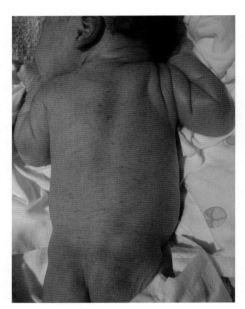

Figure 72-7 Neonatal pustular melanosis. Small hyperpigmented macules seen in a newborn. Often associated with pustules.
(Courtesy of Amy Gilliam, MD.)

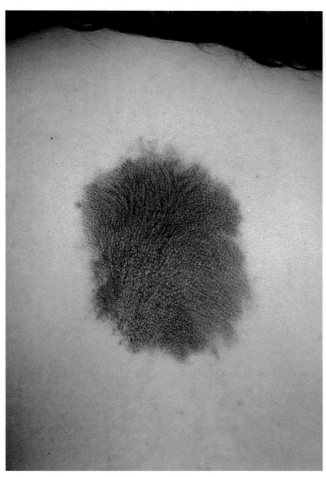

Figure 72-8 Congenital blue nevus. Bluish-discolored nevus that persists.
(Courtesy of Ilona J. Frieden, MD.)

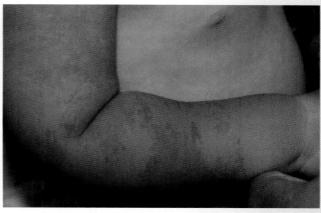

Figure 72-9 Nevoid hyperpigmentation. Previously called hypermelanosis of Ito, an irregular patterned area of hyperpigmentation.
(Courtesy of Ilona J. Frieden, MD.)

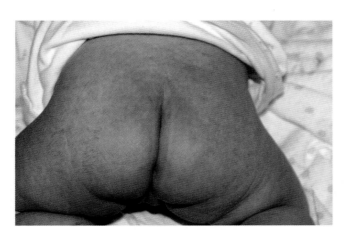

Figure 72-10 Congenital dermal melanocytosis (also called Mongolian spot). Slate gray–colored macule on back of infant.
(Courtesy of Ilona J. Frieden, MD.)

DIFFERENTIAL DIAGNOSIS

DIAGNOSIS	ICD-9	DISTINGUISHING CHARACTERISTICS	DISTRIBUTION	DURATION/ CHRONICITY
Postinflammatory Hyperpigmentation	709.00	Increased pigment in area of previous injury or inflammation	Anywhere	Acute to chronic
Acanthosis Nigricans	701.2	Velvety, hyperpigmented thickened skin in the skin folds	Frequently on neck, but can be seen in axilla, flexural surfaces	Chronic
Congenital Melanocytic Nevus (CMN)	216.x Lip, x = 0 Eyelid, x = 1 Ear, x = 2 Face, x = 3 Scalp or neck, x = 4 Trunk, x = 5 Upper limb, x = 6 Lower limb, x = 7 Other specified skin, x = 8 Skin NOS x = 9	Giant CMN >20 cm Large CMN 1.5–20 cm Small CMN <1.5 cm	Anywhere	Chronic
Café au Lait Spots	709.00	Hyperpigmented macules	Anywhere	Chronic
Tinea Versicolor	111.0	Scaly hyperpigmented or hypopigmented oval lesions that may be confluent	Usually on the chest, upper back, or shoulder	Chronic
Neonatal Pustular Melanosis	757.39	1–3 mm hyperpigmented macules with accompanying pustules	Diffuse	Acute
Blue Nevus	216	Collection of melanocytes in deep dermis Small dome-shaped nodules	Anywhere	Chronic
Nevoid Hyperpigmentation	709.00	Linear or whorled areas of hyperpigmentation	Usually on trunk	Chronic Present at birth or develops shortly afterwards May be more apparent in the first 2 yrs of life
Congenital Dermal Melanocytosis (also Called Mongolian Spot)	757.33	Blue-gray area of hyperpigmentation Caused by melanocytes in deep dermis	75% are in the sacrogluteal area but can occur elsewhere	Chronic, fades in the first 5–10 yrs of life
Freckles (Ephelis)	709.09	Red-tan macules 2–3 mm in size	Usually on face, arms, chest, and back Can occur in any sunexposed area	Chronic, first appear at age 3–5 yrs

ASSOCIATED FINDINGS	COMPLICATIONS	PRECIPITATING FACTORS	TREATMENT GUIDELINES
Healing site of injury or inflammation	Permanent hyperpigmentation	Inflammatory lesion	Treat inflammation/injury when present
Obesity	Associated with metabolic syndrome (diabetes mellitus, fatty liver, elevated cholesterol)	Obesity/overweight	Weight loss can result in improvement of appearance.
None	Cosmetic concerns Giant CMN in the head and neck region are associated with leptomeningeal melanocytosis and associated with neurological disorders such as epilepsy. Lesions over the spine can be associated with underlying spinal defects.	None	Refer to dermatology due to risk of malignant change.
Can be familial with numerous café au lait spots without other associated features Consider neurofibromatosis type I when there are more than 6 cafe au lait spots greater than or equal to I cm in size, axillary frecking, neurofibromas, or Lisch nodules. Consider McCune Albright syndrome when there are a small number of large, dark, cafe au lait spots with jagged edges.	Specific to associated conditions	Hereditary	If isolated, no further management If associated with neurofibromatosis type I or other genetic syndrome, appropriate management of underlying condition
Rare complaints of pruritus	May be difficult to treat	Infection with fungus, *Malassezia furfur* or *Microsporum sp.* Thrives in hot, humid climates	Ketoconazole shampoo or selenium sulfide 2.5% applied daily for I wk then monthly for 3 months
None	None	None	None
None	Cosmetic concerns	None	Low risk of malignant change
None	None	None	None
None	None	Common among infants of African American, Hispanic and Asian descent	None needed
Most common in children with fair skin, blue eyes, and light hair Autosomal-dominant inheritance	None	Sun exposure	None for freckles but, because these patients often have fairer skin, they should use sunscreen to prevent sunburn.

- Hormone-induced hyperpigmentation of the genitalia in normal newborns

- Xeroderma pigmentosa

- McCune-Albright syndrome

- Lentigines (such as Peutz-Jeghers syndrome)

- Other syndromes with associated café au lait spots, including Noonan syndrome, LEOPARD, Costello syndrome, and Cardio-Facio-Cutaneous syndrome

- Malignant melanoma

- Congenital melanocytic nevi have potential for malignant transformation, so they should be referred to a dermatologist for potential excision.

- Multiple café au lait spots with any associated abnormalities of the eye, seizures, developmental abnormalities, endocrine dyscrasias, or any other abnormalities should be investigated for neurofibromatosis type 1, McCune-Albright syndrome, and other associated syndromes.

- If tinea versicolor does not respond to topical treatments, consider further management with alternative topical or oral antifungal treatment.

- Children with acanthosis nigricans who are significantly overweight should be evaluated for diabetes mellitus, metabolic syndrome, or polycystic ovary syndrome. Individuals with these disorders should be evaluated by a pediatric endocrinologist.

SUGGESTED READINGS

Taïeb A, Boralevi F. Hypermelanoses of the newborn and of the infant. *Dermatol Clin*. 2007;25:327–336.

Weinberg S, Prose NS, Kristal L, eds. *Color atlas of pediatric dermatology*. 4th ed. New York, NY: McGraw Hill; 2007:267–284.

Weston WL, Lane AT, Morelli JG, eds. *Color textbook of pediatric dermatology*. 4th ed. St. Louis, MO: Mosby; 2007:309–333.

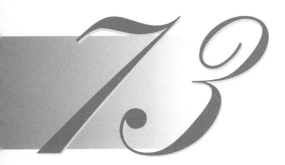

ANGELA M. ALLEVI
AND BETH A. SHORTRIDGE

Bullous Rashes

APPROACH TO THE PROBLEM

Blister-associated rashes in children are divided into two groups: *vesicular* rashes and *bullous* rashes. By definition, vesicles are raised, fluid-containing blisters in the skin or mucous membranes that are no more than 0.5 cm in diameter. Bullae are blistering lesions that are greater than 0.5 cm in diameter and may also be seen in the skin or mucous membranes. Vesicles and bullae may be round or have irregular borders. Compared with adult skin, the skin of pediatric patients is very prone to blistering. Vesicular rashes are common in the pediatric population, and are discussed in another chapter. Bullous rashes, on the other hand, are a relatively uncommon class of pediatric skin disorders.

Bullae form secondary to fluid accumulation between cells in the epidermis or between the epidermal and dermal (subepidermal) skin layers. Bullous skin disorders can be divided into *congenital* disorders, such as congenital epidermolysis bullosa; *immunologic* disorders, such as Stevens-Johnson syndrome (SJS), toxic epidermal necrolysis (TEN), and photosensitivity rashes; and *infectious* disorders, such as bullous impetigo and staphylococcal scalded skin syndrome (SSSS).

KEY POINTS IN THE HISTORY

- Systemic symptoms, such as fever, fussiness, ill appearance, and diffuse skin involvement, are associated with SJS, TEN, and SSSS.

- Epidermolysis bullosa, a congenital blistering disease, is often present at birth or during the newborn period.

- Bullae appearing in the first few days or weeks of life may be secondary to epidermolysis bullosa, bullous impetigo of the neonate, or SSSS.

- In epidermolysis bullosa, bullae form at sites of minor skin trauma or friction.

- Because they involve the epidermis only, bullous skin disorders (with the exception of TEN and rarer forms of epidermolysis bullosa) may cause temporary hyperpigmentation and lichenification and rarely cause permanent scarring.

KEY POINTS IN THE PHYSICAL EXAMINATION

- Bullous impetigo and photosensitivity rashes are seen on exposed parts of the body, primarily the face and extremities.

- In bullous impetigo, the bullae are surrounded by erythematous margins.

- Nikolsky sign—the ability to use gentle traction with a finger to separate the upper epidermis from the underlying skin in bullous lesions—is seen in a number of systemic bullous disorders, including TEN, SSSS, and epidermolysis bullosa.

- Mucous membrane involvement is seen in SJS, TEN, and in more severe forms of epidermolysis bullosa, but not in SSSS.

- In bullous impetigo, photosensitivity rashes, epidermolysis bullosa, and SSSS, bullae are seen on the skin; in SJS, they are also seen on the mucous membranes of the mouth, nares, conjunctivae, and the anorectal and perineal areas.

- Conjunctivae are involved in SSSS (erythema), SJS, and TEN (mucositis).

PHOTOGRAPHS OF SELECTED DIAGNOSES

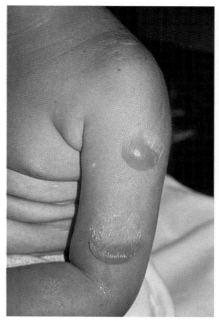

Figure 73-1 Photosensitivity. Large blisters that developed on the second day following prolonged sun exposure. (Courtesy of George A. Datto, III, MD.)

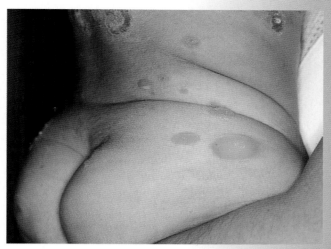

Figure 73-2 Bullous impetigo. (Used with permission from Fleisher GR, Ludwig S, Baskin MN. *Atlas of pediatric emergency medicine*. Philadelphia, PA: Lippincott Williams & Wilkins; 2004:200.)

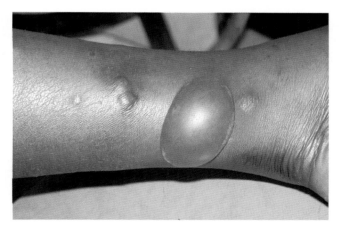

Figure 73-3 Bullous insect bite reaction. (Used with permission from Goodheart HP. *Goodheart's photoguide to common skin disorders*. 2nd ed. Philadelphia, PA: Lippincott Williams & Wilkins; 2003:3.)

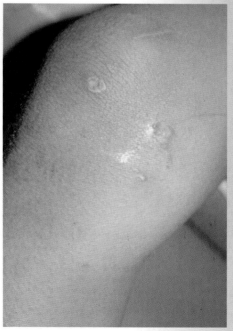

Figure 73-4 Blistering rash from streptococcal infection. (Courtesy of George A. Datto, III, MD.)

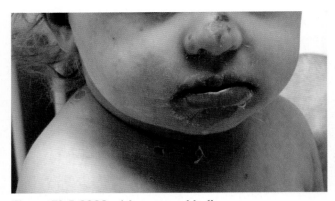

Figure 73-5 SSSS with ruptured bullae.
(Courtesy of Gary Marshall, MD.)

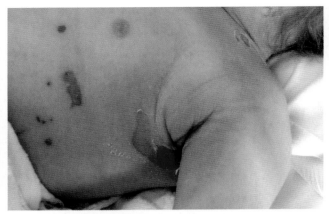

Figure 73-6 Staphylococcal scalded skin syndrome.
"Scalded" skin underlying ruptured bulla in SSSS.
(Courtesy of Gary Marshall, MD.)

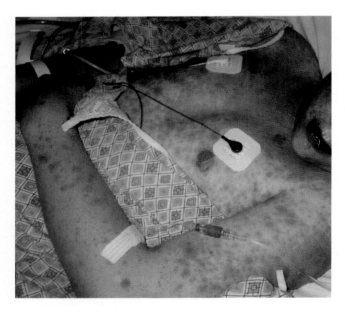

Figure 73-7 Target-like purpuric lesions of SJS.
(Courtesy of Gary Marshall, MD.)

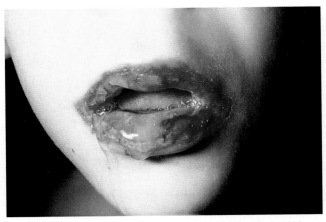

Figure 73-8 Hemorrhagic ulcerative stomatitis in SJS.
(Courtesy of Joseph Lopreiato, MD.)

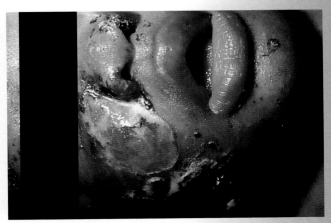

Figure 73-9 Epidermolysis bullosa. Note the ruptured
bullous lesion.
(Courtesy of Joseph Lopreiato, MD.)

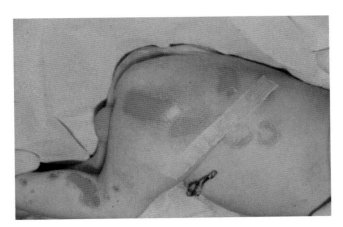

Figure 73-10 Epidermolysis bullosa congenita.
(Used with permission from the Benjamin Barankin Dermatology
Collection.)

DIFFERENTIAL DIAGNOSIS

DIAGNOSIS	ICD-9	DISTINGUISHING CHARACTERISTICS	DISTRIBUTION	ONSET/ CHRONICITY
Photosensitivity/ Photoxicity	692.72	Exaggerated sunburn Occurs in all age groups Sun-exposed areas of skin affected Vesicles and bullae in severe cases Pruritic Onset < 72 hr after sun exposure	Often involves face, upper neck ("V" portion), hands, forearms Covered and shadowed areas of body are spared.	Acute May recur
Bullous Impetigo	684	Seen most often in infants and young children Child does not appear ill. Bullae often purulent and contain *Staphylococcus aureus* Mucous membranes not involved Bullae surrounded by erythematous margins May have weeping surface under denuded bullae	Occurs on exposed areas of face and extremities, occasionally in perineal area	Acute
Staphylococcal Scalded Skin Syndrome (SSSS)	695.81	Onset in neonate frequently 3–7 days of life Vast majority of cases with onset less than 6 years of age Appears as diffuse erythema that blanches Bullae rupture leaving skin "scalded" Mucous membranes not involved Fluid inside bullae is sterile and clear. May be clinically indistinguishable from TEN	Initial lesions: small pustules in diaper area or lower abdomen or erythema with or without crusting around the mouth, diaper area, or umbilicus Spreads diffusely	Acute
Stevens-Johnson Syndrome (SJS)	695.1	Most common in children and young adults Viral-like prodrome, then rapid development of rash and bullae (within 24 hr) Bullae found on mucous membranes, and in severe cases on skin (SJS–TEN continuum) Target lesions or nonpalpable purpura Body surface area involvement <10% by some criteria, <30% in continuum criteria	May be localized to trunk, palms, and soles, or generalized Always involves mucous membranes (mouth, eyes, genitals, perianal, or anorectal area)	Acute following prodrome of 1–2 weeks Duration of oral lesions may last months.
Toxic Epidermal Necrolysis (TEN)	695.1	Occurs in all age groups but more commonly in adults May be clinically indistinguishable from SSSS in neonates Full thickness loss of epidermis: >30% of body surface area involvement	Begins with mucous membrane involvement similar to SJS, but progresses to diffuse epidermal involvement with full-thickness loss of epidermis	Acute following prodrome
Epidermolysis Bullosa	757.39	Bullae often present at birth Inherited skin disorder Three subtypes: EB simplex, junctional EB, and dystrophic EB	Most commonly involves hands and feet, but also other areas of minor trauma	Recurrent

ASSOCIATED FINDINGS	COMPLICATIONS	PREDISPOSING/ PRECIPITATING FACTORS	TREATMENT GUIDELINES
Pruritus Areas of contact dermatitis	Healing with hyperpigmentation and lichenification May see recurrence even after discontinuation of offending agent Systemic lupus erythematosus may present with photosensitivity.	Drug exposure Skin products Family history	Identification and withdrawal of suspected drug or topical agent Sun avoidance and protection Cool compresses Consider topical corticosteroids
Outbreaks in close contacts, such as family members	Recurrent folliculitis Cellulitis from progressive infection	Nasal carriage of group A strep and *S. aureus* increases risk of recurrent impetigo Bug bites Trauma	Topical antistaphylococcal antibiotics Disinfectant solutions may not be better than placebo Systemic antibiotics if systemic symptoms present
Fever Fussiness Positive Nikolsky sign Bullae and underlying skin may be extremely painful Flaking desquamation after acute phase	Sepsis Cellulitis Loss of hair and nails Osteomyelitis Pneumonia Fungal or bacterial superinfection Fluid and electrolyte disturbances Mortality higher with increasing age	Asymptomatic staphylococcal pustulosis	Multiple cultures from blood and possible sources of infection (not from sterile bullae) Systemic anti-staphylococcal antibiotics including those that cover methicillin-resistant *Staphylococcus aureus* (MRSA) Barrier emollients Stabilize fluids and electrolytes Biopsy in older children to rule out TEN Transfer to burn unit if indicated Prevention: hygiene
Weakness Lethargy Pneumonia Severe eye involvement in most cases: conjunctivitis, ulcerations, uveitis Nephritis Ulcerative/hemorrhagic stomatitis from oral lesions	Severe dehydration Secondary infection Respiratory failure Renal failure Gastric perforation Blindness Mortality <10%	Infection, including mycoplasma, Herpes Simplex Virus (HSV), and viral upper respiratory tract infections Drug exposure to antiepileptics, sulfonamides, penicillin derivatives	Transfer to burn unit if >10% body surface area (BSA) affected with blisters Stabilize and support Identify and remove or treat suspected causative agent(s) Colloidal baths/wet compresses Histamine-1 blockers Topical analgesics for oral lesions Infection prevention and treatment
See SJS Mucous membrane (of eyes, mouth) involvement Positive Nikolsky sign Painful erythematous skin	Fluid and electrolyte imbalance Ocular sequelae in 40% (including blindness) Overwhelming sepsis Mortality in up to 30%	Drug exposure, most commonly to analgesics Nonsteroidal anti-inflammatory agents, antibiotics, antifungal medications, and antiepileptics Idiopathic etiology more common in children	Same as SJS Transfer to burn unit Pain management Cyclosporine Plasma exchange transfusions Enteral feedings
Severe forms: Scarring at previously involved sites Oral involvement Nail dystrophy Palmar and plantar hyperkeratosis	Hyperpigmentation Superinfection Sepsis In severe forms scarring, contractures	Family history Bullae form at sites of minor trauma	Avoid mechanical trauma and friction Padding Cool environment Emollients Debridement as needed Prevent bacterial infection Treat for bacterial infection as needed Genetic counseling

OTHER
DIAGNOSES
TO CONSIDER

- Pemphigus

- Bullous pemphigoid

- Linear IgA bullous dermatosis

- Epidermolytic hyperkeratosis (bullous ichthyosis)

- Toxic shock syndrome

- Bullous mastocytosis

- Bullous scabies

- Insect and arachnid bites

- Burn injury

WHEN TO
CONSIDER
FURTHER
EVALUATION
OR TREATMENT

- A skin biopsy is strongly recommended in atypical SSSS or SJS and in all cases of TEN.

- Patients with suspected SSSS, SJS, and TEN need close monitoring for other organ system involvement and life-threatening complications.

- Complicated SSSS, SJS, and all TEN should be managed in a burn unit.

SUGGESTED READINGS

Bhumbra NA, McCullough SG. Skin and subcutaneous infections. *Prim Care*. 2003;30(1):1–24.
George A, Rubin G. A systematic review and meta-analysis of treatments for impetigo. *Br J Gen Pract*. 2003;53(491):480–487.
McKenna JK, Leiferman KM. Dermatologic drug reactions. *Immunol Allergy Clin North Am*. 2004;24(3):399–423.
Patel GK. Staphylococcal scalded skin syndrome: diagnosis and management. *Am J Clin Dermatol*. 2003;4(3):165–175.
Spies M, Sanford AP, Low JFA, et al. Treatment of extensive toxic epidermal necrolysis in children. *Pediatrics*. 2001;108(5):162–168.
Warwick L, Morison MD. Photosensitivity. *N Engl J Med*. 2004;350:1111–1117.

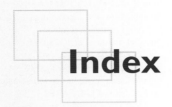

Index

glomus tympanicum, tympanic membrane
abnormalities, 154
glossitis, 208
Goldenhar syndrome, 200
ear shape/position abnormalities, 125
gonadal material palpable, female genitalia
variations and, 374
gonococcal infection
hand swelling, 306
red eye, 85
granuloma gluteale infantum
perianal/buttock redness, 438
perineal red rashes, 402
Graves disease
neck masses/swelling, 232
swelling of/around the eye, 100
griseofulvin
hairy tongue, 201
groin rashes, 397
group A beta-hemolytic streptococci
(GABHS), scarlet fever, 447
growth failure, congestive heart failure, 57
growth restriction, leg asymmetry and, 324, 329
grunting, general appearance, 54
gum abscess. see parulis
gum lesions. see focal gum lesions
gynecomastia
breast swelling/enlargement, 240, f242, 244
chest lumps, 247

H

H. influenzae, 91, 309
habit tick deformity, nail abnormalities and,
294
habitual dislocations, arm displacement and,
295
hair follicles scarring, traction alopecia, 67
hair loss
differential diagnosis, 66–67
figures, 63–65
historical points, 61
other diagnosis, 68
physical examination, 62
hair tufts, 277–284
midline back and, f279
hair, white specks in, 69–74
hairy tongue
tongue discoloration/surface changes, 201,
202, f205, 206–208
halitosis
bottle caries, 191
hairy tongue, 207
Ludwig angina, 212
hand swelling
differential diagnosis, 308–309
figures, 310
historical points, 306
other diagnosis, 311
physical examination, 306–307
hand-foot syndrome, 308–309
hand-foot-and-mouth disease, vesicular rashes,
484, f485, 488–489
Hashimoto thyroiditis, neck masses/swelling,
232
head
abnormal head shape, 25–31

head circumference, achondroplasia, 36
head lice, 69–70, 72–73
head tilt
abnormal head shape, 25
misalignment of the eyes, 117, 121
headaches
mouth sores/patches, 171
nonblanching rashes, 491
pityriasis rosea, 505
scarlet fever, 507, 512
hearing loss. see also ears
AOM/OME, 149, 153
atelectasis, 153
cholesteatoma, 149, 153
ear canal findings, 147
hemotympanum, 153
retraction pockets, 153
TM perforation, 149, 153, 154
tympanosclerosis, 149, 153
heart murmur, knee swelling and, 346
heel bisector, intoeing and, 340
helix deformity, f127, 129
hemangiomas
arm swelling and, 300, f303, 304, 305
chest lumps, 247
curvature of the back and, 270
facial rashes, 442, 448
focal red bumps, 467–468, f469–f470,
472–473, 474
lumps on the face, f77, 80–81
midline back and, 277, f281
mouth sores/patches, 178
nasal bridge swelling, f160, 161
neck masses/swelling, 226, f228
perineal sores/lesions, 404, f407, 408–409
red patches and swellings, 456, 458–459,
460
swelling of/around the eye, f96, 98–99
swellings in the mouth, 214
hemarthrosis
leg asymmetry and, 330
nonblanching rashes, 492
hematemesis, enlarged/distended abdomen,
261
hematocolpos/hematometrocolpos
female genitalia variations, f377
vulvar swelling/masses, 411, 412, f415,
416–418
hematomas
arm swelling and, 300
fingertip swelling and, f320
neck masses/swelling, 232
vulvar swelling/masses, 418
hemiatrophy of leg, 324
leg asymmetry and, 324, f327, 328–329
hemihypertrophy, 324
leg asymmetry and, 323, 324, f325, f326,
328–329
hemolysis, enlarged/distended abdomen, 261
hemolytic disease, discoloration of/around the
eye, 107
hemolytic uremic syndrome, nonblanching
rashes, 498
hemophilia
knee swelling, 352
leg asymmetry, 330

leg bowing and knock knees, 338
nonblanching rashes, 491, f493
hemorrhagic ulcerative stomatitis
bullous rashes, f531
hemorrhoids
perianal/buttock swelling, 427–428, f429,
430–432
perirectal skin tag, 431
hemotympanum
ear trauma, 135
tympanic membrane abnormalities, 153
Henoch-Schönlein purpura (HSP)
ear swelling, 136
foot swelling and, 360, 363
hand swelling and, 311
knee swelling and, 346
nonblanching rashes, 491, f494, 496–497
perineal red rashes, 398, 402
scrotal swelling, 424
vulvar swelling/masses, 418
hepatic disease, discoloration of/around the
eye, 102
hepatic encephalopathy
general appearance, 58
hepatitis B virus
Gianotti-Crosti syndrome, 481
knee swelling and, 352
viral arthritis and, 308
hepatomegaly
abdominal distention, f263
congestive heart failure, 56
enlarged/distended abdomen, f263, 264–265
Gianotti-Crosti syndrome, 481
infectious mononucleosis, 221, 481
hepatosplenomegaly
enlarged/distended abdomen, f263
JIA and, 309
hereditary angioedema, swelling of/around the
eye, 98–99
hermaphroditism, inguinal hernia, 417
hernia
abdominal midline bulge, 255–256, 260
inguinal, 411, 412, f413, 416–418, 419–420,
f421, 423
herpangina, f217
mouth sores/patches, f173, 176–177
throat redness, 216
herpes
herpetic whitlow and, 319, 321
skin abnormalities, 43
herpes gingivostomatitis, mouth sores/patches,
172
herpes keratoconjunctivitis, f87, 90–91
herpes simplex virus, 447
herpes labialis, vesicular rashes, f486, 488–489
herpes simplex. see also herpes simplex virus
atopic dermatitis, 505
perineal red rashes, 402
skin abnormalities, 44
herpes simplex neonatorum
skin abnormalities in newborn, 50
herpes simplex virus (HSV)
facial lesions, 24
facial rashes, 442, 446–447
herpes keratoconjunctivitis, 447
mouth sores/patches, f173